Beverage Consumption Habits around the World: Association with Total Water and Energy Intakes

Special Issue Editors

Lluis Serra-Majem

Mariela Nissensohn

MDPI • Basel • Beijing • Wuhan • Barcelona • Belgrade

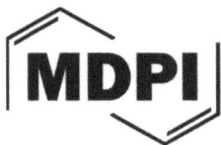

MDPI

Special Issue Editors

Lluis Serra-Majem
University of Las Palmas
de Gran Canaria
Spain

Mariela Nissensohn
University of Las Palmas
de Gran Canaria
Spain

Editorial Office
MDPI AG
St. Alban-Anlage 66
Basel, Switzerland

This edition is a reprint of the Special Issue published online in the open access journal *Nutrients* (ISSN 2072-6643) from 2016–2017 (available at: http://www.mdpi.com/journal/nutrients/special_issues/energy_intakes).

For citation purposes, cite each article independently as indicated on the article page online and as indicated below:

Author 1; Author 2. Article title. *Journal Name* **Year**, *Article number*, page range.

First Edition 2017

ISBN 978-3-03842-634-9 Pbk)
ISBN 978-3-03842-635-6 (PDF)

Table of Contents

About the Special Issue Editors

Lluis Serra-Majem, Doctor in Medicine and Nutrition and specialist in Preventive Medicine and Public Health, he is the Director of the Nutrition Research Group and Director of the Research Institute of Biomedical and Health Sciences at the Department of Clinical Sciences at the University of Las Palmas de Gran Canaria. He is also the Founder and President of the Spanish Academy of Nutrition and Food Science (AEN), the Foundation for Nutrition Research (FIN), the NGO Nutrition Without Borders and the International Foundation for the Mediterranean Diet (IFMeD). Author of more than 800 scientific publications, with 70 books and more than 500 indexed scientific articles, in the last 25 years he has participated and directed numerous national and European projects. He is also Group Coordinator of the Center for Biomedical Research in Network (CIBER) of Obesity and Nutrition Pathophysiology of the Carlos III Health Institute, integrating the PREDIMED and the PREDIMED PLUS studies and Director of the International Chair for Advanced Studies on Hydration (CIEAH), with headquarters at the University of Las Palmas de Gran Canaria, Spain. Its scientific and academic trajectory places him as one of the leadership scientists with the highest productivity national and international in the field of nutrition and public health, the Mediterranean diet, prevention of childhood obesity and hydration.

Mariela Nissensohn, PhD in Public Health Nutrition from the University of Las Palmas de Gran Canaria. Degree in Nutrition from the University of Buenos Aires (UBA), Argentina. Master in Clinical Nutrition by the Universidad Autónoma de Madrid. Researcher of the Nutrition Group of the Research Institute of Biomedical and Health Sciences (IUIBS), University of Las Palmas de Gran Canaria and of the International Chair for Advanced Studies on Hydration (CIEAH). Member of the CIBER OBN, Biomedical Research Networking Center for Physiopathology of Obesity and Nutrition, Carlos III Health Institute. She is Professor of the Nutrition Degree at the Fernando Pessoa University of Las Palmas de Gran Canaria, Spain. She has participated in several lines of research both in the field of Clinical Nutrition and Nutritional Epidemiology in national and international projects as EURRECA (European micronutrient Recommendations Aligned), omega 3 fatty acids & biomarkers, hypertension & Mediterranean Diet, different aspects of hydration in the framework of the European Hydration Institute, the ANIBES Study (Anthropometry, Ingestion and Energy Balance in Spain), Predimed Plus Study, etc. She is author and co-author of many nutrition articles published in several international scientific journals and has made several book chapters.

Preface to "Beverage Consumption Habits around the World: Association with Total Water and Energy Intakes"

Dehydration occurs when the body loses more water than is taken in. It is often accompanied by disturbances in the body's mineral salt or electrolyte balance, especially in the concentrations of sodium and potassium.

Populations at particular risk of hypohydration are the very young, those engaged in professions where fluid homeostasis is regularly challenged and the elderly. Limited data are available on the prevalence of hypohydration, but there is evidence to suggest that this may be relatively common among the western elderly populations [1]. The percentage of population with inadequate intake of water may vary from 5% to 35% in the different European countries [2].

The burden of disease from lack of access to clean water, poor sanitation and inadequate personal and food hygiene is well known, but consequences of inadequate water intake worldwide are far from being well understood. Recent research [3] into the risk of disease (bowel, metabolic and kidney diseases), disability (cognitive function, physical performance, headache, falls and accidents) and death is confirming the importance of poor hydration to overall disease burden and quality of life in a worldwide perspective. Moreover, the number of hospitalizations for dehydration has steadily increased in recent decades. In this case, dehydration increases the healthcare burden in a direct way, as a disease itself. However, sometimes, dehydration appears as a comorbidity condition in a number of diseases. Dehydration has been defined as the second most common comorbidity, occurring in 14% of all hospitalizations [4].

In addition to its individual clinical impact; dehydration also represents an important public health issue by imposing a significant economic burden. Depending on the degree or magnitude of the dehydration in hospitalized patients, costs may increase by 7% to 8.5% [5]. Higher cost will be associated with an increase in hospital mortality, as well as with an increase in the utilization of intense short and long term care facilities, readmission rates and hospital resources, especially among those with moderate to severe hypernatraemia. Dehydration represents a potential target for intervention to reduce healthcare expenditures and improve patients' quality of life [6]. However, the higher cost of dehydration is not only in hospitalized patients. Dehydration is one of the major factors limiting athletic performance and even mild dehydration can have a significant impact on working capacity and productivity [7]. Some studies have suggested a possible link between dehydration and the rise in industrial accidents during the summer, when workers are presumably thirstier [8]. A study published in 2004 found it had a real impact on performance in physical fields such as forestry, with slightly dehydrated workers being about 12% less productive than their fully hydrated peers [9].

Improving drinking habits during working and leisure time and developing comprehensive hydration guidelines for healthcare professionals and patients would be a cost-effective means of addressing the burden of hypohydration in developed countries.

Given the extent of the problem and its under-acknowledgment, will governments engage in research and awareness-raising strategy on the burden of hypohydration in the different countries and regions? Will governments address the burden of dehydration in the elderly as part of its action plan on active ageing to be proposed in the near future?

On the other side, a rising number of studies assert that sugar-containing drinks may play a key role in the etiology of overweight and obesity in children and adults [10]. However, whether this association is causa still remains controversial [11,12]. Public policy initiatives to reduce sugar in beverages consumption are the subject of current debate and different initiatives are actually developed worldwide. These should consider both, promoting an adequate water intake and a reduction in sugar and energy intake from beverages, across the different age and socioeconomic groups, all within the broader context of improving overall diet quality.

At this stage, the current Issue has received a great welcome from the scientific community which has responded to the proposal with huge interest. However, although the number of the papers published in the present book is really impressive (around 20), the needs for these kinds of studies have not decreased. The studies included were developed in different settings and different populations around the world; the diversity methodologies employed in the quantitative assessment of beverages consumption and all the details that the results of the studies have shown may eventually help to adequately address their policies worldwide. Broadly, the papers in the present volume provide a valuable milestone on our journey to understand the impacts of the hydration on health and disease and they will be helpful for those planning future studies. Our main interest has been to gradually increase the general interest placed on this emerging and fascinating area of study.

As we move forward, our progress will continue to depend heavily on beverage intake assessment methods, and underpinning this is the need to further refine and document the validity of our methods.

Again, those of us engaged in nutrition research will be highly appreciative of the great efforts of our colleagues who have produced this volume documenting our progress to date.

Lluis Serra-Majem and Mariela Nissensohn
Special Issue Editors

References

1.   Watson, P.; Whale, A.; Mears, S.A.; Reyner, L.A.; Maughan, R.J. Mild hypohydration increases the frequency of driver errors during a prolonged, monotonous driving task. *Physiol. Behav.* **2015**, *147*, 313–318.

2.   Nissensohn, M.; Castro-Quezada, I.; Serra-Majem, L. Beverage and water intake of healthy adults in some European countries. *Int. J. Food Sci. Nutr.* **2013**, *64*, 801–805.

3.   Benton, D.; Braun, H.; Cobo, J.C.; Edmonds, C.; Elmadfa, I.; El-Sharkawy, A.; Feehally, J.; Gellert, R.; Holdsworth, J.; Kapsokefalou, M.; et al. Executive summary and conclusions from the European Hydration Institute expert conference on human hydration, health, and performance. *Nutr. Rev.* **2015**, *73* (Suppl. 2), 148–150.

4.   Elixhauser, A.; *Yu, K.; Steiner, C.; Bierman, A.S.* Hospitalizations in the United States. AHRQ. 1997. Available online: http://archive.ahrq.gov/data/hcup/factbk1/ (accessed on 17 May 2016).

5.   Callahan, M.A.; Do, H.T.; Caplan, D.W.; Yoon-Flannery, K. Economic impact of hyponatremia in hospitalized patients: A retrospective cohort study. *Postgrad. Med.* **2009**, *12*, 186–191.

6.   Frangeskou, M.; Lopez-Valcarcel, B.; Serra-Majem, L. Dehydration in the elderly: A review focused on economic burden. *J. Nutr. Health Aging* **2015**, *19*, 619–627.

7.   Faraco, G.; Wijasa, T.S.; Park, L.; Moore, J.; Anrather, J.; Iadecola, C. Water deprivation induces neurovascular and cognitive dysfunction through vasopressin-induced oxidative stress. *J. Cereb. Blood Flow Metab.* **2014**, *34*, 852–860.

8.   Kenefick, R.W.; Sawka, M.N. Hydration at the work site. *J. Am. Coll. Nutr.* **2007**, *26* (Suppl. 5), 597S–603S.

9.   Wästerlund, D.S.; Chaseling, J.; Burström, L. The effect of fluid consumption on the forest workers' performance strategy. *Appl. Ergon.* **2004**, *35*, 29–36.

10.   Hu, F.B. Resolved: There is sufficient scientific evidence that decreasing sugar-sweetened beverage consumption will reduce the prevalence of obesity and obesity-related diseases. *Obes. Rev.* **2013**, *14*, 606–619.

11. Kaiser, K.; Shikany, J.; Keating, K.; Allison, D. Will reducing sugar-sweetened beverage consumption reduce obesity? Evidence supporting conjecture is strong, but evidence when testing effect is weak. *Obes. Rev.* **2013**, *14*, 620–633.

12. Gibson, S. Sugar-sweetened soft drinks and obesity: A systematic review of the evidence from observational studies and interventions. *Nutr. Res. Rev.* **2008**, *21*, 134–147.

nutrients

MDPI

Article

Beverage Consumption Habits and Association with Total Water and Energy Intakes in the Spanish Population: Findings of the ANIBES Study

Mariela Nissensohn [1,2], Almudena Sánchez-Villegas [1,2], Rosa M. Ortega [3], Javier Aranceta-Bartrina [2,4], Ángel Gil [2,5], Marcela González-Gross [2,6], Gregorio Varela-Moreiras [7,8] and Lluis Serra-Majem [1,2,*]

[1] Research Institute of Biomedical and Health Sciences, University of Las Palmas de Gran Canaria, Las Palmas de Gran Canaria 35016, Spain; marienis67@hotmail.com (M.N.); almudena.sanchez@ulpgc.es (A.S.-V.)

[2] CIBER OBN, Biomedical Research Networking Center for Physiopathology of Obesity and Nutrition, Carlos III Health Institute, Madrid 28029, Spain; jaranceta@unav.es (J.A.-B.); agil@ugr.es (A.G.); marcela.gonzalez.gross@upm.es (M.G.-G.)

[3] Department of Nutrition, Faculty of Pharmacy, Madrid Complutense University, Madrid 28040, Spain; rortega@ucm.es

[4] Department of Preventive Medicine and Public Health, University of Navarra, Pamplona 31008, Spain

[5] Department of Biochemistry and Molecular Biology II and Institute of Nutrition and Food Sciences, University of Granada, Granada 18100, Spain

[6] ImFINE Research Group, Department of Health and Human Performance, Technical University of Madrid, Madrid 28040, Spain

[7] Department of Pharmaceutical and Health Sciences, Faculty of Pharmacy, CEU San Pablo University, Madrid 28668, Spain; gvarela@ceu.es

[8] Spanish Nutrition Foundation (FEN), Madrid 28010, Spain

* Correspondence: lluis.serra@ulpgc.es; Tel.: +34-928-453-477; Fax: +34-928-451-416

Received: 28 January 2016; Accepted: 12 April 2016; Published: 20 April 2016

Abstract: Background: Inadequate hydration is a public health issue that imposes a significant economic burden. In Spain, data of total water intake (TWI) are scarce. There is a clear need for a national study that quantifies water and beverage intakes and explores associations between the types of beverages and energy intakes. **Methods:** The Anthropometry, Intake and Energy Balance Study ANIBES is a national survey of diet and nutrition conducted among a representative sample of 2285 healthy participants aged 9–75 years in Spain. Food and beverage intakes were assessed in a food diary over three days. Day and time of beverage consumption were also recorded. **Results:** On average, TWI was 1.7 L (SE 21.2) for men and 1.6 L (SE 18.9) for women. More than 75% of participants had inadequate TWI, according to European Food Safety Authority (EFSA) recommendations. Mean total energy intake (EI) was 1810 kcal/day (SE 11.1), of which 12% was provided by beverages. Water was the most consumed beverage, followed by milk. The contribution of alcoholic drinks to the EI was near 3%. For caloric soft drinks, a relatively low contribution to the EI was obtained, only 2%. Of eight different types of beverages, the variety score was positively correlated with TWI ($r = 0.39$) and EI ($r = 0.23$), suggesting that beverage variety is an indicator of higher consumption of food and drinks. **Conclusions:** The present study demonstrates that well-conducted surveys such as the ANIBES study have the potential to yield rich contextual value data that can emphasize the need to undertake appropriate health and nutrition policies to increase the total water intake at the population level promoting a healthy Mediterranean hydration pattern.

Keywords: ANIBES; total water intake; energy intake; beverages; Spain

1. Introduction

Dehydration occurs when the body loses more water than is taken in. It is often accompanied by disturbances in the body's mineral salt or electrolyte balance, especially in concentrations of sodium and potassium. Populations at particular risk of hypohydration are children, those engaged in professions where fluid homeostasis is regularly challenged, and older adults [1]. Limited data are available on the prevalence of hypohydration, but there is evidence to suggest that it may be relatively common among older populations [2]. The percentage of the population with inadequate water intake varies from 5% to 35% among European countries [3]. Whereas the burden of disease from inadequate water intake is well known, its consequences in Europe are far from being well understood. Recent research into the risk of disease (from falls and accidents and bowel, metabolic, and kidney diseases), disability (cognitive function, physical performance, and headaches), and death has confirmed the importance of poor hydration with respect to the overall disease burden and quality of life in Europe [4]. Therefore, the significant economic burden dehydration represents makes it an important public health issue. Depending on the degree or magnitude of dehydration in hospitalized patients, costs may be increased by 7%–8.5%. Dehydration represents a potential target for intervention to reduce healthcare expenditures and improve patient quality of life [5].

On the other hand, scientific literature recognizes that the "adequate intake" value of beverages (AI) is a variable event, in which differences are in part due to the inter-individual variation for water needs in response to different health status, metabolism, and environmental factors such as ambient temperature and humidity, as well as individual factors such as age, body size, and level of physical activity. Furthermore, the water needs also depend partially on overall diet and the water contained in food. About 80% of the required daily intake is provided by drinks, including water; the rest is acquired through solid food. Identifying the variety of drinks consumed and establishing the percentage of energy provided by each beverage to the diet allows us to set the pattern of individual or population-level beverage consumption. Understanding the contribution of each fluid type to the total fluid intake will allow us to draw conclusions about the adequacy of drinking habits.

In Spain, the influence of the Mediterranean Diet is widespread. This pattern of consumption also includes the hydration pattern of the population. Traditionally, this pattern included water as a main drink, along with daily but moderate consumption of wine or beer with the principal meal, and the intake of a group of beverages elaborated with fresh vegetables (Gazpacho, Salmorejo, *etc.*). However, in the last decades [6], the adherence to the Mediterranean pattern has been decreasing, especially in children and young people. The actual beverage pattern also included the occasional consumption of soft drinks, which was associated with leisure time. Furthermore, total water intake (TWI) data of Spain are scarce. There are no recent epidemiological studies that focus exclusively on beverage intake. Most available hydration data focuses on alcohol consumption. Apart from the Spanish National Survey on Dietary Intake (ENIDE) [7] in 2011, we are unaware of other research investigating beverage intake among the Spanish population. According to ENIDE data, the average beverage consumption was 1646.5 mL/day, which reflects insufficient fluid intake for that study population.

Given the extent of the problem and its poor recognition, there is the clear need for a national study to update the existing data. The aim of this study was to quantify the total water and beverage intake, and to explore associations between the types of beverage consumed and energy intake. The ANIBES study, a national survey of diet and nutrition conducted in 2013 among a representative random sample of 2285 healthy participants aged 9–75 years, provides us the likely best source of detailed information on the diet of normal individuals in Spain. Characteristics of ANIBES include a food and beverages record list (in grams) of each item consumed per participant and a record of the time of consumption. These study attributes provide a rich resource for exploring patterns of consumption according to age and gender, thereby permitting us to reach conclusions about whether or not drinking a variety of beverages helps to increase fluid intake to a level that meets current guidelines.

2. Materials and Methods

The design, protocol, and methodology of the ANIBES study have been described in detail elsewhere [8–10].

2.1. Sample

The ANIBES study is a cross-sectional study conducted using stratified multistage sampling. To guarantee better coverage and representativeness, the fieldwork was performed at 128 sampling points across Spain. The design of the ANIBES study aims to define a sample size that is representative of all individuals living in Spain, aged 9–75 years, and residing in municipalities of at least 2000 inhabitants. The initial potential sample consisted of 2634 individuals. For all analyses, we eliminated participants with anomalous values of energy intake (EI) (men, <800 or >4000 kcal/day; women, <500 or >3500 kcal/day) [11] to avoid introducing bias to the analysis. The final sample comprised 2007 individuals (1011 men, 50%; 996 women, 50%). In addition, for the youngest age groups (9–12, 13–17, and 18–24 years), an "augment sample" was included to provide at least $n = 200$ per age group (error $\pm$ 6.9%). The augment sample is the process of increasing the amount of interviews for a particular subgroup within the population in order to achieve an adequate number of interviews to allow analysis of population subgroups or segments that wouldn't normally yield a sufficient number of interviews in a main random survey, without the expense of increasing the sample size for the whole survey. Therefore, the random sample plus augment sample comprised 2285 participants.

The sample quotas according to the following variables were: age groups (9–12, 13–17, 18–64, and 65–75 years), gender (men/women), and geographical distribution (Northeast, Levant, Southwest, North–Central, Barcelona, Madrid, Balearic, and Canary Islands). Additionally, other factors for sample adjustment were considered: unemployment rate, percentage of foreigners (immigrant population), physical activity level assessed by The International Physical Activity questionnaire (IPAQ) [12], tobacco use and education or economic level. Finally, participants' weight, height, and waist circumference were measured and body mass index was also calculated.

The fieldwork for the ANIBES study was conducted from mid-September 2013 to mid-November 2013, and two previous pilot studies were also performed. To equally represent all days of the week, study subjects participated during two weekdays and one weekend day. The final protocol was approved by the Ethical Committee for Clinical Research of the Region of Madrid, Spain [9].

2.2. Food and Beverage Record

Study participants were provided with a tablet device (Samsung Galaxy Tab 2 7.0, Samsung Electronics, Suwon, South Korea) and trained in recording information by taking photos of all food and drinks consumed during the 3 days of the study, both at home and outside the home. Photos were to be taken before beginning to eat and drink, and again after finishing, so as to record the actual intake. Additionally, a brief description of meals, recipes, brands, and other information was recorded using the tablet. Participants who declared or demonstrated that they were unable to use the tablet device were offered other options, such as using a digital camera and paper record and/or telephone interviews. A total 79% of the sample used a tablet, 12% a digital camera, and 9% opted for a telephone interview. As no differences in the percentage of misreporting were found according to the type of device used to assess dietary intake, we used the measurements of the three assessment methods in the analysis. In addition to details of what and how much was eaten, for each eating/drinking event, participants recorded where they were, who they were eating with, and whether they were watching television and/or sitting at a table. After each survey day, participants recorded if their intake was representative for that day (or the reason why if it was not), and details of any dietary supplements taken. The survey also contained a series of questions about participants' customary eating habits (e.g., the type of milk usually consumed) to facilitate further coding. Food records were returned from the field in real time, to be coded by trained coders who were supervised by dieticians.

An *ad hoc* central server software/database was developed for this purpose, to work in parallel with the codification and verification processes. Food, beverage, and energy and nutrient intakes were calculated from food consumption records using VD-FEN 2.1 software, a Dietary Evaluation Program from the Spanish Nutrition Foundation (FEN), Spain, which was newly developed for the ANIBES study by the FEN and is based mainly on Spanish food composition tables [13], with several expansions and updates. Data obtained from food manufacturers and nutritional information provided on food labels were also included. A food photographic atlas was used to assist in assigning gram weights to portion sizes. The VD-FEN 2.1 software was developed to receive information from field tablets every 2 s, and the database was updated every 30 min. Energy distribution objectives for the Spanish population were used to analyze the overall quality of the diet [9,14].

2.3. Data Preparation and Analysis

The present analysis focused on the TWI of all food and drink, determined from food composition tables with several adaptations and updates [13]. Metabolic water (water derived from oxidation of substrates) was not included so as to focus on comparisons with dietary water requirements.

Beverages were combined into eight categories for further analysis: (1) hot beverages, including hot tea and coffee (iced teas in cans or bottles were considered caloric soft drinks); (2) milk (all types of milk without separation by fat percentage); (3) fruit and vegetable juices (including nectars, juice–milk blends, 100% fruit juices, and some typical Spanish beverages: horchata, gazpacho, salmorejo, and white garlic); (4) caloric soft drinks (including colas, tonic water, sodas, ginger ale, fruit flavored drinks, iced teas in cans or bottles, sports drinks such as isotonic drinks with mineral salts, and caffeinated energy drinks); (5) diet soft drinks (including the same beverages as in the caloric soft drinks group but with artificial sweetener); (6) alcoholic drinks, including two groups: (a) low-alcohol grade (mostly beer, wine, and cider); and (b) high-alcohol grade (including brandies, liqueurs, tequila, vodka, whisky, *etc.*); (7) water (including tap water and bottled water); and (8) other beverages (including soy-based beverages, non-alcoholic beer and wine, and others).

Additionally, a variety score was created as the sum of the different beverages used in our classification with a minimum value of 0 and a maximum value of 8.

To investigate daily trends, beverage consumption events were aggregated into six time periods, approximately corresponding to breakfast (up to 10:00 a.m.), mid-morning (10:00 a.m.–1:00 p.m.), lunch (1:00 p.m.–4:00 p.m.), mid-afternoon (4:00 p.m.–7:00 p.m.), dinner (7:00 p.m.–10:00 p.m.), and other times.

TWI was compared with the European Food Safety Authority (EFSA) Dietary Reference Values (DRV) for the Adequate Intake (AI) of water for men and women from 14 years of age onward (2.5 L and 2.0 L, respectively), and for boys and girls from 9 to 13 years of age (2.1 L and 1.9 L, respectively) [15]. Furthermore, Nordic and German-speaking countries take the approach that water intake is considered inadequate when it is less than 1 g per kilocalorie of energy requirement [15]. Therefore, we used three different approaches to define water intake adequacy to provide a more comprehensive estimate of the proportion of participants who consume low amounts of water [16]. First, a classification based on the AI value, defined by the EFSA as criterion 1. The second (criterion 2), a ratio between TWI (water from food and beverages in grams) and EI in kcal higher than 1; and the combination of both as final criterion.

2.4. Statistical Analyses

Owing to reported differences in water consumption and recommended intakes between male and female individuals, all analyses were carried out separately by gender. Crude differences in TWI and beverage consumption between groups were assessed through an analysis of variance test or *t*-tests with Bonferroni correction for multiple comparisons. Chi-squared tests were used for categorical variables. All analyses were two-tailed, with statistical significance set at $p < 0.05$.

Partial Correlations between water intake, energy intake, and beverage consumption adjusted for age, gender, body weight, and physical activity were calculated by the use of a variety score.

Multivariable linear regression models included adjustment for gender, age, weight, and physical activity level. Multiple linear regression models were fitted to assess the effect of varying the type of beverages consumed (caloric *vs.* non-caloric) on EI while controlling for the effect of confounders (gender, age, weight, and physical activity). The effect of replacing 100 g of caloric beverages with 100 g of non-caloric beverages was estimated by including caloric beverages (as a percentage of total beverage weight) as the main independent variable, with total beverage weight (g) held constant. This necessarily implies an equal and opposite change in other beverages. A further model included energy from food, thus disallowing compensation (reduction in calories from food). Finally, we used within-person daily consumption data to explore the effect of changes in daily beverage consumption, with each person acting as their own control. The independent variables represent the standard deviation of the mean of the three different measurements (3-day records) for each type of beverage collected for each participant. The outcome (change in EI) was derived using the same methodology (deviation from participants' 3-day mean in energy intake) [16].

3. Results

The ANIBES sample was of 2285 healthy subjects aged 9 to 75 years, of which 50% of the population was men and the other 50% were women. The study sample reflects the distribution of male and female individuals in the general population of Spain [17] (Statistics National Institute (INE) 2011). A more detailed description of the ANIBES study population is given in Table 1 [13]. There was no statistically significant difference in the education or economic level between men and women. However, men smoked more but engaged in more sport than women. Regarding the measures of overweight and obesity, the data of ANIBES study were representative of the Spanish adult population, according to the Spanish National Health Survey 2011–2012 [18]: 37% and 32% of men and women, respectively, were overweight, and 21% and 19%, respectively, were obese.

Figure 1 shows the frequency distribution of TWI (g/day) over a three-day recording period, organized by gender. On average, the TWI was 1.7 L (SE 21.2) for men and 1.6 L (SE 18.9) for women, far less than the EFSA AI recommendations for adults (2.5 L and 2.0 L, respectively).

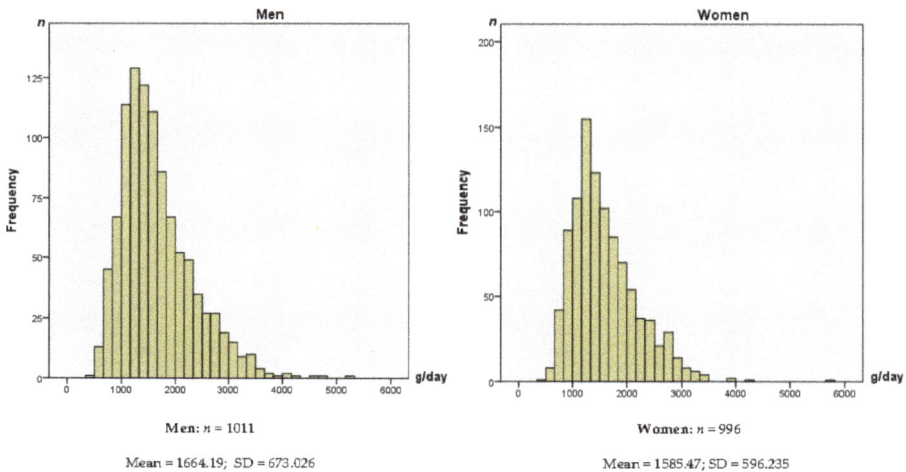

Figure 1. Frequency distribution of total water intake (g/day) over three days by gender.

Percentages of total weight consumed (g/day), daily EI (kcal/day), and water intake (g/day) are presented in Table 2. Beverages were separated by category, with most consumed in similar amounts by participants of both genders. However, men consumed exactly two times more alcoholic beverages than women. The mean total EI was 1809 kcal/day (SE 11.1), and the relative contribution to total EI from beverages was 12% (13% for men, 12% for women). Furthermore, 68% of the TWI came from beverages and 32% from food. Those amounts coincided with EFSA recommendations (70%–80% provided by beverages of all types and the remaining 20%–30% from food).

Table 1. Statistical description of the sample ANIBES.

			Total	%	Male	%	Female	%
		Total	2007	100	1011	50.4	996	49.6
Age Group	9–12	Count	100	5	62	6.1	38	3.8
	13–17	Count	123	6.1	84	8.3	39	3.9
	18–39	Count	777	38.7	387	38.3	390	39.2
	40–64	Count	810	40.4	385	38.1	425	42.7
	65–75	Count	197	9.8	93	9.2	104	10.4
Unemployed		Count	270	13.5	184	18.2	86	8.6
Foreigners (immigrant population)	Spanish	Count	1933	96.3	975	96.4	958	96.2
	Foreign	Count	74	3.7	36	3.6	38	3.8
Level of physical activity	Inactive	Count	884	44.0	389	38.5	495	49.7
	Active	Count	1123	56.0	622	61.5	501	50.3
Level of education	Primary or less	Count	743	37.0	378	37.4	365	36.6
	Secondary	Count	858	42.8	434	42.9	424	42.6
	Tertiary or University	Count	406	20.2	199	19.7	207	20.8
Economical level	1000 € or less	Count	397	19.8	191	18.9	206	20.7
	From 1000 to 2000 €	Count	795	39.6	393	38.9	402	40.4
	Over 2000 €	Count	320	15.9	163	16.1	157	15.8
	No income	Count	7	0.3	4	0.4	3	0.3
	No answer	Count	488	24.3	260	25.7	228	22.9
Geographical distribution	Northwest	Count	152	7.6	77	7.6	75	7.5
	North Central	Count	161	8.0	79	7.8	82	8.2
	Northeast + Barcelona AAMM	Count	368	18.3	177	17.5	191	19.2
	Center + Madrid AAMM	Count	455	22.7	240	23.7	215	21.6
	Levante	Count	335	16.7	176	17.4	159	16.0
	South	Count	443	22.1	218	21.6	225	22.6
	Canarias	Count	93	4.6	44	4.4	49	4.9
Tabaco	Yes	Count	602	30.0	338	33.4	264	26.5
	No	Count	1182	58.9	527	52.1	655	65.8
Weight (kg)		Mean (SE)	72.30 (0.39)		78.40 (0.56)		66.10 (0.46)	
Height (cm)		Mean (SE)	166.20 (0.23)		172.10 (0.31)		160.20 (0.22)	
Waist Circumference		Mean (SE)	87.70 (0.34)		91.90 (0.48)		83.40 (0.45)	
BMI class (kg/m^2)	Underweight	Count	27	1.34	5	0.5	22	2.2
	Normal weight	Count	880	43.84	417	41.2	463	46.5
	Overweight	Count	694	34.57	375	37.1	319	32.0
	Obese	Count	406	20.22	214	21.2	192	19.3

Table 2. Contribution of food and beverages to total water and energy intake.

		Total Weight Consumed (g/Day) GRAMS			Contribution to Energy Intake (kcal/Day) KCAL			Contribution to Water Intake (g/Day) WATER		
	Count	Total 2007	Men 1011	Women 996	Total 2007	Men 1011	Women 996	Total 2007	Men 1011	Women 996
All food and drink	Mean (SE)	2071.55 15.87	2136.35 23.81	2005.77 20.74	1809.01 11.15	1955.68 16.43	1660.15 13.52	1625.12 14.22	1664.19 21.17	1585.47 18.89
Food only	Mean (SE)	45.0% 0.3%	45.5% 0.4%	44.6% 0.4%	87.8% 0.1%	87.2% 0.2%	88.4% 0.2%	32.2% 0.3%	32.4% 0.3%	32.1% 0.4%
Beverages only	Mean (SE)	55.0% 0.3%	54.5% 0.4%	55.4% 0.4%	12.2% 0.1%	12.8% 0.2%	11.6% 0.2%	67.8% 0.3%	67.6% 0.3%	67.9% 0.4%
Hot beverages	Mean (SE)	6.1% 0.1%	5.5% 0.2%	6.6% 0.2%	0.4% 0.0%	0.4% 0.0%	0.5% 0.0%	7.7% 0.2%	7.0% 0.2%	8.3% 0.3%
Milk	Mean (SE)	10.0% 0.2%	9.5% 0.2%	10.6% 0.2%	5.6% 0.1%	5.1% 0.1%	6.0% 0.1%	11.8% 0.2%	11.3% 0.3%	12.3% 0.3%
Fruit & Vegetable Juices	Mean (SE)	2.4% 0.1%	2.6% 0.2%	2.2% 0.1%	1.3% 0.1%	1.4% 0.1%	1.2% 0.1%	2.8% 0.1%	3.0% 0.2%	2.5% 0.2%
Caloric soft drink	Mean (SE)	5.1% 0.2%	5.8% 0.3%	4.4% 0.2%	2.2% 0.1%	2.4% 0.1%	2.0% 0.1%	6.1% 0.2%	6.9% 0.4%	5.2% 0.3%
Diet soft drink	Mean (SE)	1.8% 0.1%	1.4% 0.1%	2.1% 0.2%	0.0% 0.0%	0.0% 0.0%	0.0% 0.0%	2.3% 0.1%	1.8% 0.2%	2.7% 0.2%
Alcohol	Mean (SE)	4.6% 0.2%	6.2% 0.3%	3.0% 0.2%	2.7% 0.1%	3.5% 0.2%	1.9% 0.1%	5.7% 0.2%	7.6% 0.4%	3.7% 0.2%
Water	Mean (SE)	24.8% 0.4%	23.3% 0.5%	26.3% 0.5%	-- --	-- --	-- --	31.2% 0.4%	29.5% 0.6%	32.9% 0.6%
Other non-alcoholic beverages	Mean (SE)	0.2% 0.0%	0.3% 0.1%	0.2% 0.0%	0.0% 0.0%	0.0% 0.0%	0.0% 0.0%	0.3% 0.0%	0.3% 0.1%	0.2% 0.0%

On average, the percentage of total beverage consumption from water over the three-day study period was 46% for women and 41% for men (Figure 2). Water was the most frequently consumed beverage, followed by milk, for both genders. Among men, the decreasing order of consumption was alcoholic drinks, caloric soft drinks, and hot beverages, with similar percentages (11%, 11%, and 10%, respectively). For women, the decreasing order was hot beverages (12%), caloric soft drinks (8%), and alcohol (5%). Fruit and vegetable juices and diet soft drinks were consumed in lower amounts by both genders.

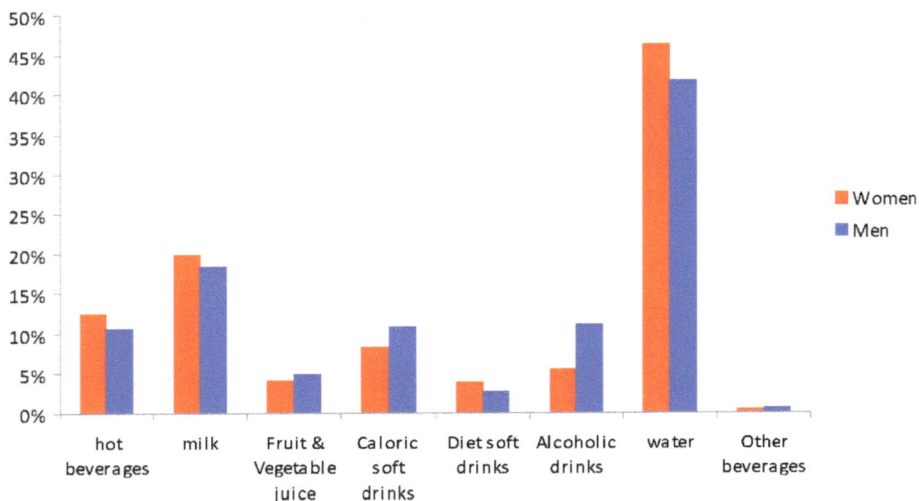

Figure 2. Percentage of beverages consumed over a three-day period by gender.

In general (Table 3), the contribution of water intake from food increased with age, from 434 g/day (SE 13.9) among younger participants (13–17 years) to 584 g/day (SE 24.8) among older adults (65–75 years). This finding is likely owing to lower consumption of fruits and vegetables, which are rich in water, for the youngest participants. The water contribution from beverages declined from 1202 g/day (SE 21.6) among adults (18–64 years) to 1002 g/day (SE 44.0) among older adults.

For adolescents, the mean consumption of caloric soft drinks was 167 g/day (SE 19.1) for men, and 139 g/day (SE 15.9) for women (equivalent to about three cans per week for each). However, consumption was lower among adults, with 114 g/day (SE 6.3) for men and 82.1 g/day (SE 4.6) for women. Consumption of alcoholic drinks for adult men and women averaged 160 g/day (SE 9.0) and 71 g/day (SE 4.8), respectively. The intake of alcoholic drinks among the oldest participants (65–75 years) averaged 143 g/day (SE 19.0) for men and 53 g/day (SE 9.8) for women.

The principal sources of total dietary water, by gender and age group, are shown in Figure 3. For both men and women, the main source was water, followed by milk. Children and adolescents consumed higher amounts of water from milk and juices than adults, for both genders; however, adolescents consumed less water from hot beverages and diet soft drinks than adults. Adults and older adults had a lower intake of caloric soft drinks and juices but consumed greater amounts of hot beverages and alcohol, for both men and women.

Table 3. Total water intake and beverage consumption (g/day) by sex and age group (n = 2281).

	Men						Women					
	Base	Age Group				p¹	Base	Age Group				p¹
		9-12	13-17	18-64	65-75			9-12	13-17	18-64	65-75	
	(A)	(B)	(C)	(D)	(E)		(F)	(G)	(H)	(I)	(J)	
Base	1156	125	136	796	99		1125	87	74	857	107	
Total Water intake from food & beverage Mean (SE)	1638.63 (19.40)	1440.20 [a] (45.47)	1398.04 [b] (43.29)	1717.49 (24.69)	1585.57 (57.75)	<0.001	1559.94 (17.53)	1334.55 [h] (46.58)	1235.51 [f,g] (40.07)	1608.35 (20.97)	1579.77 (48.94)	<0.001
Water from Food Mean (SE)	503.90 (6.07)	443.62 [a,c] (13.72)	433.60 [b,d] (13.96)	515.60 [e] (7.41)	583.72 (24.81)	<0.001	476.31 (5.67)	440.18 (19.42)	403.67 [g,i] (17.83)	475.75 [i] (6.45)	560.47 (19.59)	<0.001
Water from beverages only Mean (SE)	1134.73 (16.74)	997.58 [a] (39.33)	964.44 [b] (36.31)	1201.89 [e] (21.61)	1001.85 (44.03)	<0.001	1083.62 (15.55)	894.37 [h] (40.30)	831.84 [f] (33.16)	1132.60 (18.72)	1019.31 (42.33)	<0.001
Total beverages Consumption Mean (g/day) (SE)	1181.00 (16.94)	1058.60 [a] (40.39)	1026.43 [b] (37.54)	1244.72 [e] (21.86)	1035.52 (44.79)	<0.001	1121.62 (15.65)	943.92 [i] (41.27)	881.93 [f] (33.59)	1169.24 (18.85)	1050.49 (42.78)	<0.001
OF WHICH (g/day)												
Hot beverages Mean (g/day) (SE)	107.14 (3.60)	41.20 [a,c] (4.26)	54.43 [b,d] (7.37)	120.95 (4.55)	151.82 (12.91)	<0.001	123.93 (3.96)	41.85 [h,i] (6.12)	37.15 [f,g] (6.81)	134.00 (4.33)	170.00 (19.02)	<0.001
Milk Mean (g/day) (SE)	204.48 (4.52)	309.73 [a,c] (12.00)	274.67 [b,d] (16.00)	175.69 (4.94)	206.64 (15.24)	<0.001	202.55 (3.85)	249.77 [h] (14.51)	201.86 (15.43)	196.82 (4.28)	210.45 (14.12)	0.003
Fruit & Vegetable Juices Mean (g/day) (SE)	58.22 (3.15)	91.56 [a,c] (11.83)	87.67 [b,d] (11.31)	50.94 (3.51)	34.25 (7.74)	<0.001	45.05 (2.42)	91.76 [h,i] (12.08)	93.35 [h,i] (17.17)	37.46 (2.27)	34.42 (6.66)	<0.001
Caloric soft drink Mean (g/day) (SE)	112.76 (5.25)	113.02 [c] (14.76)	166.97 [b,d] (19.06)	114.19 [e] (6.32)	26.43 (6.57)	<0.001	79.17 (3.86)	67.32 (11.10)	138.94 [g] (15.91)	82.15 [i] (4.59)	23.66 (6.18)	<0.001
Diet soft drink Mean (g/day) (SE)	28.81 (2.70)	12.09 [a,c] (3.17)	21.65 [b] (6.41)	35.25 [d] (3.68)	7.98 (3.13)	0.003	40.26 (3.56)	20.90 (6.48)	18.56 (9.28)	46.88 (4.48)	17.91 (6.16)	0.011
Alcohol Mean (g/day) (SE)	122.36 (6.72)	-	1.14 [b,d] (1.14)	159.66 (9.05)	143.45 (19.00)	<0.001	59.03 (3.88)	-	2.93 (2.34)	70.64 (4.85)	52.82 (9.78)	<0.001
Water Mean (g/day) (SE)	542.12 (14.81)	491.00 (35.99)	419.88 [b] (33.19)	582.15 (19.15)	452.69 (40.51)	<0.001	568.75 (14.17)	472.31 (39.27)	389.14 [f] (34.77)	597.92 (17.03)	537.72 (40.88)	<0.001
Other non alcoholic beverages (g/day) (SE)	5.11 (1.11)	-	-	5.90 (1.49)	12.26 (5.05)	0.034	2.90 (0.55)	-	-	3.347 (0.67)	3.52 (2.14)	0.195

p¹ value obtained through ANOVA test; [a] BD; [b] CD; [c] BE; [d] CE; [e] DE; [f] HI; [g] HJ; [h] GI; [i] GJ; [j] IJ = Significant.

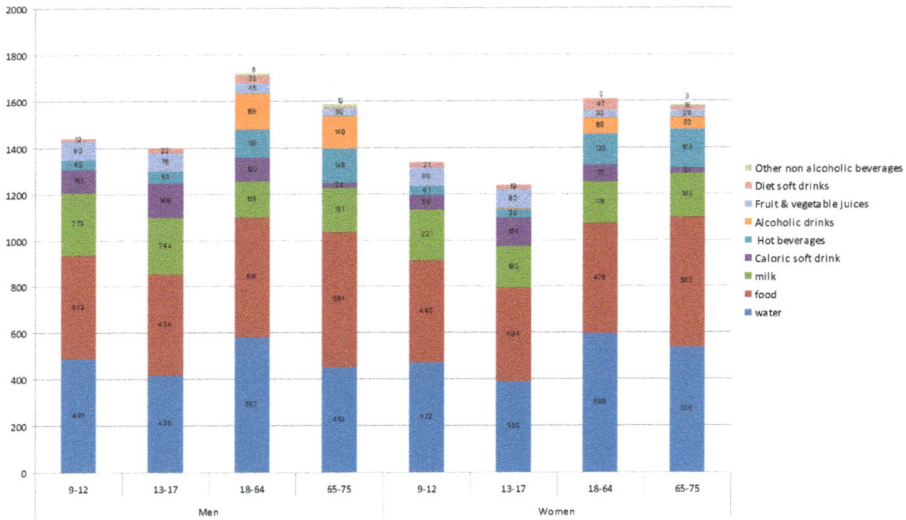

Figure 3. Daily Water intakes (g/day) from beverage/food categories by age and gender among ANBIES population.

TWI was highly correlated with beverage weight and water from beverages ($r = 0.95$), and was more weakly correlated with food intake ($r = 0.54$, Table 4). Caloric soft drinks and alcoholic drinks had a moderate correlation with total energy from beverages ($r = 0.47$ and 0.49, respectively), whereas coefficients were lowest for hot beverages and diet soft drinks.

Regarding beverage variety of eight types of beverages in our classification, the variety score was positively correlated with TWI ($r = 0.39$, $p < 0.001$) and with EI ($r = 0.23$, $p < 0.001$), suggesting that beverage variety is an indicator of a higher consumption of food and drinks.

Figure 4 represents the influence of day of the week on beverage consumption. The total amount of beverage intake (g) was slightly higher on Fridays among men and on Saturdays among women than on other days of the week. This appears to be attributable to a higher consumption of alcoholic drinks on the weekends for both groups. Consumption of water, milk, fruit and vegetable juices, hot beverages, and diet soft drinks did not vary greatly by day of the week. With respect to beverage consumption according to the time of day, over a 24 h period, in general, no significant differences were found by age or time of day in either men or women (Table 5). One exception was seen in differences in the amount of beverages consumed by males during lunch when comparing children and adolescents to adults, the consumption is higher in 18–64 year-old subjects.

Table 4. Partial correlations between water intake, energy intake and beverage consumption. (3 days mean data adjusted for age, gender, body weight and physical activity).

	Total Water (from Food & Beverages) (g/Day)	Total Water from Beverages (g/Day)	Total Water from Food (g/Day)	Total Food Weight (g/Day)	Total Beverages Weight (g/Day)	Total Energy (kcal)	Total Energy from Food (kcal)	Total Energy (kcal) from Beverages
Total Water (g/day) (from food and beverages)	1	0.952 **	0.524 **	0.542 **	0.950 **	0.411 **	0.376 **	0.258 **
Total Water (g/day) from beverages	0.952 **	1	0.239 **	0.271 **	0.999 **	0.315 **	0.256 **	0.301 **
Total Water (g/day) from food	0.524 **	0.239 **	1	0.966 **	0.233 **	0.428 **	0.480 **	−0.017
Total Food weight (g/day)	0.542 **	0.271 **	0.966 **	1	0.268 **	0.594 **	0.647 **	0.042
Total Beverages weight (g/day)	0.950 **	0.999 **	0.233 **	0.268 **	1	0.331 **	0.264 **	0.335 **
Total energy (kcal)	0.411 **	0.315 **	0.428 **	0.594 **	0.331 **	1	0.962 **	0.477 **
Total Energy (kcal) from food	0.376 **	0.256 **	0.480 **	0.647 **	0.264 **	0.962 **	1	0.219 **
Total Energy (kcal) from beverages	0.258 **	0.301 **	−0.017	0.042	0.335 **	0.477 **	0.219 **	1
(1) Hot beverages (g/day)	0.241 **	0.220 **	0.153 **	0.145 **	0.214 **	0.001	0.008	−0.022
(2) Milk (g/day)	0.160 **	0.170 **	0.036	0.069 **	0.189 **	0.199 **	0.111 **	0.356 **
(3) Fruit & vegetable juice (g/day)	0.086 **	0.093 **	0.015	0.028	0.113 **	0.154 **	0.074 **	0.315 **
(4) Caloric soft drink (g/day)	−0.028	0.009	−0.115 **	−0.072 **	0.038	0.273 **	0.157 **	0.471 **
(5) Diet soft drink (g/day)	0.068 **	0.096 **	−0.052 *	−0.040	0.093 **	0.000	0.023	−0.074 **
(6) Alcohol (g/day)	0.271 **	0.304 **	0.014	0.031	0.304 **	0.193 **	0.061 **	0.494 **
(7) Water (g/day)	0.830 **	0.857 **	0.249 **	0.256 **	0.843 **	0.127 **	0.171 **	−0.097 **
(8) Other non alcoholic beverages (g/day)	0.064 **	0.056 *	0.049 *	0.048 *	0.054 *	0.015	0.021	−0.015
Variety of beverages consumed in day (out of 8)	0.392 **	0.401 **	0.130 **	0.156 **	0.408 **	0.229 **	0.143 **	0.360 **

** Correlation is significant at the 0.01 level (bilateral); * Correlation is significant at the 0.05 level (bilateral).

Table 5. Beverage consumption according to time of day (hour interval), by age and gender.

Amount of Beverages (g/Day) Consumed between	Men						Women					
	Age Group						Age Group					
	9–12 (A)	13–17 (B)	18–64 (C)	65–75 (D)	Total	p^1	9–12 (A)	13–17 (B)	18–64 (C)	65–75 (D)	Total	p^1
Breakfast <10:00 Mean (SE)	231.90 (6.84)	233.10 (9.50)	223.50 (4.45)	238.70 (12.47)	226.90 (3.50)	0.532	217.70 (10.54)	194.10 [d] (10.24)	233.50 (4.47)	256.40 (13.47)	232.00 (3.81)	0.01
Mid-morning 10:00 to 13:00 Mean (SE)	160.50 (17.28)	153.60 (17.17)	173.90 (6.98)	140.50 (13.23)	167.50 (5.66)	0.301	120.40 (11.25)	126.40 (13.68)	149.10 (6.19)	149.30 (14.86)	146.10 (5.20)	0.436
Lunch 13:00 to 16:00 Mean (SE)	283.90 [a] (12.72)	295.70 [b] (14.02)	344.80 (6.32)	303.40 (16.00)	328.80 (5.09)	<0.001	248.30 (14.33)	268.50 (12.20)	285.10 (5.15)	274.50 (12.42)	280.10 (4.32)	0.116
Snack 16:00 to 19:00 Mean (SE)	166.30 (12.66)	135.00 (8.71)	167.00 (6.79)	134.40 (14.28)	160.60 (5.10)	0.1	147.10 (12.22)	124.40 (10.73)	138.80 (5.15)	172.10 (14.23)	142.00 (4.32)	0.096
Dinner 19:00 to 22:00 Mean (SE)	248.30 [a] (9.86)	278.00 (14.16)	301.70 (6.02)	259.10 (13.85)	289.50 (4.77)	<0.001	229.80 (13.37)	252.40 (20.04)	248.20 (4.72)	237.80 (14.76)	246.00 (4.20)	0.593
Other moments Mean (SE)	237.80 [a] (34.62)	309.80 (50.88)	444.20 [c] (25.25)	218.70 (37.67)	392.40 (19.78)	<0.001	180.80 [a] (27.13)	140.50 [b] (11.01)	397.90 (17.71)	311.50 (47.13)	364.10 (15.19)	<0.001

p^1 value obtained through ANOVA test. (a) AC; (b) BC; (c) CD; (d) BD = significant.

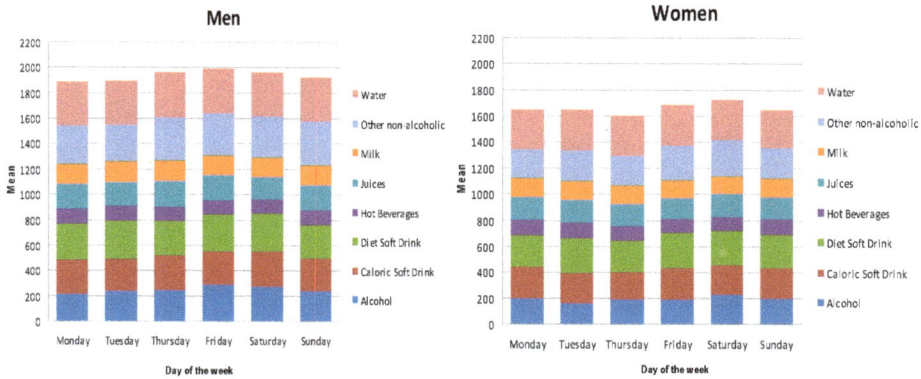

Figure 4. Amount and types of beverages consumed according to day of the week (mean g/day), separated by gender.

Appendix Table A1 shows a multiple regression model including four covariates (gender, age, weight, and physical activity) as well as total beverage intake, which is mathematically equivalent to substituting caloric beverages (sum of hot beverages, milk, fruit and vegetable juices, caloric soft drinks, and alcoholic drinks) with an equal weight of non-caloric beverages (diet soft drinks and water). The predicted effect of replacing 100 g of caloric beverages with 100 g of non-caloric drinks was associated with a reduction in EI of 50 kcal (Model 1). When food EI was constrained as a constant (*i.e.*, disallowing compensation), the net impact of 100 g of caloric beverages was estimated at 40 kcal (Model 2). Further adjustment for level of education, economic level, employment, *etc.* did not change the reported results.

The second regression model analysis (Appendix Table A2) used a within-person change model to address whether a change in a participants' beverage consumption habits on any day could be associated with a change in their total EI (compared with their three-day mean). Modeling each beverage separately, with total beverage weight held constant, each of the above two non-caloric beverages (diet soft drink and water) was negatively associated with energy (as were hot beverages), whereas the five caloric beverages mentioned above were positively associated with energy (Model 3). When combining caloric beverages, the final models (Models 4 and 5) gave an estimated effect of 43 kcal per 100 g of caloric drinks substituted, or 34 kcal if EI from food was held constant.

Participants who fulfilled the EFSA AI recommendations of TWI for men and women (2.5 L and 2.0 L, respectively) were classified as Criterion 1. Participants with ratios of water/energy intake >1.0 were included as Criterion 2 (considering a value of 1 g of water per 1 kcal of energy intake). Finally, participants who met both definitions (Criteria 1 and 2) were classified as Criterion 3. For children 9–13 years old, the EFSA AI is 2.1 L for boys and 1.9 L for girls. Following this analysis, Table 6 shows that for both genders, more than 75% of women, about 80% of men, and nearly 90% of children did not meet the AI recommendation for water consumption.

Table 6. Combined classification for the Total water intake (TWI) following established criteria.

EFSA 2.5 L Men, 2.0 L Women (14 a 75 Years) n = 2023	Men	Women
CRITERION 1: n (%)	241 (12)	431 (21)
CRITERION 2: n (%)	538 (27)	805 (40)
CRITERION 3 (1 and 2): n (%)	202 (10)	370 (18)
EFSA 2.1 L Boys, 1.9 L Girls (9 a 13 Years) n = 258	**Boys**	**Girls**
CRITERION 1: n (%)	28 (11)	28 (11)
CRITERION 2: n (%)	25 (10)	28 (11)
CRITERION 3 (1 and 2): n (%)	13 (5)	18 (7)

EFSA: European Food Safety Authority. (1) Criterion 1: TWI >2.5 L men, >2 L women (aged 14 to 75 years) >2.1 L boys, >1.9 L girls (ages 9 to 13 years); (2) Criterion 2: Ratio of total water/total energy intakes >1; (3) Criterion 3: Both criteria.

4. Discussion

This study provides analyses of total water intakes from all sources among a nationally representative sample of the Spanish population aged 9–75 years, included in the 2013 ANIBES study database. To our knowledge, the present analyses represent one of the few explorations of the consumption of water and beverages in Spain, as well as the association with energy intake, consumption according to time of day and day of the week, the association between beverage variety and increased fluid intake, and compliance with current AI recommendations, by gender and age.

The main findings of this study indicate that for the entire sample, TWI was 1625 g/day (SE 14.2). In general, and as expected, male individuals had statistically higher intakes than female individuals for both food and beverages. However, neither men nor women consumed sufficient amounts of water (1664 g/day for men, 1585 g/day for women), according to EFSA AI reference values [15]. Men consumed approximately 33% less than the AI and women nearly 21% less.

Most of the data analysis in this work was based on an earlier survey by Gibson and Shirreffs [16], who analyzed the weighed dietary records from the National Diet and Nutrition Survey (2000/2001) of 1724 British adults. Contrary to our findings, mean TWI in that population was nearly identical to the EFSA reference AI for both genders.

The comparison is difficult to do when we want to compare American and Spanish populations. The NHANES study, developed in the US between 2005 and 2010, used the proposal by the Institute of Medicine of the United States of America (IOM) as reference value, set as 3.7 L/day for men and 2.7 L/day for women [19]. This leads us to consider the need to investigate why the recommendations of the EFSA and the IOM are so different if both recommendations include the water from both food and beverage sources. The clarification of this issue deserves further study.

Mean daily EI was 1809 kcal/day (SE 11.1), of which 12% was provided by the beverages, close to the 10% proposed by some international authorities (EFSA, WHO) [15,20] who recommended that no more than 10% of the daily calorie intake should come from beverages. In the NHANES study [21], the proportion of energy from beverages was 21%, while it was 16% in the British study [16]. Regarding this issue, in recent years, the impact of caloric soft drink consumption on obesity and metabolic disorders has come under intense scrutiny and debate worldwide [22–25], and large differences between countries have been observed. The present study showed that for the entire Spanish population, caloric soft drinks contributed only 2% of the total EI, or 41.4 kcal/day (SE 1.5) out of a total EI of 1809 kcal/day (SE 11.1). Lower consumption was seen in older adults, at 26.5 g/day (SE 6.6). Higher consumption was found among adolescents, at 167 g/day (SE 19.1), followed by adults and children, with similar mean consumptions of 114.2 g/day (SE 6.3) and 113 g/day (SE 14.8), respectively). This finding is perhaps one of the most interesting findings of our study. The relatively low contribution of caloric soft drinks to the EI could be attributable to the Mediterranean pattern of consumption that this society keeps. By contrast, the NHANES study of the United States [21] has the highest contribution to EI from sweetened beverages. For adults, soda accounted for near 6% of energy intake.

On the other hand, beverage consumption is uneven throughout the day; in this study, it tended to be concentrated at lunchtime and was slightly higher on Fridays in men and on Saturdays in women. Although we did not find large variation, these findings reflect certain cultural trends of consumption that appear to be attributable to a higher intake of alcoholic beverages on weekends among both genders. The contribution of alcoholic drinks to the diet in the ANIBES study (135.7 g/day, SE 7.5) was slightly higher than that in the ENIDE dietary survey of Spanish adults in 2011 (117 g/day) [7]. It is important to note that beverages with lower alcohol content (beer, wine, and cider) represented over 90% of the energy contribution in adult and older populations. Furthermore, although these data are of the highest quality obtainable, alcohol intake is one of the dietary components for which underreporting may occur, especially among women and participants with higher education and socioeconomic levels [26,27]. In fact, the reported amount of alcohol consumed by men was twice that reported by women in this study. Anyway, this relatively high consumption of alcohol shown could also be attributable to the Mediterranean dietary pattern that certainly remains rooted in Spanish society. The Spanish Society of Community Nutrition (SENC) recommends the maximum consumption of 1 to 1.5 servings/day of alcoholic beverages in women and 2 to 2.5 servings/day for adult males in the context of a Mediterranean balanced diet. Consumption of alcoholic beverages is associated with a more or less healthy dietary pattern. The types of alcoholic beverages that are closer to the Mediterranean environment are [28] fermented drinks, wine, beer, and cider consumed during the principal meals.

The strengths of this study include the careful design, protocol, and methodology used in the ANIBES study. The present analysis can be used to inform approaches to improving the overall quality of diet and hydration status of the Spanish population.

Two important limitations of this study must be noted. This study is a cross-sectional design, which provides evidence for association but not causal relationships. The second limitation is that, for logistical reasons, there was no inclusion of a hydration biomarker, which would allow assessment of dietary beverage intake and hydration status without the bias of self-reported dietary intake and also intra-individual variability. This biomarker should be included in further studies.

5. Conclusions

The present study shows clearly that neither men nor women consumed adequate TWI when compared with EFSA reference values. The ANIBES study demonstrated that well-conducted national surveys have the potential to yield rich contextual value data that can emphasize the need to undertake appropriate health and nutrition policies to increase the total water intake at the population level, promoting a healthy Mediterranean hydration pattern.

Acknowledgments: The ANIBES study was supported by Coca-Cola Iberia through an agreement with the Spanish Nutrition Foundation (FEN) who assisted with the technical advice. The current analysis included in this paper was financially supported by a Grant from the European Hydration Institute to the Canarian Foundation Science and Technology Park of the University of Las Palmas de Gran Canaria. The funding sponsors had no role in the design of the study, the collection, analysis, or interpretation of the data, writing of the manuscript, or in the decision to publish the results.

Author Contributions: M.N., A.S.V. and L.S.M. analyzed the data. M.N. also drafted and wrote the manuscript. L.S.M. contributed to the analysis and wrote the manuscript. This author is a member of the Scientific Advisory Board of the ANIBES study and, together with the other members, was responsible for careful review of the protocol, design, and methodology. This author provided continuous scientific advice for the study and for interpretation of the results. J.A.B., A.G., R.M.O. and M.G.G. are members of the Scientific Advisory Board of the ANIBES study and were responsible for careful review of the protocol, design, and methodology. These authors provided continuous scientific advice for the study and for the interpretation of results. These authors also critically reviewed the manuscript. G.V.M., Principal Investigator of the ANIBES study, was responsible for the design, protocol, methodology, and follow-up checks of the study. All authors approved the final version of the manuscript.

Conflicts of Interest: The authors declare no conflict of interest.

Appendix

Table A1. Regression model estimating change in energy intake associated with adding caloric beverages in place of non-caloric beverages.

Model 1		B	*p* Value	95% Confidence Interval for B	
				Lower	Upper
(Constant)		1597.476	<0.001	1507.809	1687.144
Gender	men	253.295	<0.001	211.937	294.653
Age (years)		−4.715	<0.001	−5.931	−3.499
Weight (kg)		−2.722	<0.001	−3.956	−1.488
Physical activity	active	−34.556	0.092	−74.704	5.592
Total beverages (100 g/day)		18.191	<0.001	14.541	21.841
5caloricbeverages (100 g) *		49.817	<0.001	42.757	56.877

Model 2: Keeping Food Constant		B	*p* Value	95% Confidence Interval for B	
				Lower	Upper
(Constant)		46.798	<0.001	27.063	66.533
Gender	men	22.655	<0.001	15.224	30.085
Age (years)		−0.969	<0.001	−1.182	−0.755
Weight (kg)		−0.286	0.009	−0.502	−0.070
Physical activity	active	3.582	0.316	−3.424	10.589
Food (Kcal)		1.005	<0.001	0.997	1.012
Total beverages (100 g)		−0.889	<0.008	−1.542	−0.235
5caloricbeverages (100 g) *		40.079	<0.001	38.845	41.312

* "5caloricbeverages" = sum of hot beverages, milk, fruit & vegetable juice, caloric soft drinks and alcoholic drinks.

Table A2. Within-person change Model: estimated change in energy intake associated with beverage substitution.

Model 3: Estimated Effect of Substituting Each Beverage Type *			95% Confidence Interval for B	
Changes in:	B	*p* Value	Lower	Upper
Hot beverages (100 g)	−29.080	0.016	−52.833	−5.326
Milk (100 g)	6.539	0.506	−12.726	25.804
Fruit & vegetable juice (100 g)	47.147	0.030	4.578	89.716
Caloric soft drink (100 g)	17.681	0.155	−6.706	42.069
Diet soft drink (100 g)	−35.621	0.069	−73.997	2.755
Alcoholic drinks (100 g)	18.612	0.027	2.128	35.096
Water (100 g)	−34.139	<0.0001	−42.263	−26.014

Model 4: Estimated Effect of Caloric Beverages Replacing Non-Caloric Beverages	B	*p* Value	95% Confidence Interval for B	
			Lower	Upper
Change in total beverages (100 g)	−6.083	0.007	−10.485	−1.682
Change in caloric beverages (100 g)	43.387	<0.0001	34.702	52.071

Model 5: Estimated Effect of Caloric Beverages Replacing Caloric Beverages, Holding Food Energy Constant	B	*p* Value	95% Confidence Interval for B	
			Lower	Upper
Change in food energy (100 kcal)	103.626	<0.0001	102.587	104.666
Change in total beverages (100 g)	−7.718	<0.0001	−8.701	−6.735
Change in caloric beverages (100 g)	34.232	<0.0001	32.292	36.173

* Model 6 is a composite of 7 regressions, one for each beverage, adjusted for change in total beverages.

References

1. Maughan, R. Impact of mild dehydration on wellness and on exercise performance. *Eur. J. Clin. Nutr.* **2003**, *57*, S19–S23. [CrossRef] [PubMed]
2. Watson, P.; Whale, A.; Mears, S.A.; Reyner, L.A.; Maughan, R.J. Mild hypohydration increases the frequency of driver errors during a prolonged, monotonous driving task. *Physiol. Behav.* **2015**, *147*, 313–318. [CrossRef] [PubMed]
3. Nissensohn, M.; Castro-Quezada, I.; Serra-Majem, L. Beverage and water intake of healthy adults in some European countries. *Int. J. Food Sci. Nutr.* **2013**, *64*, 801–805. [CrossRef] [PubMed]
4. Serra-Majem, L. Opening remarks: The burden of disease attributable to hydration in Europe. *Nutr. Hosp.* **2015**, *32*, 10260. [PubMed]
5. Frangeskou, M.; Lopez-Valcarcel, B.; Serra-Majem, L. Dehydration in the Elderly: A Review Focused on Economic Burden. *J. Nutr. Health Aging* **2015**, *19*, 619–627. [CrossRef] [PubMed]
6. Bach-Faig, A.; Fuentes-Bol, C.; Ramos, D.; Carrasco, J.L.; Roman, B.; Bertomeu, I.F.; Cristià, E.; Geleva, D.; Serra-Majem, L. The Mediterranean diet in Spain: Adherence trends during the past two decades using the Mediterranean Adequacy Index. *Public Health Nutr.* **2011**, *14*, 622–628. [CrossRef] [PubMed]
7. Spanish Agency for Food Safety and Nutrition (AESAN). ENIDE: Encuesta Nacional de Ingesta Dietética Española 2011. Available online: http://www.aesan.msc.es (accessed on 12 January 2015).
8. Ruiz, E.; Ávila, J.M.; Castillo, A.; Valero, T.; del Pozo, S.; Rodriguez, P.; Aranceta Bartrina, J.; Gil, A.; González-Gross, M.; Ortega, R.M.; et al. The ANIBES study on energy balance in Spain: Design, protocol and methodology. *Nutrients* **2015**, *7*, 970–998. [CrossRef] [PubMed]
9. Ruiz, E.; Ávila, J.M.; Valero, T.; Del Pozo, S.; Rodriguez, P.; Aranceta-Bartrina, J.; Gil, Á.; González-Gross, M.; Ortega, R.M.; Serra-Majem, L.; et al. Energy intake, profile, and dietary sources in the Spanish population: Findings of the ANIBES study. *Nutrients* **2015**, *12*, 4739–4762. [CrossRef] [PubMed]
10. Varela Moreiras, G.; Ávila, J.M.; Ruiz, E. Energy Balance, a new paradigm and methodological issues: The ANIBES study in Spain. *Nutr. Hosp.* **2015**, *31*, 101–112. [PubMed]
11. Willet, W.C. *Issues in Analysis and Presentation of Dietary Data. Nutritional Epidemiology*, 2nd ed.; Oxford University Press: New York, NY, USA, 1998.
12. Roman-Viñas, B.; Serra-Majem, L.; Hagströmer, M.; Ribas-Barba, L.; Sjöström, M.; Segura-Cardona, R. International physical activity questionnaire: Reliability and validity in a Spanish population. *Eur. J. Sport Sci.* **2010**, *10*, 297–304. [CrossRef]
13. Moreiras, O.; Carbajal, A.; Cabrera, L.; Cuadrado, C. *Tablas de Composición de Alimentos/Guía de Prácticas*, 16th ed.; Ediciones Pirámide: Madrid, Spain, 2013.
14. Sociedad Española de Nutrición Comunitaria (SENC). Objetivos nutricionales para la población española. Consenso de la Sociedad Española de Nutrición Comunitaria, 2011. *Rev. Esp. Nutr. Comunitaria* **2011**, *17*, 178–199.
15. EFSA Panel on Dietetic Products, Nutrition, and Allergies (NDA). Scientific opinion on dietary reference values for water. *EFSA J.* **2010**, *8*, 1459.
16. Gibson, S.; Shirreffs, S.M. Beverage consumption habits "24/7" among British adults: Association with total water intake and energy intake. *Nutr. J.* **2013**, *10*, 9. [CrossRef] [PubMed]
17. INE 2011: Instituto Nacional de Estadística: Censos de Población y Viviendas, 2011. Available online: http://www.ine.es/censos2011_datos/cen11_datos_inicio.htm (accessed on 2 November 2015).
18. Encuesta Nacional de Salud 2011–2012. Available online: http://www.msssi.gob.es/estadEstudios/estadisticas/encuestaNacional/encuesta2011.htm (accessed on 12 January 2015).
19. Institute of Medicine. Dietary reference intakes for water, potassium, sodium, chloride and sulfate. In *Food and Nutrition Board*; The National Academies Press: Washington, DC, USA, 2004.
20. WHO/FAO. *Diet, Nutrition and the Prevention of Chronic Diseases*; Report No. 916; World Health Organization: Geneva, Switzerland, 2002.
21. Drewnowski, A.; Rehm, C.D.; Constant, F. Water and beverage consumption among adults in the United States: Cross-sectional study using data from NHANES 2005–2010. *BMC Public Health* **2013**, *12*, 1068. [CrossRef] [PubMed]
22. Lustig, R.; Schmidt, L.; Brindis, C. The toxic truth about sugar. *Nature* **2012**, *482*, 27–29. [CrossRef] [PubMed]

23. Johnson, R.J.; Segal, M.S.; Sautin, Y.; Nakagawa, T.; Feig, D.I.; Kang, D.H.; Gersch, M.S.; Benner, S.; Sánchez-Lozada, L.G. Potential role of sugar (fructose) in the epidemic of hypertension, obesity and the metabolic syndrome, diabetes, kidney disease, and cardiovascular disease. *Am. J. Clin. Nutr.* **2007**, *86*, 899–906. [PubMed]

24. Johnson, R.K.; Appel, L.J.; Brands, M.; Howard, B.V.; Lefevre, M.; Lustig, R.H.; Sacks, F.; Steffen, L.M.; Wylie-Rosett, J. American Heart Association Nutrition Committee of the council on Nutrition, Physical Activity, and Metabolism and the Council on Epidemiology and Prevention. Dietary sugars intake and cardiovascular health: A scientific statement from the American Heart Association. *Circulation* **2009**, *24*, 1011–1020.

25. Malik, V.S.; Popkin, B.M.; Bray, G.A.; Despres, J.P.; Hu, F.B. Sugar-sweetened beverages, obesity, type 2 diabetes mellitus, and cardiovascular disease risk. *Circulation* **2010**, *121*, 1356–1364. [CrossRef] [PubMed]

26. Johansson, L.; Solvoli, K.; Gunn-Elin, A.B.; Drevon, C.A. Under- and overreporting of energy intake related to weight status and lifestyle in a nationwide sample. *Am. J. Clin. Nutr.* **1998**, *68*, 266–274. [PubMed]

27. Rasmussen, L.B.; Matthiessen, J.; Biltoft-Jensen, A.; Tetens, I. Characteristics of misreporters of dietary intake and physical activity. *Public Health Nutr.* **2007**, *10*, 230–237. [CrossRef] [PubMed]

28. Serra-Majem, L.; Bach-Faig, A.; Raidó-Quintana, B. Nutritional and cultural aspects of the Mediterranean diet. *Int. J. Vitam. Nutr. Res.* **2012**, *82*, 157–162. [CrossRef] [PubMed]

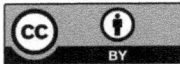

nutrients

MDPI

Article

Water Intake and Hydration Indices in Healthy European Adults: The European Hydration Research Study (EHRS)

Olga Malisova [1], Adelais Athanasatou [1], Alex Pepa [1], Marlien Husemann [2], Kirsten Domnik [2], Hans Braun [2], Ricardo Mora-Rodriguez [3], Juan F. Ortega [3], Valentin E. Fernandez-Elias [3] and Maria Kapsokefalou [1,*]

[1] Unit of Human Nutrition, Department of Food Science and Human Nutrition, Agricultural University of Athens, 75 Iera Odos Str., Athens 11855, Greece; olgamalisova@yahoo.gr (O.M.); dathanasatou@gmail.com (A.A.); alekspepa@gmail.com (A.P.)
[2] Institute of Biochemistry, German Sport University, Cologne 50993, Germany; m.husemann@biochem.dshs-koeln.de (M.H.); kirsten.domnik@gmx.de (K.D.); h.braun@dshs-koeln.de (H.B.)
[3] Exercise Physiology Lab at Toledo, University of Castilla-la Mancha, Toledo 13071, Spain; ricardo.mora@uclm.es (R.M.-R.); juanfernando.ortega@uclm.es (J.F.O.); valentin.fernandez@uclm.es (V.E.F.-E.)
* Correspondence: kapsok@aua.gr; Tel.: +30-210-529-4708

Received: 29 January 2016; Accepted: 30 March 2016; Published: 6 April 2016

Abstract: Hydration status is linked with health, wellness, and performance. We evaluated hydration status, water intake, and urine output for seven consecutive days in healthy adults. Volunteers living in Spain, Germany, or Greece ($n = 573$, 39 ± 12 years (51.1% males), 25.0 ± 4.6 kg/m^2 BMI) participated in an eight-day study protocol. Total water intake was estimated from seven-day food and drink diaries. Hydration status was measured in urine samples collected over 24 h for seven days and in blood samples collected in fasting state on the mornings of days 1 and 8. Total daily water intake was 2.75 ± 1.01 L, water from beverages 2.10 ± 0.91 L, water from foods 0.66 ± 0.29 L. Urine parameters were: 24 h volume 1.65 ± 0.70 L, 24 h osmolality 631 ± 221 mOsmol/kg H$_2$O, 24 h specific gravity 1.017 ± 0.005, 24 h excretion of sodium 166.9 ± 54.7 mEq, 24 h excretion of potassium 72.4 ± 24.6 mEq, color chart 4.2 ± 1.4. Predictors for urine osmolality were age, country, gender, and BMI. Blood indices were: haemoglobin concentration 14.7 ± 1.7 g/dL, hematocrit 43% $\pm$ 4% and serum osmolality 294 ± 9 mOsmol/kg H$_2$O. Daily water intake was higher in summer (2.8 ± 1.02 L) than in winter (2.6 ± 0.98 L) ($p = 0.019$). Water intake was associated negatively with urine specific gravity, urine color, and urine sodium and potassium concentrations ($p < 0.01$). Applying urine osmolality cut-offs, approximately 60% of participants were euhydrated and 20% hyperhydrated or dehydrated. Most participants were euhydrated, but a substantial number of people (40%) deviated from a normal hydration level.

Keywords: hydration status; water intake; hydration indices; urine; blood; seasonality; country

---

1. Introduction

The evaluation of hydration status in the general population in free-living and/or under special conditions such as in disease or in the work environment is of unequivocal importance for public health. This is because dehydration is linked with reduced physical and cognitive performance [1] or disease [2,3].

Hydration status reflects the balance between water intake and loss. Water intake includes, approximately, 20% contribution of water from solid foods and 80% contribution of water from beverages and drinking water [4–6]. It follows that water intake, although mostly driven by thirst, depends on a variety of factors such as eating and drinking habits and preferences or availability of foods and beverages [7–9]. Water loss consists mainly from excretion of water in urine, respiratory water, feces and sweat [10]. Since the contribution of sweat in water loss is higher in a physically active person and in hot weather [11], water loss is affected by physical activity levels and season. Therefore, water loss is highly variable, even in healthy individuals, depending on the lifestyle of the individual and on environmental conditions or geographical location.

Data on water intake in relation to hydration status in population groups in free-living conditions are scarce. This constitutes a knowledge gap and consequently an obstacle in supporting initiatives for improving the hydration of the population. There is an urgent need to build databases on the estimation of water intake and of hydration status in the population.

Selecting the appropriate research tools for evaluating water intake and hydration status is crucial. Seven day diaries, in which all foods and beverages consumed are recorded, may present advantages in reflecting intake [12] compared with other tools, such as 24 h recall or food frequency questionnaires [13]. A synthesis of indices in urine and blood samples [3,12,14–17] is necessary for the evaluation of hydration status of individuals or population groups, as there is no single index to reflect hydration status [12,18,19]. Yet, measuring a series of hydration indices in samples collected over seven days instead of spot urine [20] may provide advantages since this approach incorporates factors that fluctuate during the week and affect hydration status, such as eating and drinking habits, physical activity, and environmental conditions.

The objectives of the study were to assess hydration status, water intake and urine output in summer and winter over seven days in a sample of healthy adults in three European countries.

2. Materials and Methods

Participating centers were the Agricultural University of Athens, Greece (GR), the German Sport University, Cologne (GER), Germany, and the University of Castilla La Mancha, Spain (ESP). The study was conducted in population living in the metropolitan areas of Athens, Cologne, and Toledo, respectively, in parallel and following identical protocols during winter (1–3/2013, 12/2013, 1–2/2014) and summer (6–8/2013, 6–7/2014). Five hundred and seventy three subjects aged 20–60 (39 ± 12 years) (51.1% males) with a BMI 25.5 ± 4.2 kg/m^2 for males and 24.5 ± 4.9 kg/m^2 for females were enrolled in the study. Subjects were adults aged 20–60 years with approximately equal numbers in each decade of life. Demographic factors such as ethnic origin, living conditions, marital status, and other were not considered to further stratify the sample.

The study protocol was approved by the Research Ethics Committee in each center involved (197/27-02-2012 for Agricultural University of Athens, Greece, 4/02/213-18 for University of Castilla La Mancha, Spain, 1/26-11-2012 for German Sport University, German). Written informed consent was obtained from all subjects. Exclusion criteria were disease (diabetes insipidus, renal disease, liver disease, gastrointestinal diseases or problems, cardiac or pulmonary diseases, disease that limits mobility including muscle-skeletal diseases, or orthopedic problems), pregnancy, lactation, hypertensive under severe salt restriction, taking drugs that are, or contain, diuretics, phenytoin, lithium, demeclocycline, or amphotericin, and following a high-protein and/or hypocaloric diet. Subjects were rescheduled or omitted if they caught flu (cold) or had fever, vomiting, and/or diarrhea or menstruation during the data collection period. Data from subjects who lost or gained more than 2% of body mass between day 1 and 8 were discarded. Additionally, data from subjects with values of creatinine excretion rate (CER) >3500 mg/day or <350 mg/day were revealing inaccurate 24 h urine collection [21], consequently four subjects who had CER >3500 mg/day were excluded from the analyses. Twenty-eight subjects did not complete the protocol (13 in winter, 15 in summer) for personal reasons.

2.1. Recruitment

Recruitment started two weeks before, and continued throughout, the study period. Recruitment strategy included invitations (a) sent by email to the non-academic and academic personnel of the three study centers; (b) uploaded on social media and published in local newspapers; (c) uploaded on internet sites related to nutrition; (d) distributed in paper at various non-academic places; (e) sent by email to other academic and social work institutions in the greater area of the centers involved (f) distributed at any seminar that the research teams were giving. Volunteers expressing interest for participating to the study completed a screen questionnaire in order to detect any of the exclusion criteria. If admitted to the study, subjects received the study protocol in writing, verbal responses to any questions they had on the purpose of the study, detailed instructions on study procedures including recording of food, drink and urination, and signed an informed consent form.

2.2. Study Protocol

Subjects entering the study received a small back pack containing instruction sheet for study protocol; a diary for recording urine volume; a kitchen scale readable to 1 g; a urine collection container; eight Zip-loc bags, seven of them containing 10 screw cap tubes (10 mL) for urine sampling, each labeled with subject code number, day, and urination time and one Zip-loc bag containing one screw cap tube (10 mL) for urine sampling in the morning of the eighth day. Additionally, subjects received a styrofoam box (30 × 50 × 20 cm) and/or ice packs for the storage of samples. Furthermore, each subject received (a) a seven day diary (7DD) to report in detail foods, drinks, water, wake up time, bed time; (b) a physical activity questionnaire (Short version of the International Physical Activity Questionnaires; IPAQ) [22] for each day of the week; and (c) a questionnaire including a series of questions regarding the profile of the individual, behavior and knowledge about hydration. A mini interview on motives and barriers to good hydration was conducted on the first day of the study period of each individual.

Subjects entered the study on different days of the week in order to achieve a reasonable distribution of starting days over the week. On study day 1 subjects arrived fasted at the study center between 7:00 and 9:30, bringing a weighted sample of their first morning urine void. Upon arrival, participants' body height was measured was with mechanical sliding scale (Seca 711 Mechanical Sliding Weight Beam Scale) and mass measured with electronic digital scale (TANITA, Body Composition Analyser, TBF 300) wearing underwear and no shoes. They were also instructed to sit for approximately 15–20 min while filling in study questionnaires. Subsequently, a blood sample (5 mL) from a vein in the forearm was collected without stasis.

On days 1–7, while going about their normal daily routine, subjects recorded their food and drink consumption based on portion sizes and/or package information, collected and recorded the weight of each urination and of time of collection and retained a sample in a numbered tube, as instructed. Subjects stored the urine tubes in their refrigerator or in the styrofoam box using ice packs until arrival to the refrigerator. On day 8, following an overnight fast, subjects visited the laboratory, delivered their first morning urine sample, blood samples were taken and body mass was measured as on day 1. Urine collection of each day was from 00:00 to 24:00. A reconstituted sample of 10 mL for each day consisted of samples from all samples that were collected during the 24 h period. The ratio of the volume of each urination per 24 h volume was calculated. The contribution of each urination to the reconstituted sample of 10 mL was calculated so that the volume ratio of each urination per 10 mL was the same to that of the volume ratio of each urination per the 24 h volume. Urine color was determined via the eight-point urine color chart developed by Armstrong (1994), urine and serum osmolality were measured in duplicate using freezing-point osmometer (Cryoscopic Osmometer, Osmomat 030, Gonotec). Urine and serum sodium and potassium were measured by ion selective electrode methods and urine creatinine was measured by the Jaffe enzymatic colorimetric method (Cobas Integra 400 plus). Urine specific gravity was measured with a pen refractometer (Master Reftractometer, Atago, cat. No. 2771). Urine volume was measured with an electronic digital scale (Soehnle Fiesta 65106). Hematocrit was determined via Micro Hematocrit

Centrifuge (model, KHT-400), hemoglobin via spectrophotometer absorption (Pointe Scientific Inc. Hemoglobin Reagent Set, Canton, MI, USA). Finally, 7DD were analyzed with Diet Analysis plus version 6.1 (ESHA Research, Wadsworth Publishing Co. Inc., Salem, OR, USA) for the Greek population, PCN CESNID version 1.0 (Centre D'Ensenyament Superior De Nutricio I Dietetica, University of Barcelona, Barcelona, Spain) for the Spanish population and EBIS pro (German Food Database 3.1, University of Hohenheim, Stuttgart, Germany) for the German population.

Meteorological conditions (minimum and maximum temperature; relative humidity, precipitation) were provided by the nearest weather station of the center on each of the sampling days.

2.3. Statistical Analysis

Continuous variables are expressed as mean ± standard deviation for variables following normal distribution. Normal distribution of all continuous variables was tested with the parametric test Shapiro–Wilk or graphically assessed by histograms. Correlations between variables were evaluated using Pearson's or Spearman's correlation coefficient. Differences between genders and seasons (P1–P4) were derived through Student's *t*-test for normally distributed variables. Differences among countries (P5) and among hyperhydrated, euhydrated, and dehydrated subjects were derived through One Way Anova test for normally distributed variables. *Post hoc* comparisons among countries were performed using Bonferroni test. The multivariate associations between variables were assessed using linear regression models, adjusted for all biologically plausible confounders. Subjects with missing some day value in one variable were not excluded from the analysis; the average of the week value was calculated from the remaining data. Statistical analysis was performed by SPSS package, version 16.1 (SPSS Inc., Chicago, IL, USA). We deemed statistical significance at $\alpha = 0.05$.

3. Results

The population of the study that completed the protocol consisted of 573 subjects (age 39 ± 12 years; 280 females). 297 subjects (age 39 ± 12 years; 155 females) completed the protocol in the summer period. The mean BMI of males was 25.5 ± 4.2 kg/m^2 and females 24.5 ± 4.9 kg/m^2 ($p = 0.012$).

3.1. 24 h Urine Samples

Mean hydration indices (sodium, potassium, osmolality, urine volume, specific gravity, color) for 24 h urine samples from the seven days collection for males and females in winter and summer period and for each country are presented in Table 1.

Urine samples of men were more concentrated, as they had higher osmolality, specific gravity, and darker color. Women's lower osmolality values are in agreement with the finding that quantities of sodium, potassium, and creatinine over a 24 h period ($p < 0.001$) are lower in women. There were also significant sex differences in summer period for most urine indices; females produced less concentrated urine of lower osmolality ($p < 0.001$) and excreted lower quantities of sodium and potassium ($p < 0.001$ and $p = 0.016$, respectively). Differences were observed in all urinary hydration indices ($p < 0.001$) among countries.

Table 1. 24 h urine hydration indices of participants in winter and summer.

		Sodium (mEq/Day)	Potassium (mEq/Day)	Creatinine (mg/Day)	Urine Osmolality (mOsmol/kg: H_2O)	Urine Volume (L)	USG	Color
Winter	Male	178.4 ± 51.5	76.0 ± 20.1	1738.4 ± 523.0	652 ± 211	1.66 ± 0.62	1.018 ± 0.005	4.4 ± 1.4
	Female	162.9 ± 56.7	68.8 ± 21.8	1335.6 ± 404.1	571 ± 197	1.70 ± 0.72	1.016 ± 0.005	4.1 ± 1.3
	Total	171.4 ± 54.4	72.7 ± 21.2	1555.2 ± 512.8	615 ± 209	1.68 ± 0.66	1.017 ± 0.005	4.2 ± 1.4
Summer	Male	181.9 ± 50.1	76.2 ± 25.7	1820.6 ± 451.6	698 ± 192	1.61 ± 0.70	1.018 ± 0.005	4.6 ± 1.2
	Female	145.6 ± 53.1	68.5 ± 28.3	1290.0 ± 474.4	596 ± 251	1.63 ± 0.77	1.015 ± 0.006	3.9 ± 1.6
	Total	162.8 ± 54.7	72.2 ± 27.3	1543.7 ± 533.6	645 ± 230	1.62 ± 0.73	1.017 ± 0.006	4.2 ± 1.5
	P1	0.021	0.005	<0.001	0.001	0.586	0.003	0.069
	P2	<0.001	0.016	<0.001	<0.001	0.789	<0.001	<0.001
	P3	0.065	0.789	0.795	0.111	0.370	0.679	0.983
Winter & Summer	Total Male	180.1 ± 50.8	76.1 ± 22.9	1779.1 ± 489.9	675 ± 203	1.63 ± 0.66	1.018 ± 0.005	4.5 ± 1.3
	Total Female	153.2 ± 55.3	68.6 ± 25.6	1310 ± 444.7	585 ± 229	1.66 ± 0.74	1.015 ± 0.006	4.0 ± 1.5
	Total Sample	166.9 ± 54.7	72.4 ± 24.6	1549.1 ± 523.4	631 ± 221	1.65 ± 0.70	1.017 ± 0.005	4.2 ± 1.4
	P4	<0.001	<0.001	<0.001	<0.001	0.619	<0.001	<0.001
Country	German	162.2 ± 50.3 *,#	77.9 ± 24.1 #	1454.0 ± 401.0 *	492 ± 170 *,#	2.13 ± 0.76 *,#	1.014 ± 0.005 *,#	4.4 ± 1.3 #
	Spain	192.8 ± 51.7 +	74.0 ± 27.8 +	1807.9 ± 621.2 +	753 ± 180 +	1.40 ± 0.49	1.019 ± 0.004 +	4.4 ± 1.5 +
	Greece	143.8 ± 51.0	64.4 ± 18.7	1377.9 ± 415.3	658 ± 224	1.36 ± 0.50	1.017 ± 0.006	4.0 ± 1.5
	P5	<0.001	<0.001	<0.001	<0.001	<0.001	<0.001	0.008

p-values derived through Student's *t*-test for differences between genders and season; and one-way ANOVA among countries; * significant difference between German and Spain; # significant difference between German and Greece; + significant difference between Spain and Greece; P1 refers to comparisons between gender for winter, P2 refers to comparisons between gender for summer, P3 refers to comparisons between summer and winter for the total sample (males and females together); P4 refers to comparisons between males and females (winter and summer together); P5 refers to comparisons between countries.

3.2. Blood Indices

Differences in serum osmolality ($p = 0.001$), hemoglobin and hematocrit were observed between genders ($p < 0.001$; Table 2). All indices were within the physiological ranges. In the summer population no differences were observed in serum glucose ($p = 0.081$), serum sodium ($p = 0.166$), and serum potassium ($p = 0.092$) between males and females.

Table 2. Blood and serum hydration indices of participants in winter and summer.

		Hb (g/dL)	Htc (%)	Glucose (mmol/L)	Serum Osmolality (mOsmol/kg H_2O)	Sodium (mEq/L)	Potassium (mEq/L)
Winter	Male	15.3 ± 1.5	45 ± 3	4.67 ± 0.46	297 ± 10	143.0 ± 4.9	4.4 ± 0.4
	Female	14.1 ± 1.6	42 ± 4	4.73 ± 0.52	294 ± 10	141.6 ± 3.9	4.4 ± 0.4
	Total	14.7 ± 1.7	43 ± 4	4.70 ± 0.49	296 ± 10	142.4 ± 4.5	4.4 ± 0.4
Summer	Male	15.5 ± 1.5	45 ± 3	5.02 ± 1.09	293 ± 7	143.3 ± 5.1	4.5 ± 0.5
	Female	14.0 ± 1.6	41 ± 4	4.88 ± 1.59	291 ± 8	144.7 ± 11.3	4.6 ± 0.6
	Total	14.7 ± 1.7	43 ± 4	4.94 ± 1.37	292 ± 8	144.0 ± 8.9	4.6 ± 0.6
	P1	<0.001	<0.001	0.339	0.015	0.020	0.580
	P2	<0.001	<0.001	0.388	0.081	0.166	0.064
	P3	0.824	0.397	0.005	<0.001	0.005	<0.001
Winter & Summer	Total Male	15.4 ± 1.5	45 ± 3	4.84 ± 0.85	295 ± 9	143.1 ± 5.0	4.5 ± 0.5
	Total Female	14.0 ± 1.6	42 ± 4	4.81 ± 1.24	292 ± 9	143.3 ± 8.9	4.5 ± 0.5
	Total Sample	14.7 ± 1.7	43 ± 4	4.83 ± 1.06	294 ± 9	143.2 ± 7.2	4.5 ± 0.5
	P4	<0.001	<0.001	0.724	0.001	0.717	0.159
Country	German	14.3 ± 1.3 *	43 ± 3 *,#	4.52 ± 1.43 *,#	298 ± 11*,#	141.0 ± 1.7 #	4.5 ± 0.4 #
	Spain	15.2 ± 1.3[+]	46 ± 3 [+]	4.96 ± 0.39	289 ± 8 [+]	141.2 ± 2.6 [+]	4.4 ± 0.5 [+]
	Greece	14.6 ± 2.3	41 ± 4	5.07 ± 0.97	294 ± 6	148.5 ± 11.4	4.6 ± 0.6
	P5	<0.001	<0.001	<0.001	<0.001	<0.001	<0.001

p-values derived through Student's *t*-test for differences between genders and season; and one-way ANOVA among countries; * significant difference between German and Spain; # significant difference between German and Greece; [+] significant difference between Spain and Greece; P1 refers to comparisons between gender for winter, P2 refers to comparisons between gender for summer, P3 refers to comparisons between summer and winter for the total sample (males and females together), P4 refers to comparisons between males and females (winter and summer together), and P5 refers to comparisons between countries.

3.3. Total Water Intake

Total water intake, water from beverages, water from foods, total energy intake, and energy from beverages are presented by gender, season, and country (Table 3). Water intake from beverages is correlated positively with total water intake (rho = 0.955, $p < 0.001$), energy intake (rho = 0.297, $p < 0.001$), and energy intake from beverages (rho = 0.576, $p < 0.001$). Daily water intake and water intake from beverages were higher in the summer compared to the winter period ($p = 0.019$ and $p = 0.027$ respectively). Differences were also observed between genders; when compared to females, males recorded higher total water (2.93 ± 1.10 L/day) and energy intake (2329 ± 686 kcal/day), consumed more water from beverages (2.27 ± 1.02 L/day) and received more calories from beverages (320 ± 219 kcal/day) ($p < 0.001$). Water intake derived from foods was higher in males compared to females totally ($p = 0.027$), but no differences were observed between seasons.

Table 3. Daily intake of water from all sources, from beverages and foods, separately of participants in winter and summer periods.

		Total Water Intake (L/Day)	Water from Beverages (L/Day)	Water from Foods (L/Day)	Total Energy Intake (kcal/Day)	Energy from Beverages (kcal/Day)
Winter	Male	2.77 ± 1.10	2.12 ± 1.09	0.67 ± 0.31	2248 ± 659	302 ± 203
	Female	2.49 ± 0.80	1.89 ± 0.71	0.61 ± 0.25	1913 ± 477	258 ± 143
	Total	2.64 ± 0.98	2.01 ± 0.94	0.64 ± 0.29	2093 ± 605	282 ± 179
Summer	Male	3.09 ± 1.07	2.41 ± 0.93	0.69 ± 0.29	2413 ± 706	338 ± 233
	Female	2.61 ± 0.91	1.97 ± 0.75	0.64 ± 0.29	1989 ± 580	254 ± 141
	Total	2.84 ± 1.02	2.18 ± 0.87	0.68 ± 0.29	2192 ± 676	294 ± 195
	P1	0.014	0.034	0.075	<0.001	0.038
	P2	<0.001	<0.001	0.152	<0.001	0.001
	P3	0.019	0.027	0.339	0.068	0.430
Winter & Summer	Total Male	2.93 ± 1.10	2.27 ± 1.02	0.68 ± 0.30	2329 ± 686	320 ± 219
	Total Female	2.55 ± 0.86	1.93 ± 0.73	0.63 ± 0.27	1955 ± 537	256 ± 142
	Total Sample	2.75 ± 1.01	2.10 ± 0.91	0.66 ± 0.29	2148 ± 644	288 ± 188
	P4	<0.001	<0.001	0.027	<0.001	<0.001
Country	German	3.29 ± 0.98 *,#	2.49 ± 0.87 *,#	0.81 ± 0.27 *,#	2412 ± 609 *,#	358 ± 240 *,#
	Spain	2.55 ± 0.98	1.96 ± 0.95	0.61 ± 0.29 +	2214 ± 633 +	296 ± 145 +
	Greece	2.35 ± 0.77	1.82 ± 0.74	0.54 ± 0.23	1777 ± 512	203 ± 113
	P5	<0.001	<0.001	<0.001	<0.001	<0.001

p-values derived through Student's *t*-test for differences between genders and season; and one-way ANOVA among countries; * significant difference between German and Spain; # significant difference between German and Greece; + significant difference between Spain and Greece; P1 refers to comparisons between genders for winter, P2 refers to comparisons between gender for summer, P3 refers to comparisons between summer and winter for the total sample (males and females together), P4 refers to comparisons between males and females (winter and summer together), and P5 refers to comparisons between countries.

3.4. Classification of Subjects

Subjects were further classified as hyperhydrated, euhydrated, and dehydrated according to reference values of 24 h urine osmolality for men and women [16,17]; classification is presented in summary in Figure 1, and in detail in Table 4.

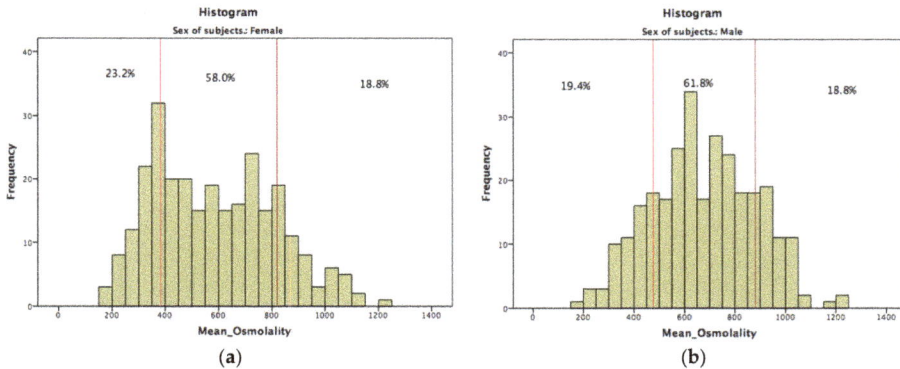

Figure 1. Distribution of hyperhydrated, euhydrated, and dehydrated (**a**) females and (**b**) males.

Table 4. Water intake and 24 h urine indices of females and males, according to the categories of hydration status based to urine osmolality.

	Categories of Hydration Status According to Urine Osmolality (mOsm/kg H_2O)			
	Hyperhydrated	**Euhydrated**	**Dehydrated**	*p*
	(<383)	(383 to 810)	(>810)	
Females, % (n)	23.2 (64)	58.0 (160)	18.8 (52)	
Total water intake (L/day)	3.36 ± 1.02	2.42 ± 0.61	2.02 ± 0.65	<0.001
Water from beverages (L/day)	2.60 ± 0.91	1.81 ± 0.49	1.53 ± 0.57	<0.001
24 h urine volume (L)	2.51 ± 0.73	1.54 ± 0.52	1.00 ± 0.25	<0.001
24 h urine specific gravity	1.009 ± 0.002	1.016 ± 0.004	1.023 ± 0.003	<0.001
24 h urine color	3.0 ± 1.2	3.9 ± 1.2	5.5 ± 1.2	<0.001
24 h urine Na (mEq/day)	129.4 ± 37.1	158.7 ± 59.1	166.3 ± 54.2	<0.001
24 h urine K (mEq/day)	73.9 ± 36.5	67.6 ± 21.6	65.4 ± 20.1	0.153
24 h urine creatinine (mg/day)	1137.6 ± 249.1	1362.5 ± 494.0	1363.6 ± 429.6	0.002
	(<475)	(475 to 880)	(>880)	
Males, % (n)	19.4 (55)	61.8 (181)	18.8 (54)	
Total water intake (L/day)	3.59 ± 1.04	2.8 ± 0.99	2.64 ± 1.25	<0.001
Water from beverages (L/day)	2.83 ± 1.00	2.15 ± 0.86	2.08 ± 1.31	<0.001
24 h urine volume (L)	2.45 ± 0.69	1.56 ± 0.46	1.00 ± 0.24	<0.001
24 h urine specific gravity	1.011 ± 0.002	1.018 ± 0.003	1.025 ± 0.02	<0.001
24 h urine color	3.6 ± 1.4	4.3 ± 1.1	5.9 ± 1.0	<0.001
24 h urine Na (mEq/day)	156.4 ± 50.0	187.7 ± 46.4	180.1 ± 59.5	<0.001
24 h urine K (mEq/day)	76.9 ± 19.9	77.7 ± 24.4	69.8 ± 20.2	0.091
24 h urine creatinine (mg/day)	1517.7 ± 399.02	1862.9 ± 483.3	1771.2 ± 522.1	<0.001

Results are presented as mean ± SD; *p*-values derived through one-way ANOVA for the normally distributed variables.

It was observed that 23.2%, 58.0%, and 18.8% of females and 19.4%, 61.8%, and 18.8% of males classified to the hyperhydrated, euhydrated, and dehydrated categories, respectively. Subjects that were classified to the hyperhydrated category also had higher total water intake ($p < 0.001$), greater urine volume ($p < 0.001$), lower specific gravity ($p < 0.001$), lighter color ($p < 0.001$), lower sodium and creatinine concentration ($p < 0.001$), and higher water intake from beverages ($p < 0.001$).

3.5. Linear Regression Model

Age (Beta = −4.033, $p < 0.001$), country (Beta = 81.196, $p < 0.001$), sex of subjects (Beta = 90.447, $p < 0.001$) and BMI (Beta = 9.146, $p < 0.001$) were significant predictors of 24 h urine osmolality while season and physical activity were not. The overall model fit was $R^2 = 0.208$.

The age (Beta = 0.007, $p = 0.009$) and the country (Beta = −0.396, $p < 0.01$) of the subjects were predictors of 24 h urine volume. The overall model fit was $R^2 = 0.224$. Country (Beta = −0.244, $p = 0.001$), sex of subjects (Beta = 0.473, $p < 0.01$), age (Beta = −0.013, $p = 0.018$), and BMI (Beta = 0.046, $p = 0.002$) were significant predictors of 24 h urine color. The overall model fit was $R^2 = 0.068$.

4. Discussion

For the first time, a series of urine hydration indices from 24 h samples collected over seven consecutive days and blood hydration indices were measured in a sample of 573 healthy participants in three European countries and compared with water intake from seven day dietary records. The study contributes with new data to the literature referring to European hydration issues, allowing the observation of associations between water intake and hydration biomarkers.

Data in large populations groups of hydration indices are rare. Urine and blood hydration indices provide information that reflect water intake, water losses, and physiological processes. The present study is the first that measures fluid intake and urine output in a sample of the population from three countries at the same time using alike methodology. A demanding protocol for the collection of water intake information and urine samples, incorporates fluctuations in intake, and indices within the day and the week.

Urine hydration indices (24 h osmolality, volume, and color) were associated with age, gender, BMI, and country.

Country, gender, and age were found to be significant predictors of 24 h urine osmolality. This finding is in accordance with the review from Manz and Wentz [23], that describes large intercultural differences in 24 h urine osmolality values (from 360 to 860 mosm/kg). In our study values of 24 h urine osmolality, specific gravity, and color were significantly lower in the German population compared with the Spanish or Greek ($p < 0.05$ in all cases), while 24 h urine volume was significantly higher ($p < 0.05$). Total water intake and water intake from beverages was significantly higher in the German population than the Spanish or Greek populations. These differences may be attributed to dietary habits observed in the regions studied, partly related to the availability of local foods or beverages.

Regarding gender, women, in comparison to men had better hydration status. This may reflect different hydration, dietary and/or lifestyle choices between men and women. In general, women exhibit a more virtuous pattern of eating and food choices than men [24]. A study conducted in 23 countries showed that men's dietary choices were less healthy, because health is less important motivation to them in the food domain [25]. Women seem to be more reflective about health issues and foods. Therefore, when it comes to adopting hydration guidelines there may be analogies with adopting nutritional guidelines in men and in women.

Age was a significant predictor for 24 h urine osmolality; as age increases urine osmolality decreases. This finding is in accordance with the study of Manz, *et al.* [26] where age related decrease in urine osmolality was observed. In the present study we found that country (Greece, Spain or Germany) was a significant predictor for 24 h urine volume. In a previous study conducted in adults ($n = 10,079$) large differences of mean 24-h urine volume identified between 52 centers all over the world [27]. It may be that lifestyle choices, environmental conditions, and other factors associated with living in different countries affect hydration status of the populations.

Using cutoffs for 24 h urine osmolality [16,17] approximately 60% of the subjects from three European countries were euhydrated. The distribution of hyperhydrated and dehydrated was similar for males and females. Hyperhydrated subjects consumed more fluids on daily basis (about 3.5 L/day), voided larger volumes (2.5 L/day) and provided urine samples that were less concentrated.

It must be noted that results presented herein derive from a volunteer sample of subjects from three countries and may not be generalizable to the entire European population. Further analysis of data by country of origin, age group, physical activity level, *etc.*, may reveal the influence of these factors to the hydration status of the studied group.

In our study the mean total water intake was 2.75 ± 1.01 L/day. Previous studies [23,28] have reported daily fluid intake using Food Frequency Questionnaires (FFQ) or 24 h recall. These tools may underestimate water intake [29]. Gibson and Shirreffs [30] found that total water intake from foods and beverages was 2270 g/day in UK population and observed fluctuations in water intake during a week, recording higher consumption of drinks on Fridays and Saturdays. A seven-day fluid specific record given in 13 different countries found that mean daily water intake was 1980 mL/day, with highest fluid intake recorded in Germany (2.47 L/day) and the lowest in Japan (1.50 L/day) [31]. Water intake guidelines are frequently complex and not always harmonized. For example, D-A-CH suggests the intake of water from 1 mL/kcal of energy intake for adults [32], European Food Safety Authority (EFSA) suggests 2.5 and 2.0 L/day from males and females [4], and I.O.M. suggests 3.7 and 2.7 L/day for males and females respectively [5]. Recommendations for the Europeans are lower than US population and refer to water intake from all sources.

The contribution of foods in water intake was 24% (approximately 700 mL) with no differences reported between genders. This finding is similar to those provided in the scientific opinion of EFSA [4] and in previous studies [3,33].

The daily intake of beverages (2.1 ± 0.91 L/day) contributes approximately 290 kcal (13% of energy intake). Data of total energy intake are in accordance with previous published studies. In particular, total energy intake in the EPIC study was 2508 (2167, 2950) kcal for men and 1999 (1741, 2348) kcal for women and in the ATTICA study was 2595 ± 877 kcal for men and 2132 ± 658 kcal for women [34,35]. In the present study 24 h total water intake is strong and positively correlated with 24 h water intake from beverages ($r = 0.955$, $p < 0.001$) and energy intake from beverages ($r = 0.543$, $p < 0.001$). Moreover, differences were observed in the total water intake between seasons ($p = 0.019$). This difference could be explained due to high temperatures in summer period compared to winter, which reflects higher fluid intake and sweat loss. However, this difference of 200 mL/day between seasons is lower than a previous study in Greece [33]. This difference could be explained due to different environmental conditions (temperature, humidity) and alternative lifestyle choices of the participants [20].

5. Conclusions

In conclusion, in a free-living population from German, Spain, and Greece approximately 60% were euhydrated while approximately 20% were hyperhydrated and 20% dehydrated on average over a seven-day period. Differences observed on urine and blood hydration indices, total water intake, and water intake from beverages and foods suggest that a variety of dietary or lifestyle factors that may be associated with improving hydration status.

Acknowledgments: The study was supported by a grant from the European Hydration Institute. We also thank Demosthenes B. Panagiotakos and Ekavi Georgousopoulou, Harokopio University in Athens, for their statistical assistance.

Author Contributions: M.K., H.B. and R.M.R. conceived and designed the experiments; O.M., A.A., A.P., M.H., K.D., H.B., R.M.R., J.O., V.F.E., M.K. performed the experiments, analyzed the data, contributed reagents/materials/analysis tools, wrote the paper.

Conflicts of Interest: The authors declare no conflict of interest.

References

1. EFSA. Scientific opinion on the substantiation of health claims related to water and maintenance of normal physical and cognitive functions (id **1102**, *1209*, 1294, 1331), maintenance of normal thermoregulation (id 1208) and "basic requirement of all living things" (id 1207) pursuant to article 13(1) of regulation (ec) no 1924/2006. *EFSA J.* **2011**, *9*, 2075–2091.
2. Tack, I. Effects of water consumption on kidney function and excretion. *Nutr. Today* **2010**, *45*, S37–S40. [CrossRef]
3. Perrier, E.; Vergne, S.; Klein, A.; Poupin, M.; Rondeau, P.; Le Bellego, L.; Armstrong, L.E.; Lang, F.; Stookey, J.; Tack, I. Hydration biomarkers in free-living adults with different levels of habitual fluid consumption. *Br. J. Nutr.* **2013**, *109*, 1678–1687. [CrossRef] [PubMed]
4. EFSA. Scientific opinion on dietary reference values for water. *EFSA J.* **2010**, *8*, 1459–1507.
5. Medicine, I.O. *Panel on Dietary Reference Intakes for Electrolytes and Water: Dietary Reference Intakes for Water, Potassium, Sodium, Chloride and Sulfate*; National Academies Press: Washington, DC, USA, 2005.
6. Popkin, B.M.; D'Anci, K.E.; Rosenberg, I.H. Water, hydration, and health. *Nutr. Rev.* **2010**, *68*, 439–458. [CrossRef] [PubMed]
7. Perrier, E.; Demazieres, A.; Girard, N.; Pross, N.; Osbild, D.; Metzger, D.; Guelinckx, I.; Klein, A. Circadian variation and responsiveness of hydration biomarkers to changes in daily water intake. *Eur. J. Appl. Physiol.* **2013**, *113*, 2143–2151. [CrossRef] [PubMed]
8. Lemaire, J.B.; Wallace, J.E.; Dinsmore, K.; Lewin, A.M.; Ghali, W.A.; Roberts, D. Physician nutrition and cognition during work hours: Effect of a nutrition based intervention. *BMC Health Serv. Res.* **2010**, *10*, 241. [CrossRef] [PubMed]
9. McKiernan, F.; Houchins, J.A.; Mattes, R.D. Relationships between human thirst, hunger, drinking, and feeding. *Physiol. Behav.* **2008**, *94*, 700–708. [CrossRef] [PubMed]

10. Malisova, O.; Bountziouka, V.; Panagiotakos, D.B.; Zampelas, A.; Kapsokefalou, M. The water balance questionnaire: Design, reliability and validity of a questionnaire to evaluate water balance in the general population. *Int. J. Food Sci. Nutr.* **2012**, *63*, 138–144. [CrossRef] [PubMed]
11. Cotter, J.D.; Thornton, S.N.; Lee, J.K.; Laursen, P.B. Are we being drowned in hydration advice? Thirsty for more? *Extreme Physiol. Med.* **2014**, *3*, 18. [CrossRef] [PubMed]
12. Perrier, E.; Rondeau, P.; Poupin, M.; Le Bellego, L.; Armstrong, L.E.; Lang, F.; Stookey, J.; Tack, I.; Vergne, S.; Klein, A. Relation between urinary hydration biomarkers and total fluid intake in healthy adults. *Eur. J. Clin. Nutr.* **2013**, *67*, 939–943. [CrossRef] [PubMed]
13. Schatzkin, A.; Kipnis, V.; Carroll, R.J.; Midthune, D.; Subar, A.F.; Bingham, S.; Schoeller, D.A.; Troiano, R.P.; Freedman, L.S. A comparison of a food frequency questionnaire with a 24-h recall for use in an epidemiological cohort study: Results from the biomarker-based observing protein and energy nutrition (OPEN) study. *Int. J. Epidemiol.* **2003**, *32*, 1054–1062. [CrossRef] [PubMed]
14. Cheuvront, S.N.; Ely, B.R.; Kenefick, R.W.; Sawka, M.N. Biological variation and diagnostic accuracy of dehydration assessment markers. *Am. J. Clin. Nutr.* **2010**, *92*, 565–573. [CrossRef] [PubMed]
15. Cheuvront, S.N.; Fraser, C.G.; Kenefick, R.W.; Ely, B.R.; Sawka, M.N. Reference change values for monitoring dehydration. *Clin. Chem. Lab. Med.* **2011**, *49*, 1033–1037. [CrossRef] [PubMed]
16. Armstrong, L.E.; Johnson, E.C.; Munoz, C.X.; Swokla, B.; Le Bellego, L.; Jimenez, L.; Casa, D.J.; Maresh, C.M. Hydration biomarkers and dietary fluid consumption of women. *J. Acad. Nutr. Diet.* **2012**, *112*, 1056–1061. [CrossRef] [PubMed]
17. Armstrong, L.E.; Pumerantz, A.C.; Fiala, K.A.; Roti, M.W.; Kavouras, S.A.; Casa, D.J.; Maresh, C.M. Human hydration indices: Acute and longitudinal reference values. *Int. J. Sport Nutr. Exerc. Metab.* **2010**, *20*, 145–153. [PubMed]
18. Armstrong, L.E. Assessing hydration status: The elusive gold standard. *J. Am. Coll. Nutr.* **2007**, *26*, 575S–584S. [CrossRef] [PubMed]
19. Kavouras, S.A. Assessing hydration status. *Curr. Opin. Clin. Nutr. Metab. Care* **2002**, *5*, 519–524. [CrossRef] [PubMed]
20. Vergne, S. Methodological aspects of fluid intake records and surveys. *Nutr. Today* **2012**, *47*, S7–S10. [CrossRef]
21. Ix, J.H.; Wassel, C.L.; Stevens, L.A.; Beck, G.J.; Froissart, M.; Navis, G.; Rodby, R.; Torres, V.E.; Zhang, Y.L.; Greene, T.; *et al.* Equations to estimate creatinine excretion rate: The CKD epidemiology collaboration. *Clin. J. Am. Soc. Nephrol.* **2011**, *6*, 184–191. [PubMed]
22. Craig, C.L.; Marshall, A.L.; Sjostrom, M.; Bauman, A.E.; Booth, M.L.; Ainsworth, B.E.; Pratt, M.; Ekelund, U.; Yngve, A.; Sallis, J.F.; *et al.* International physical activity questionnaire: 12-country reliability and validity. *Med. Sci. Sports Exerc.* **2003**, *35*, 1381–1395. [PubMed]
23. Manz, F.; Wentz, A. 24-h hydration status: Parameters, epidemiology and recommendations. *Eur. J. Clin. Nutr.* **2003**, *57*, S10–S18. [CrossRef] [PubMed]
24. Beards, A.; Bryman, A.; Keil, T.; Goode, J.; Haslam, C.; Lanchashire, E. Women, men and food: The significance of gender for nutritional attitudes and choices. *Br. Food J.* **2002**, *104*, 470–491. [CrossRef]
25. Wardle, J.; Haase, A.M.; Steptoe, A.; Nillapun, M.; Jonwutiwes, K.; Bellisle, F. Gender differences in food choices: The contribution of health beliefs and dieting Ann. *Behav. Med.* **2004**, *27*, 107–116. [CrossRef]
26. Manz, F.; Johner, S.A.; Wentz, A.; Boeing, H.; Remer, T. Water balance throughout the adult life span in a german population. *Br. J. Nutr.* **2012**, *107*, 1673–1681. [CrossRef] [PubMed]
27. Intersalt cooperative research group. Intersalt: An international study of electrolyte excretion and blood pressure. Results for 24 h urinary sodium and potassium excretion. *BMJ* **1988**, *297*, 319–328.
28. Hedrick, V.E.; Comber, D.L.; Estabrooks, P.A.; Savla, J.; Davy, B.M. The beverage intake questionnaire: Determining initial validity and reliability. *J. Am. Diet. Assoc.* **2010**, *110*, 1227–1232. [CrossRef] [PubMed]
29. Ma, G.; Zhang, Q.; Liu, A.; Zuo, J.; Zhang, W.; Zou, S.; Li, X.; Lu, L.; Pan, H.; Hu, X. Fluid intake of adults in four Chinese cities. *Nutr. Rev.* **2012**, *70*, S105–S110. [CrossRef] [PubMed]
30. Gibson, S.; Shirreffs, S.M. Beverage consumption habits "24/7" among british adults: Association with total water intake and energy intake. *Nutr. J.* **2013**, *12*, 9. [CrossRef] [PubMed]
31. Ferreira-Pego, C.; Guelinckx, I.; Moreno, L.A.; Kavouras, S.A.; Gandy, J.; Martinez, H.; Bardosono, S.; Abdollahi, M.; Nasseri, E.; Jarosz, A.; *et al.* Total fluid intake and its determinants: Cross-sectional surveys among adults in 13 countries worldwide. *Eur. J. Nutr.* **2015**, *54*, 35–43. [PubMed]

32. Wolfram, G. New reference values for nutrient intake in germany, austria and switzerland (dach-reference values). *Forum Nutr.* **2003**, *56*, 95–97. [PubMed]
33. Malisova, O.; Bountziouka, V.; Panagiotakos, D.; Zampelas, A.; Kapsokefalou, M. Evaluation of seasonality on total water intake, water loss and water balance in the general population in greece. *J. Hum. Nutr. Diet.* **2013**, *26*, 90–96. [CrossRef] [PubMed]
34. Manios, Y.; Panagiotakos, D.B.; Pitsavos, C.; Polychronopoulos, E.; Stefanadis, C. Implication of socio-economic status on the prevalence of overweight and obesity in greek adults: The attica study. *Health Policy* **2005**, *74*, 224–232. [CrossRef] [PubMed]
35. Trichopoulou, A.; Gnardellis, C.; Lagiou, A.; Benetou, V.; Naska, A.; Trichopoulos, D. Physical activity and total energy intake selectively predict the waist-to-hip ratio in men but not in women. *Am. J. Clin. Nutr.* **2011**, *74*, 574–578.

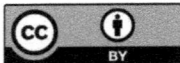

nutrients

MDPI

Article

Influence of Physical Activity and Ambient Temperature on Hydration: The European Hydration Research Study (EHRS)

Ricardo Mora-Rodriguez [1,*], Juan F. Ortega [1], Valentin E. Fernandez-Elias [1],
Maria Kapsokefalou [2], Olga Malisova [2], Adelais Athanasatou [2], Marlien Husemann [3],
Kirsten Domnik [3] and Hans Braun [3]

[1] Exercise Physiology Lab at Toledo, University of Castilla-La Mancha, Toledo 45071, Spain;
Juanfernando.ortega@uclm.es (J.F.O.); valentin.fernandez@uclm.es (V.E.F.-E.)

[2] Department of Food Science and Human Nutrition, Agricultural University of Athens,
Athens 11855, Greece; kapsok@aua.gr (M.K.); olgamalisova@yahoo.gr (O.M.);
dathanasatou@gmail.com (A.A.)

[3] Institute of Biochemistry, German Sport University, Cologne 50993, Germany;
m.husemann@biochem.dshs-koeln.de (M.H.); k.domnik@biochem.dshs-koeln.de (K.D.);
H.Braun@dshs-koeln.de (H.B.)

* Correspondence: ricardo.mora@uclm.es; Tel.: +34-925-268-800

Received: 17 February 2016; Accepted: 25 April 2016; Published: 27 April 2016

Abstract: This study explored the effects of physical activity (PA) and ambient temperature on water turnover and hydration status. Five-hundred seventy three healthy men and women (aged 20–60 years) from Spain, Greece and Germany self-reported PA, registered all food and beverage intake, and collected 24-h urine during seven consecutive days. Fasting blood samples were collected at the onset and end of the study. Food moisture was assessed using nutritional software to account for all water intake which was subtracted from daily urine volume to allow calculation of non-renal water loss (*i.e.*, mostly sweating). Hydration status was assessed by urine and blood osmolality. A negative association was seen between ambient temperature and PA ($r = -0.277$; $p < 0.001$). Lower PA with high temperatures did not prevent increased non-renal water losses (*i.e.*, sweating) and elevated urine and blood osmolality ($r = 0.218$ to 0.163 all $p < 0.001$). When summer and winter data were combined PA was negatively associated with urine osmolality ($r = -0.153$; $p = 0.001$). Our data suggest that environmental heat acts to reduce voluntary PA but this is not sufficient to prevent moderate dehydration (increased osmolality). On the other hand, increased PA is associated with improved hydration status (*i.e.*, lower urine and blood osmolality).

Keywords: hydration status; physical activity; urine osmolality; 24-h urine volume

1. Introduction

Water intake comes from drinking fluids (water and other beverages), moisture in food and water produced by the body during oxidation. In turn, body water losses occur via urine, feces, sweat and insensible loss through the skin and by evaporation from the respiratory tract. Hydration status is the result of the balance between water intake and body water loss. When body water losses are higher than fluid intake, hypohydration results. In this paper, we will refer to the acute process of loss of body water as dehydration [1] and to the maintained body fluid deficit as hypohydration. Hypohydration has been linked to negative long-term health outcomes. Inadequate hydration together with elevated ingestion of calcium and sodium are related to nephrolithiasis [2]. A low intake of plain water is also associated with a higher prevalence of chronic kidney disease [3]. Furthermore, low water intake is associated with increased risk of developing hyperglycemia [4] and may increase the risk of developing type II diabetes [5]. Prospective studies measuring the impact of increased water intake on the development of these diseases are still in a preliminary phase [6].

Adequate fluid intakes (AI) representing population median consumption in apparently healthy sedentary adults under temperate climate have been reported [7,8]. The Institute of Medicine guidelines for adequate intake of total water for USA and Canada is 3.7 and 2.7 L/day for men and women, respectively [8]. However, the European Food Safety Authority (EFSA; [7]) has lower total water intake recommendations of 2.5 and 2.0 L/day for adult men and women, respectively. The EFSA adequate intake calculations attempted to incorporate hydration status into the recommendation and account for the maintenance of daily urine osmolality below a certain threshold (<500 mOsmol$\cdot$kg^{-1}; [7]). Although general recommendations for adults exist, both organizations recognize that individual requirements could widely vary depending on personal characteristics (age, size, body composition, physical activity) and environment.

The effects of physical activity on fluid intake and loss in free-living adults has been previously investigated in a small sample of healthy young lean subjects in The Netherlands [8]. In that study a sample of 42 women and 10 men were tested for water intake (weighted record of foodstuff and beverage) and physical activity (difference between total and resting energy expenditure) in summer and winter [9]. The study revealed that in men, water loss was proportional to physical activity, but in women water loss was higher in summer but was unrelated to physical activity [9]. In another study, a comparison of water turnover in rural and urban women in Kenya revealed that BMI was the stronger predictor of water loss but the addition of physical activity (measured by accelerometry) explained an additional 12% of the variance [10]. Thus, the influence of physical activity level on water loss/intake is not readily evident from the available literature. Furthermore, no measure of hydration status (changes in blood or urine concentration) was reported in these studies. In addition, the interplay between climate and physical activity and its consequences for water loss and intake are largely unknown in the European population.

Some studies suggest that the fluctuations in climate, food and water availability linked to seasons may be an important risk factors for malnutrition and other disorders [11]. The identification of seasonal differences in fluid intake [12], and the effect of environmental temperature on fluid loss could be relevant for the implementation of season-specific strategies to improve the hydration habits of the population if deficiencies are detected. Body water needs are highly individualized and depend upon body size and composition, resting metabolic rate, physical activity, dietary osmotic load and climate among others [13]. The purpose of this study was to assess the influence of physical activity and environmental temperature (linked to season) on water intake, water losses and hydration status in a large sample of healthy men and women aged 20–60 years from one northern (Germany) and two southern (Spain and Greece) European countries. We used a series of objective (body weight, blood and urine chemistry) and subjective (questionnaires and diaries) measures to assess hydration status and water intake and output, respectively. A novel characteristic of our study is that we followed subjects during seven consecutive days in an attempt to increase accuracy and spread possible spurious reporting into a more extensive data collection set.

2. Experimental Section

2.1. Participants

Between winter 2013 and summer 2014, a sample of 573 men and women from Germany, Spain and Greece were studied during seven consecutive days of free-living. Subjects were healthy and not disabled according to a pre-participation medical questionnaire, not undergoing a diet, not taking medicines that could affect the outcome measures (diuretics, phenytoin, lithium, demeclocycline or amphotericin B) and women were non-pregnant or breastfeeding and were tested out of their proliferative menstrual phase. Subject recruitment was oriented to reach a quota of 25 subjects in each of the following age groups in each country; 20–30; 31–40; 41–50; 50–60 years old. This subject recruitment scheme (100 per country) was repeated in winter and summer with a goal of 200 subjects tested per country. All centers obtain ethical approval from their local Institutional Review Board and all subjects signed an informed consent form were the study was detailed (197/27-02-2012 for Agricultural University of Athens, Greece, 4/02/2013-18 for University of Castilla-La Mancha, Spain, 1/26-11-2012 for German Sport University, Germany).

2.2. Study Design

Upon recruitment, subjects were instructed on dietary and fluid intake data logging and 24-h urine collection procedures and were given the materials necessary for these tasks. On the morning of the first and the last day of testing (day 1 and day 8) subjects arrived at the laboratory after an overnight fast and were weighed with only their underwear using a sensitive scale (±0.05 kg) before a blood sample was collected. For the remaining of the week subjects collected all urine produced, logged every foodstuff and beverage ingested at the time when it occurred and filled in a questionnaire that summarized their physical activity at the end of every day.

2.3. Food and Water Intake Diary

Total water intake corresponded to the sum of beverages and water in food recorded from the dietary records of each day of the testing week. Water content in the food was analyzed with nutritional software specific for each population (*i.e.*, CESNID, Barcelona, Spain; ESHA Research, Wadsworth Publishing Co Inc, Salem, OR, USA for Greece; and EBIS pro German Food Database 3.1, University of Hohenheim, Stuttgart, Germany).

2.4. Physical Activity Diary

Physical activity was evaluated using the short version of the International Physical Activity Questionnaire (IPAQ) [14]. The questionnaire requires recording of the minutes per day of vigorous, moderate, walk or sitting time and the days per week of each activity. The questionnaire was filled out daily, but was reduced to four questions by suppressing the frequency questions (*i.e.*, days per week) since data was collected every day. IPAQ data was processed in a continuous mode [14,15] accounting for 3.3 metabolic equivalent of a task (MET) for walking, 4.0 METs for moderate activities and 8.0 METs for vigorous activities. The units were expressed as METs-min per week as recommended by the investigators who validated the questionnaire [14,16,17].

2.5. Urine and Blood Biomarkers

Subjects arrived at the laboratory in the morning of the first day of testing after an overnight fast. Subjects provided a sample of their first morning urine and were weighed. After 15 min in a seated or a reclined position a 5 mL blood sample was drawn from an antecubital vein. A 0.5 mL aliquot was immediately analyzed for hemoglobin (ABL-520, Radiometer, Bronshoj, Denmark) hematocrit in duplicate by microcentrifugation (Biocen, Alresa; Barcelona, Spain). The remaining blood was allowed to clot in serum tubes (Z Serum Sep Clot Activator, Vacuette, Kremsmunster, Austria) centrifuged at 2000 g for 10 min (MPW-350R, Medical Instruments, Warsaw, Poland). The so obtained serum portion was analyzed for osmolality by freeze point depression (Advanced Instruments, Norwood, MA, USA) and the remaining stored at $-30\ °C$ for further analyses. Serum sodium and potassium concentrations were analyzed using an ion selective analyzer (Easylyte Plus, Medica Corporation, Bedford, MA, USA) and glucose concentration by spectrophotometry using glucose oxidase to produce gluconate from glucose (Thermo Scientific, Waltham, MA, USA). Subjects were then dispatched and advised to proceed with their normal life routines during the following 7 days while recording all food and fluid ingested and collecting all urine produced. On the morning of day 8, subjects returned to the lab for body weight, blood sampling and morning urine void. During the seven days of urine collection, subjects weighed and recorded every void with the aid of a collection vessel and a portable scale (±1 g accuracy). Then, they saved in a plastic bag a representative aliquot (~3 mL) of every void, labeled with the date, time of day and subject initials. The bag with the aliquots were kept refrigerated by the subjects. Urine from each day was reconstituted in proportion to the volume urinated and analyzed for osmolality, sodium and potassium using the same instruments described for blood analyses. Only one laboratory analyzed serum osmolality within 1 hour of blood collection and before freezing the serum samples while blood storage was the norm in the other two laboratories. Since variability due to different analyses time was a concern [18,19] we calculated serum osmolality according to the following formulae:

$$\text{Calculated Osmolality} = 2 \times ([\text{Na}^+] + [\text{K}^+]) + ([\text{Glucose}]) \tag{1}$$

where all concentrations are in mmol/L.

2.6. Hydration Status Calculations

We assumed that our subjects were in water balance and therefore total water intake matched total water losses. Any cumulative discrepancy would have resulted in a change in body mass that should have been apparent in a change in body mass measured on day 8. The difference between water intake from the dietary records and 24-h urine volume represented non-renal water losses (NRWL) composed of sweat, respiratory and fecal water. We calculated the 7 days average NRWL as follows [20]:

$$\text{NRWL (L/day)} = \text{average total water intake (L/day)} - \text{average } 24-\text{h urine volume (L/day)} \tag{2}$$

The excretion of solutes by the kidneys per day is the product of the average urine osmolality (mOsm/kg) multiplied by urine volume in liters per day. Since our subjects weighed their urine voids for this calculation, we assumed that 1 kg urine corresponds to 1 L and that errors introduced by the variable specific gravity of urine will be small. Obligatory urine volume (OUV) is the water volume necessary to excrete all urine solutes. To calculate OUV, a threshold of maximum urine osmolality of 830 mOsm/kg is used for a 20 years old individual [21]. Since aging reduces the renal capacity to concentrate urine [21], 3.4 mOsm/kg are subtracted from that threshold value per year above 20 years. The calculation then is as follows [22]:

$$\text{OUV (L/day)} = \text{average } 24-\text{h urine solutes (mOsm/day)}/[830 - 3.4 \times (\text{age} - 20)] \tag{3}$$

Free-water reserve (FWR) is the difference between the actual 24-h urine volume and the calculated obligatory urine volume [23]:

$$\text{FWR (L/day)} = 24-\text{h urine volume (L/day)} - \text{obligatory urine volume (L/day)} \tag{4}$$

Positive FWR values reflects euhydration and negative values hypohydration. In a population, euhydration is ensured if at least 97% of the subjects show positive values of free-water-reserve [22]. We also categorized subjects as hypohydrated if their urine osmolality exceeded the 500 mOsm/kg threshold based on EFSA recommendations [7].

2.7. Statistical Analysis

Normality of data distribution was evaluated for each variable using parametric Shapiro-Wilk test. Data collected during seven consecutive days (urine output, fluid intake, peak ambient temperature and physical activity) were averaged in each subject. Subjects missing some day value in one variable were not excluded from the analysis and the average of the week value was calculated from the remaining data. Subjects missing more than two values in a given variable were removed from the analysis in that variable. Data collected at the beginning and end of the experiment (morning of day 1 and day 8) were also averaged (body weight and blood chemistry) after checking for variability (Table 1). Discrete variables with two levels (gender, season, free water reserve) were analyzed using student's *T*-test for unpaired samples. Discrete variables with more than two levels (country, age group) were analyzed using ANOVA. Upon a significant *F* value Tukey's post-hoc was used to identify differences between groups. Cohen's formula for effect size (ES) [24] was used, and the results were based on the following criteria; >0.70 large effect; 0.30–0.69 moderate effect; ⩽0.30 small effect. Associations between continuous variables were tested using Pearson product-moment correlation coefficient (*r*). Partial correlation was used to adjust for age as a covariate. All tests were performed with SPSS software version 18 (IBM Software, Chicago, IL, USA). Data are presented as mean ± SD. All statistical test were two-tailed and statistical significance level was set at *p* < 0.05.

Table 1. Effects of gender, season, site, age group and hydration on physical activity and 24-h water intake/fluid loss.

	IPAQ (MET-min/Week)	Max Air Temp (°C)	Water Intake (L/Day)	Urine Volume (L/Day)	Non-Renal Water Loss (L/Day)	Urine Osmol (mOsmol/kg)
Female	2356 ± 1774	22 ± 9	2.57 ± 0.89	1.66 ± 0.74	0.89 ± 0.56	585 ± 228
Male	2141 ± 1475	21 ± 9	2.93 ± 1.00 *	1.64 ± 0.66	1.31 ± 0.94 *	674 ± 203 *
Winter	2571 ± 2018	14 ± 6	2.64 ± 0.98	1.67 ± 0.66	0.99 ± 0.87	615 ± 208
Summer	1942 ± 1087 *	29 ± 4 *	2.85 ± 1.03 *	1.62 ± 0.73	1.21 ± 0.71 *	646 ± 230
Germany	2945 ± 2053	17 ± 8	3.29 ± 0.98	2.13 ± 0.75	1.16 ± 0.62	492 ± 170
Spain	2088 ± 988 *	24 ± 8 *	2.56 ± 1.01 *	1.40 ± 0.49 *	1.14 ± 1.00	754 ± 179 *
Greece	1422 ± 1200 *,†	25 ± 8 *	2.34 ± 0.77 *	1.35 ± 0.49 *	1.02 ± 0.72	658 ± 224 *,†
20–30 years old	2103 ± 1196	21 ± 9	2.68 ± 1.12	1.49 ± 0.72	1.18 ± 0.81	686 ± 220
30–40 years old	2327 ± 1782	23 ± 8	2.75 ± 0.91	1.69 ± 0.71	1.07 ± 0.65	613 ± 226 *
40–50 years old	2176 ± 1810	22 ± 9	2.86 ± 0.96	1.70 ± 0.69 *	1.18 ± 0.75	621 ± 224 *
50–60 years old	2420 ± 1722	22 ± 8	2.71 ± 1.05	1.74 ± 0.63 *	0.96 ± 0.95	590 ± 199 *
Urine >500 (mOsm/kg)	2086 ± 1408	23 ± 9	2.53 ± 0.94	1.35 ± 0.46	1.19 ± 0.85	750 ± 155
Urine <500 (mOsm/kg)	2563 ± 1984 *	20 ± 8 *	3.20 ± 1.01 *	2.25 ± 0.72 *	0.94 ± 0.65 *	377 ± 79 *
(−) FWR	1983 ± 1137	25 ± 8	2.38 ± 1.02	1.10 ± 0.31	1.24 ± 0.94	891 ± 104
(+) FWR	2362 ± 1787 *	21 ± 9 *	2.92 ± 0.98 *	1.87 ± 0.69 *	1.04 ± 0.73 *	520 ± 153 *

Data represents average of 7 days data collection ± SD; *, different from the first value listed in that cell; †, different from the value above in cells that contain more than two values (*i.e.*, country and age group); all *p* < 0.05; FWR, stands for Free Water Reserve.

3. Results

Table 2 depicts the number of subjects for each discrete category in the main variables of interest in this study, *i.e.*, physical activity and maximal air temperature. An average of 536 of the 573 subjects that completed the study (93%) had data in these two variables. In addition, data were well balanced between the category levels such as gender, season, country, age group (see percentages in Table 2). We analyzed the variability, one week apart, for body weight and some blood parameters. After one week of data collection, blood hemoglobin (14.7 ± 1.7 *vs.* 14.7 ± 1.6 g/L) and glucose (4.8 ± 1.8 *vs.* 4.7 ± 0.6 mmol/L) remained unchanged (*P* > 0.05). Body weight (74.6 ± 15.4 *vs.* 74.4 ± 15.3 kg), blood sodium (143 ± 8 *vs.* 141 ± 6 mmol/L) and potassium (4.50 ± 0.52 *vs.* 4.46 ± 0.46 mmol/L) were slightly but significantly reduced after one week of testing (*p* < 0.05). However, the differences were very small judging by Cohen's effect size calculation (⩽0.30 small effect). Thus, we feel entitled to average data during the seven consecutive days of testing to improve the power analysis and data consistency.

Table 2. Sample size in categorical variables and percentage in each category.

	Physical Activity (% Subjects)	Maximal Air Temp °C (% Subjects)
Gender		
Female	249 (50%)	282 (50%)
Male	252 (50%)	284 (50%)
Total	501	566
Season		
Winter	240 (47%)	272 (47%)
Summer	266 (53%)	301 (53%)
Total	506	573
Country		
Germany	188 (37%)	201 (36%)
Spain	192 (38%)	193 (34%)
Greece	126 (25%)	170 (30%)
Total	506	564
Age groups		
20–30 years' old	140 (28%)	155 (27%)
30–40 years' old	123 (25%)	139 (25%)
40–50 years' old	125 (25%)	138 (24%)
50–60 years' old	113 (22%)	132 (24%)
Total	501	564
Urine Osmol		
>500 mOsmol/kg	343 (68%)	384 (67%)
<500 mOsmol/kg	162 (32%)	187 (33%)
Total	505	571

Average sample size of 536 individuals.

Physical activity (PA) in METs-min per week was not affected by gender ($p = 0.065$; ES = 0.132; Table 1) or age group ($p = 0.410$). However PA was lower in the summer ($p < 0.001$; ES = 0.388) and higher in individuals better hydrated with urine osmolality below 500 mOsmol/kg ($p = 0.008$; ES = 0.249) and positive free water reserve ($p = 0.019$; ES = 0.259). There was also a marked country effect on physical activity with Germans reporting higher levels than Spaniards and Greeks (both $p = 0.001$; ES = 0.532 and 0.905, respectively). In turn, Spaniards reported higher physical activity than Greeks did ($p = 0.001$; ES = 0.605; Table 1). Physical activity data was positively associated with urine volume and water intake while negatively associated with urine, blood osmolality and maximal air temperature (Tables 3 and 4).

Table 3. Correlation (*r* Pearson) among physical activity, maximal air temperature, 24-h water intake/fluid loss and urine osmolality.

	IPAQ (MET-min/Week)	Max Air Temp (°C)	Water Intake (L/Day)	Urine Volume (L/day)	Non-Renal Water Loss (L/Day)	Urine Osmolality (mOsmol/kg)
IPAQ (MET-min/week)	——	−0.283 $p < 0.001$	0.145 $p < 0.001$	0.158 $p < 0.001$	NS	−0.151 $p = 0.001$
Max Air Temp (°C)		——	NS	−0.222 $p < 0.001$	0.147 $p < 0.001$	0.218 $p < 0.001$
Water Intake (L/day)			——	0.623 $p < 0.001$	0.716 $p < 0.001$	−0.349 $p < 0.001$
Urine Volume (L/day)				——	−0.095 $p = 0.024$	−0.736 $p < 0.001$
Non-Renal Water Loss (L/day)					——	0.208 $p < 0.001$
Urine Osmolality (mOsmol/kg)						——

r correlation values are listed in bold and *p* values below; NS, stands for non-significant.

Table 4. Correlation (*r* Pearson) between blood variables and physical activity, air temperature and 24-h water intake/ fluid loss.

	IPAQ (MET-min/Week)	Max Air Temp (°C)	Water Intake (L/Day)	Urine Volume (L/Day)	Non-Renal Loss (L/Day)
Serum [Na⁺] (mEq/L)	−0.145 $p < 0.003$	0.189 $p < 0.001$	−0.118 $p = 0.006$	−0.115 $p < 0.005$	NS
Serum [K⁺] (mEq/L)	−0.098 $p = 0.040$	0.154 $p < 0.001$	NS	NS	NS
Blood Glucose (mmol/L)	−0.125 $p = 0.023$	0.194 $p < 0.001$	NS	−0.115 $p = 0.007$	NS
Serum Osmolality calculated (mOsmol/kg)	−0.137 $p = 0.004$	0.163 $p < 0.001$	−0.123 $p = 0.008$	−0.112 $p = 0.015$	NS
Blood hemoglobin (g/L)	NS	NS	NS	NS	0.174 $p < 0.001$

r correlation values are listed in bold and *p* values below, NS, stands for non-significant.

As expected, the maximal seven day average air temperature was higher in the summer than in winter ($p < 0.001$; ES = 2.827; Table 1). Maximal temperatures were lower in Germany than in Spain and Greece (both $p = 0.001$; ES = 0.751 and 0.877, respectively) without differences between these two south European countries. Maximal air temperature was lower in the better-hydrated subjects, those with urine osmolality below 500 mOsmol· kg⁻¹ ($p < 0.001$; ES = 0.337) and in positive free water reserve ($p < 0.001$; ES = 0.430; Table 1). Maximal average air temperature was positively correlated with non-renal fluid loss (*i.e.*, sweating) and urine osmolality (*r* = 0.147 and 0.218, respectively; $p < 0.001$) and negatively with urine volume (*r* = −0.222; $p < 0.001$; Table 3).

Average 24-h water intake was higher in men and in all subjects during the summer (Table 1). Furthermore, water intake was lower in Spain and Greece than in Germany but not different among age groups (Table 1). Interestingly, water intake was positively correlated with physical activity, urine volume, non-renal water losses (*i.e.*, NRWL) and negatively correlated with urine osmolality (*r* = −0.349; $p < 0.001$; Table 3). Likewise, with 24-h water intake, average 24-h urine volume was higher in the German subjects than in the Spaniards and Greeks. We observe that increases in age are associated to an increase in urine volume (from 40 to 60 years' old) and a reduction in urine osmolality (Table 1). Urine volume was positively correlated with physical activity (*r* = 0.152; $p < 0.001$) and water intake (*r* = 0.623; $p < 0.001$) and negatively with maximal air temperature (*r* = −0.222; $p < 0.001$) NRWL and urine osmolality (*r* = −0.736; $p < 0.001$; Table 3).

NRWL were higher in males and in the summer (Table 1). NRWL were positively associated with maximal temperature (*r* = 0.147; $p < 0.001$), water intake (*r* = 0.716; $p < 0.001$), negatively with urine volume (*r* = −0.095; $p < 0.024$) and positively with urine osmolality (0.208; $p < 0.001$; Table 3). However, NRWL was not associated with physical activity or serum osmolality.

Average 24-h urine osmolality (an index of hydration, [25]) was higher in males, lower in the German sample and as mentioned above decreasing with the increases in age group (see last column of Table 1). Based on urine osmolality we calculated obligatory urine volume and the difference with the actual urine volume collected to result in the calculation of free water reserve (*i.e.*, FWR). FWR was negative in 29% of the sample (163 out of 558 subjects with this variable) which suggests hypohydration in an important portion of our sample. Subjects with negative FWR (*i.e.*, hypohydrated) ingested less fluid on a daily basis, had lower urine output, lived in higher environmental temperatures, had higher NRWL (*i.e.*, sweat) and higher urine osmolalities (Table 1).

4. Discussion

There are several studies in the literature using dietary and activity logs to determine water intake and physical activity levels in different populations [9,10,26–28]. The novelty of our data is that although we use these subjective measurements of physical activity and water intake we followed subjects during seven consecutive days in an attempt to increase accuracy and spread possible spurious reporting into a more extensive data collection set. Subjects were instructed to carry with them their meal and beverage log and to report their physical activity at the end of every day by completing four simple questions modified from the international physical activity questionnaire (*i.e.*, short version IPAQ, [14,17,29,30]). Expectedly, the differences between weekend and weekdays in physical activity, fluid and meal ingestion were normalized by the full week collecting period with subjects starting data collection at different days of the week. In addition, subjects collected 24-h urine output during those seven consecutive days and a fasting blood sample was drawn in the morning of day 1 and day 8. These biological samples provide us with objective data to determine body hydration based on urine and blood osmolality. Using urine output in conjunction with water intake diaries we calculated non-renal water losses (NRWL) assuming that subjects were in fluid balance during the week of testing. Based on average urine osmolality we also calculated obligatory urine volume and free water reserve (FWR; see methods) to enhance our ability to detect dehydration using different indexes.

4.1. Effects of Physical Activity on Water Intake/Fluid Loss and Hydration

We found that physical activity estimated by seven days average IPAQ, is negatively associated with elevations in dehydration indexes (urine and blood osmolality; Tables 3 and 4). This suggests that high levels of physical activity does not increase the risk of hypohydration. Conversely, our less physically active individuals are more likely to be hypohydrated based on urine osmolality. Physical activity seems to increase water turnover since we also found a positive association between physical activity and water intake and urine volume (Table 3). The transitory dehydration that accompanies increases in physical activity triggers the release of hormones like arginine vasopressin, which in turn stimulates thirst to regain fluid balance. In our data, 24-h water intake was strongly correlated with non-renal water loss (*i.e.*, sweating; $r = 0.716$; $p < 0.001$) which suggest that increased levels of physical activity are met by increased water intake in a voluntary or thirst-induced response to restore the water deficit created by exercise. Seemingly, elevated levels of physical activity result in a higher water loss compensated with higher fluid intake, which prevents from dehydration and even seems to promote a better hydration status (lower urine and blood osmolalities). There may be non-physiological influences for the observed increased water consumption in people with higher levels of physical activity. Among those, consumer education throughout advertisement that permeates and convince exercise enthusiast to increase hydration beyond their thirst drive.

It is well known that repeated bouts of vigorous physical activity results in hemodilution [31] due to plasma volume expansion [32]. However, it is unclear if the moderately-intense physical activity of most of our subjects (grand mean of 2241 MET-min· week^{-1}) could result in plasma volume expansion. Plasma volume expansion results if physical activity is followed by thermally induced profuse sweating (*i.e.*, sauna, [33]). Thus, it is possible that the combination of moderately-intense physical activity of our subjects and the exposure to high ambient temperatures in the summer could have resulted in some degree plasma volume expansion. We have recently found that exercise training expands not only blood plasma but also water within the exercised muscles [34]. Thus, the finding that people with increased physical activity show reduced urine osmolality could be explained by this exercise training adaptations that raise body water content. Suggesting plasma volume expansion, blood concentration of sodium, potassium, glucose and calculated blood osmolality were also lower in people with the highest levels of physical activity (Table 4).

4.2. Effects of Climate on Physical Activity, Water Intake/Fluid Loss and Hydration

We found an interaction effect between physical activity and climate. Physical activity (estimated by IPAQ) was reduced in the summer and this reduction was associated with increased maximal ambient temperatures ($r = -0.277$; $p < 0.001$; Table 3). In contrast, most of the available data show that physical activity increases from winter to spring or summer [35]. However, these studies were conducted in places with moderate summer temperatures like Ontario, Massachusetts, Glasgow,

Netherlands, Central Japan or Aberdeen [35]. The high temperatures in Toledo and Athens in the summer may have been responsible for the currently reported reduction summer physical activity. This environmentally mediated reduction in physical activity in the summer, did not prevent the occurrence of higher non-renal water losses likely belonging to increased sweating ($r = 0.147$; $p < 0.001$). Maximal ambient temperature was associated with reduced urine output and increased urine osmolality ($r = 0.218$; $p < 0.001$; Table 3). Blood also responded to ambient temperature with increased concentration (Table 4). Our interpretation of these data is that environmental heat acts to reduce voluntary physical activity but does not prevent higher sweat losses that in the face of an insufficient increase in water intake, results in moderate dehydration. When data is analyzed using winter-summer category instead of using the continuous maximal daily temperature, urine osmolality (dehydration index) was not higher in the summer (Table 1). One factor that could explain the lack of effect of season in urine osmolality is that while in Spain and Greece maximal temperatures during summer likely induce sweating and dehydration, in Germany summer temperatures are lower and less dehydrating. Thus, the winter-summer classification may not be ideal when testing subjects in different latitudes.

Although in the short term, physical activity results in water loss (*i.e.*, exercise induce-sweating), it is less clear what is the result of different levels of physical activity on 24-h water intake and loss. In a thorough study, Westerterp and co-workers studied 42 women and 10 Dutch men (all lean and young) during 7 days. They were tested for water intake (weighted record of foodstuff and beverage), physical activity (difference between total and resting energy expenditure) and water loss (deuterium elimination method) in summer and winter [9]. The study revealed that in men, water loss was higher in subjects with a higher physical activity regardless of the season. However, in women water loss was higher in summer but was unrelated to physical activity [9]. In another study, water turnover was measured in rural and urban women in Kenya. The authors found that that BMI was the strongest predictor of water loss. However, the addition of physical activity (measured by accelerometry) to the prediction equation accounted for an additional 12% of the variance in water loss [10]. Our study in a much larger and heterogeneous subject sample confirms a positive association between physical activity and water loss (urine volume) but also a positive association with 24-h water intake (Table 3). Seemingly this higher water turnover results in improved hydration status with lower urine and blood osmolality in the subjects with higher physical activity levels.

4.3. Effects of Aging on Hydration

Our older groups of participants (40–50 and 50–60 years' old) seemed to be able to maintain a level of physical activity similar to the younger age groups (Table 1). This project was housed in three Universities and although it was meant to reach all population segment and types from the surrounding cities (Cologne, Athens and Toledo) the socioeconomic status of the inhabitants in these urban, university-cities is moderate to high. This population receive and can better implement the health advices to promote physical activity for healthy aging than in the rural areas. From this perspective, it is not surprising the reported maintenance of physical activity in the older segments of our sample. Furthermore, the age group of 20–30 years' old tended to be the less physically active group (Table 1) likely due to high time-consuming nature of studying/starting in a new job. The similar physical activity in the older subjects did not prevent the decrease in the capacity for renal water reabsorption described in previous studies [21,22]. Reduction in the capacity to concentrate urine is supported in our result of higher urine output and lower urine osmolality with increases in age ([21]; Table 1).

4.4. Effects of Gender and Country of Residency on Hydration

Men displayed higher 24-h water intake, NRWL (*i.e.*, sweating) and urine osmolality than the women of our sample. The larger average body size linked to higher energy expenditure/consumption could explain the highest sweat loss and fluid intake in men. However, there is no ready explanation for the gender effect on urine osmolality. The chief metabolite in urine is urea, which is derived from protein catabolism. On average, men have more muscle mass, protein turnover and thus may need to clear more urea in urine. We recently found that men with higher amount of muscle mass (rugby players) have higher urine osmolality than men with lower muscle mass (endurance runners) despite similar hydration status [36]. Alternatively, men may consume more protein than women influencing urine osmolality. Thus, the higher urine osmolality in men in comparison to women (Table 1) does not necessarily mean that the men in our sample were hypohydrated in comparison to the women but rather that urine osmolality is influenced by factors apart from hydration.

We also found significant country differences the most obvious being the lower maximal temperature in Germany in comparison to Spain and Greece (17 °C *vs.* 24–25 °C when averaging summer and winter data). Our German subjects were more physically active and there was a significant correlation between higher maximal ambient temperatures and reduced physical activity. Thus, our data suggests that the higher ambient temperatures in Spain and Greece may have inhibited physical activity in comparison to Germany. Besides environmental heat, differences in city architectural design to allow physical activity engagement (*i.e.*, parks, bike-lanes, pedestrian paths) and people's knowledge of the impact of exercise in their health, could also contribute to the higher PA found in German subjects. German subjects also ingests more fluid per day and had a higher urine volume. These data corroborates our finding of a link between PA and water turnover even when data are analyzed by countries.

4.5. Limitations of the Study

There are some limitations in our study that should be kept in mind. Water intake, urine volume and physical activity were all self-reported values. These variables are subjected to participant under or over-reporting. To avoid misreporting, subjects were instructed to record drinks and food ingested immediately after it happened but some underreporting in weekends was conceivable. Subjects were instructed to collect each void in a plastic jar, and record the urine weight before disposal. Likewise than with the food and drink diary, underreporting was possible. Completeness of 24-h urine collection could have been assessed by urine analysis of the recovery of p-aminobenzoic acid previously ingested [37]. However, this biochemical analysis was not available in our facilities. Subjects recorded physical activity at night by filling out a daily log and thus this measurement was subjected to individual's recall ability. Other means to track physical activity ordered by precision are pedometers, accelerometers or double-labelled water, which were not available in our study. Lastly, our correlations (Tables 3 and 4) only point to associations between variables and manipulative studies are due to establish cause-effect among these factors. Furthermore, we ought to recognize that although significant, many correlations among variables were small ($r < 0.3$) and the conclusions based on those are tentative.

5. Conclusions

Our data compiling seven consecutive testing days on 573 men and women aged 20–60 years' old suggests an association between elevated ambient temperatures and lowering physical activity with a larger effect in the southern European countries (Spain and Greece) in comparison to northern Europe (Germany). The reduction in physical activity in summer did not prevent higher non-renal water loss (*i.e.*, mostly sweating) and hypohydration despite increased water intake. When summer and winter data were compiled, better hydration (lower urine and plasma osmolality) was associated with elevated levels of physical activity (IPAQ). This suggests that the exercise training adaptations to expand body water and improve hydration status may also occur in the general population, mostly in those with high levels of physical activity. Finally, our results confirm previous reports in that aging reduce the capacity to concentrate urine.

Acknowledgments: The authors would like to thank the participants of the study and the graduate students that processed the diets. We also thank Ekavi Georgousopoulou and Demosthenes B. Panagiotakos from the Department of Nutrition and Dietetics, Harokopio University in Athens for their excellent statistical assistance.

We also are grateful for the grant funds provided by the European Hydration Institute. The funding Institute served no other role in this work.

Author Contributions: Ricardo Mora-Rodriguez, Maria Kapsokefalou and Hans Braun designed the study, collected the data and wrote the manuscript. Juan F. Ortega, Valentin E. Fernandez-Elias, Olga Malisova, Adelais Athanasatou, Marlien Husemann and Kirsten Domnik collected the data, conducted the analyses and corrected manuscript drafts. All authors have read and approved the final manuscript.

Conflicts of Interest: The authors declare no conflict of interest.

References

1. EJCN. Summary and outlook. *Eur. J. Clin. Nutr.* **2003**, *57* (Suppl. S2), 96–100.
2. Fink, H.A.; Wilt, T.J.; Eidman, K.E.; Garimella, P.S.; MacDonald, R.; Rutks, I.R.; Brasure, M.; Kane, R.L.; Ouellette, J.; Monga, M. Medical management to prevent recurrent nephrolithiasis in adults: A systematic review for an american college of physicians clinical guideline. *Ann. Intern. Med.* **2013**, *158*, 535–543. [CrossRef] [PubMed]
3. Sontrop, J.M.; Dixon, S.N.; Garg, A.X.; Buendia-Jimenez, I.; Dohein, O.; Huang, S.H.; Clark, W.F. Association between water intake, chronic kidney disease, and cardiovascular disease: A cross-sectional analysis of nhanes data. *Am. J. Nephrol.* **2013**, *37*, 434–442. [CrossRef] [PubMed]
4. Roussel, R.; Fezeu, L.; Bouby, N.; Balkau, B.; Lantieri, O.; Alhenc-Gelas, F.; Marre, M.; Bankir, L. Low water intake and risk for new-onset hyperglycemia. *Diabetes Care* **2011**, *34*, 2551–2554. [CrossRef] [PubMed]
5. Carroll, H.A.; Davis, M.G.; Papadaki, A. Higher plain water intake is associated with lower type 2 diabetes risk: A cross-sectional study in humans. *Nutr. Res.* **2015**, *35*, 865–872. [CrossRef] [PubMed]
6. Clark, W.F.; Sontrop, J.M.; Moist, L.; Huang, S.H. Increasing water intake in chronic kidney disease: Why? Safe? Possible? *Ann. Nutr. Metab.* **2015**, *66* (Suppl. S3), 18–21. [CrossRef] [PubMed]
7. EFSA (European Food Safety Authority). Scientific opinion on dietary reference value for water. *EFSA J.* **2010**, *8*, 1459–1506.
8. IOM (Institute of medicine). *Dietary Reference Intakes for Water Potassium, Sodium, Chloride, and Sulfate*; National Academies Press: Washington, DC, USA, 2004.
9. Westerterp, K.R.; Plasqui, G.; Goris, A.H. Water loss as a function of energy intake, physical activity and season. *Br. J. Nutr.* **2005**, *93*, 199–203. [CrossRef] [PubMed]
10. Keino, S.; van den Borne, B.; Plasqui, G. Body composition, water turnover and physical activity among women in narok county, Kenya. *BMC Public Health* **2014**, *14*, 1212. [CrossRef] [PubMed]
11. Brown, K.H.; Black, R.E.; Robertson, A.D.; Becker, S. Effects of season and illness on the dietary intake of weanlings during longitudinal studies in rural bangladesh. *Am. J. Clini. Nutr.* **1985**, *41*, 343–355.
12. Malisova, O.; Bountziouka, V.; Panagiotakos, D.; Zampelas, A.; Kapsokefalou, M. Evaluation of seasonality on total water intake, water loss and water balance in the general population in Greece. *J. Hum. Nutr. Diet.* **2013**, *26* (Suppl. S1), 90–96. [CrossRef] [PubMed]
13. Jequier, E.; Constant, F. Water as an essential nutrient: The physiological basis of hydration. *Eur. J. Clin. Nutr.* **2010**, *64*, 115–123. [CrossRef] [PubMed]
14. Craig, C.L.; Marshall, A.L.; Sjostrom, M.; Bauman, A.E.; Booth, M.L.; Ainsworth, B.E.; Pratt, M.; Ekelund, U.; Yngve, A.; Sallis, J.F.; *et al.* International physical activity questionnaire: 12-country reliability and validity. *Med. Sci. Sports Exerc.* **2003**, *35*, 1381–1395. [CrossRef] [PubMed]
15. Ainsworth, B.E.; Haskell, W.L.; Whitt, M.C.; Irwin, M.L.; Swartz, A.M.; Strath, S.J.; O'Brien, W.L.; Bassett, D.R.; Schmitz, K.H.; Emplaincourt, P.O.; *et al.* Compendium of physical activities: An update of activity codes and met intensities. *Med. Sci. Sports Exerc.* **2000**, *32*, 498–504. [CrossRef]
16. Hagstromer, M.; Oja, P.; Sjostrom, M. The International Physical Activity Questionnaire (IPAQ): A study of concurrent and construct validity. *Public Health Nutr.* **2006**, *9*, 755–762. [CrossRef] [PubMed]
17. Lee, P.H.; Macfarlane, D.J.; Lam, T.H.; Stewart, S.M. Validity of the international physical activity questionnaire short form (IPAQ-SF): A systematic review. *Int. J. Behav. Nutr. Phys. Activ.* **2011**, *8*, 115. [CrossRef] [PubMed]
18. Abbadi, A.; El-Khoury, J.M.; Wang, S. Stability of serum and plasma osmolality in common clinical laboratory storage conditions. *Clin. Biochem.* **2014**, *47*, 686–687. [CrossRef] [PubMed]

19. Seifarth, C.C.; Miertschischk, J.; Hahn, E.G.; Hensen, J. Measurement of serum and plasma osmolality in healthy young humans—Influence of time and storage conditions. *Clin. Chem. Lab Med.* **2004**, *42*, 927–932. [CrossRef] [PubMed]

20. Wang, Z.; Deurenberg, P.; Wang, W.; Pietrobelli, A.; Baumgartner, R.N.; Heymsfield, S.B. Hydration of fat-free body mass: Review and critique of a classic body-composition constant. *Am. J. Clin. Nutr.* **1999**, *69*, 833–841. [PubMed]

21. Manz, F.; Johner, S.A.; Wentz, A.; Boeing, H.; Remer, T. Water balance throughout the adult life span in a german population. *Br. J. Nutr.* **2012**, *107*, 1673–1681. [CrossRef] [PubMed]

22. Manz, F.; Wentz, A. 24-h hydration status: Parameters, epidemiology and recommendations. *Eur. J. Clin. Nutr.* **2003**, *57* (Suppl. S2), 10–18. [CrossRef] [PubMed]

23. Rolls, B.J.; Phillips, P.A. Aging and disturbances of thirst and fluid balance. *Nutr. Rev.* **1990**, *48*, 137–144. [CrossRef] [PubMed]

24. Cohen, J. *Statistical Power Analysis for the Behavioural Sciences*, 2nd ed.; Lawrence Erlbaum Associates: Hillsdale, NJ, USA, 1988; p. 567.

25. Cheuvront, S.N.; Kenefick, R.W.; Charkoudian, N.; Sawka, M.N. Physiologic basis for understanding quantitative dehydration assessment. *Am. J. Clin. Nutr.* **2013**, *97*, 455–462. [CrossRef] [PubMed]

26. Park, S.; Sherry, B.; O'Toole, T.; Huang, Y. Factors associated with low drinking water intake among adolescents: The Florida Youth Physical Activity and Nutrition Survey, 2007. *J. Am. Diet. Assoc.* **2011**, *111*, 1211–1217. [CrossRef] [PubMed]

27. Polkinghorne, B.G.; Gopaldasani, V.; Furber, S.; Davies, B.; Flood, V.M. Hydration status of underground miners in a temperate australian region. *BMC Public Health* **2013**, *13*, 426. [CrossRef] [PubMed]

28. Yang, M.; Chun, O.K. Consumptions of plain water, moisture in foods and beverages, and total water in relation to dietary micronutrient intakes and serum nutrient profiles among us adults. *Public Health Nutr.* **2015**, *18*, 1180–1186. [CrossRef] [PubMed]

29. Hallal, P.C.; Victora, C.G. Reliability and validity of the international physical activity questionnaire (IPAQ). *Med. Sci. Sports Exerc.* **2004**, *36*, 556. [CrossRef] [PubMed]

30. Papathanasiou, G.; Georgoudis, G.; Papandreou, M.; Spyropoulos, P.; Georgakopoulos, D.; Kalfakakou, V.; Evangelou, A. Reliability measures of the short international physical activity questionnaire (IPAQ) in Greek young adults. *Hell. J. Cardiol.* **2009**, *50*, 283–294.

31. Convertino, V.A. Blood volume: Its adaptation to endurance training. *Med. Sci. Sports Exerc.* **1991**, *23*, 1338–1348. [CrossRef] [PubMed]

32. Convertino, V.A. Blood volume response to physical activity and inactivity. *Am. J. Med. Sci.* **2007**, *334*, 72–79. [CrossRef] [PubMed]

33. Stanley, J.; Halliday, A.; D'Auria, S.; Buchheit, M.; Leicht, A.S. Effect of sauna-based heat acclimation on plasma volume and heart rate variability. *Eur. J. Appl. Phys.* **2015**, *115*, 785–794. [CrossRef] [PubMed]

34. Mora-Rodriguez, R.; Sanchez-Roncero, A.; Fernandez-Elias, V.E.; Guadalupe-Grau, A.; Ortega, J.F.; Dela, F.; Helge, J.W. Aerobic exercise training increases muscle water content in obese middle-age men. *Med. Sci. Sports Exerc.* **2015**, *21*. [CrossRef] [PubMed]

35. Shephard, R.J.; Aoyagi, Y. Seasonal variations in physical activity and implications for human health. *Eur. J. Appl. Phys.* **2009**, *107*, 251–271. [CrossRef] [PubMed]

36. Hamouti, N.; Del Coso, J.; Avila, A.; Mora-Rodriguez, R. Effects of athletes' muscle mass on urinary markers of hydration status. *Eur. J. Appl. Phys.* **2010**, *109*, 213–219. [CrossRef] [PubMed]

37. Raman, A.; Schoeller, D.A.; Subar, A.F.; Troiano, R.P.; Schatzkin, A.; Harris, T.; Bauer, D.; Bingham, S.A.; Everhart, J.E.; Newman, A.B.; *et al.* Water turnover in 458 American adults 40–79 years of age. *Am. J. Physiol. Ren. Physiol.* **2004**, *286*, 394–401. [CrossRef] [PubMed]

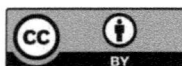

nutrients

MDPI

Article

Plain Water and Sugar-Sweetened Beverage Consumption in Relation to Energy and Nutrient Intake at Full-Service Restaurants

Ruopeng An

Department of Kinesiology and Community Health, College of Applied Health Sciences, University of Illinois at Urbana-Champaign, Champaign, IL 61820, USA; ran5@illinois.edu; Tel.: +1-217-244-0966

Received: 2 March 2016; Accepted: 27 April 2016; Published: 4 May 2016

Abstract: Background: Drinking plain water, such as tap or bottled water, provides hydration and satiety without adding calories. We examined plain water and sugar-sweetened beverage (SSB) consumption in relation to energy and nutrient intake at full-service restaurants. Methods: Data came from the 2005–2012 National Health and Nutrition Examination Survey, comprising a nationally-representative sample of 2900 adults who reported full-service restaurant consumption in 24-h dietary recalls. Linear regressions were performed to examine the differences in daily energy and nutrient intake at full-service restaurants by plain water and SSB consumption status, adjusting for individual characteristics and sampling design. Results: Over 18% of U.S. adults had full-service restaurant consumption on any given day. Among full-service restaurant consumers, 16.7% consumed SSBs, 2.6% consumed plain water but no SSBs, and the remaining 80.7% consumed neither beverage at the restaurant. Compared to onsite SSB consumption, plain water but no SSB consumption was associated with reduced daily total energy intake at full-service restaurants by 443.4 kcal, added sugar intake by 58.2 g, saturated fat intake by 4.4 g, and sodium intake by 616.8 mg, respectively. Conclusion: Replacing SSBs with plain water consumption could be an effective strategy to balance energy/nutrient intake and prevent overconsumption at full-service restaurant setting.

Keywords: plain water; sugar-sweetened beverage; diet quality; 24-h dietary recall; full-service restaurant; energy intake; added sugar; saturated fat; sodium

1. Introduction

Eating out has become an essential part of the American diet [1,2]. A long line of existing studies have documented fast-food restaurant consumption in relation to increased energy intake and elevated risk of obesity in children and adults [3–13]. Accumulating evidence suggests that full-service restaurant consumption shares similar, if not more concerning, nutrition implications as fast-food restaurant consumption [14,15]. Given that approximately one fifth of U.S. adults eat in a full-service restaurant on any given day [14], reducing energy intake and improving diet quality in full-service restaurant settings may profoundly impact Americans' nutritional and health status.

Adequate hydration is essential to body function [16]. Drinking plain water, such as tap or bottled water, delivers adequate hydration without adding calories [17]. Plain water intake has been linked to reduced energy consumption and improved body weight management [18–21]. Potential mechanisms include, but may not be limited to, plain water intake in substitution for caloric beverage consumption [22], and satiety from plain water consumption in coping with feelings of hunger and desire to eat [23]. The 2015–2020 Dietary Guidelines for Americans recommended "choosing beverages with no added sugars, such as water, in place of sugar-sweetened beverages" as an effective strategy to reduce added sugar consumption [24]. In addition, beverages are often consumed together with other foods, which jointly impact daily total calorie intake and overall diet quality. Using individual fixed-effects model based on two non-consecutive NHANES 24-h dietary recall data, An (2016) documented that in comparison to the days when no sugar-sweetened beverages (SSBs) were consumed, participants tended to consume more discretionary foods—foods that are typically low in nutrient value but high in added sugar, sodium, saturated fats, and cholesterol on days when they consumed SSBs [25].

Plain water is often available and free-of-charge at a full-service restaurant. Drinking plain water in substitution for SSBs could contribute to the reduction of total energy intake and intake of certain nutrients that are of major public health concern, such as added sugar when dining at a full-service restaurant. To our knowledge, no study has examined the nutritional implications of plain water consumption at full-service restaurant setting. Using in-person 24-h dietary recall data from a nationally-representative repeated cross-sectional health survey, this study assessed plain water and SSB consumption in relation to energy and nutrient intake at full-service restaurants among U.S. adults.

2. Materials and Methods

2.1. Survey Setting

The National Health and Nutrition Examination Survey (NHANES) is a program of studies conducted by the National Center for Health Statistics (NCHS) to assess the health and nutritional status of children and adults. The program began in the early 1960s and periodically conducted separate surveys focusing on different population groups or health topics. Since 1999, the NHANES has been conducted continuously in two-year cycles and has a changing focus on a variety of health and nutrition measurements. A multistage probability sampling design is used to select participants representative of the civilian, non-institutionalized U.S. population. Certain population subgroups are oversampled to increase the reliability and precision of health status indicator estimates for these groups. Detailed information regarding the NHANES sampling design, questionnaires, clinical measures, and individual-level data, can be found on its web portal [26].

2.2. Dietary Recall

Starting from the NHANES 1999–2000 wave, all participants were asked to complete an in-person 24-h dietary recall (a subsequent telephone-based dietary recall was added since 2001–2002 wave and data became publicly available since 2003–2004 wave). In the dietary recall, each food/beverage item and corresponding quantity consumed by a participant from midnight to midnight on the day before the recall was recorded. The in-person dietary recall was conducted by trained dietary interviewers in the Mobile Examination Center with a standard set of measuring guides. These tools aimed to help the participant accurately report the volume and dimensions of the food/beverage items consumed. Following the dietary recall, the energy and nutrient contents of each reported food/beverage item were systematically coded with the U.S. Department of Agriculture's Food and Nutrient Database for Dietary Studies (FNDDS).

Following An and McCaffrey [27] and Drewnowski et al. [28,29], this study used individual-level data from the NHANES 2005–2006, 2007–2008, 2009–2010, and 2011–2012 waves. Those waves were chosen because the collection of data on tap and bottled water consumption as a beverage only started in 2005 as part of the 24-h dietary recall, whereas in previous waves, such information was assessed via questionnaire after the 24-h dietary recall was completed.

2.3. Plain Water Consumption

Following An and McCaffrey (2016) [27] and Drewnowski et al. (2013a, b) [28,29], plain water consumption includes intake of plain tap water, water from a drinking fountain, water from a water cooler, bottled water, and spring water. In the NHANES 2005–2012 waves, the FNDDS codes 94000100 ("water, tap") and 94100100 ("water, bottled, unsweetened") were used to identify plain water consumption.

2.4. Sugar-Sweetened Beverage Consumption

SSBs include sodas, fruit drinks, energy drinks, sports drinks, and sweetened bottled waters, consistent with definitions reported by the Centers for Disease Control and Prevention (CDC) and the National Cancer Institute (NCI) [30]. In the NHANES 2011–2012 wave, SSBs consist of 48 reported beverage items. The number of reported items in the SSB category differed only slightly across survey waves.

2.5. Consumption of Other Beverage Types

In addition to plain water and SSBs, consumption of other beverage types including diet beverage, coffee, tea, alcohol, juice, and milk were summarized in descriptive statistics. Diet beverage includes calorie-free and low-calorie versions of sodas, fruit drinks, energy drinks, sports drinks, and carbonated water consistent with definitions reported by the CDC, NCI, and the Food and Drug Administration food labeling guidelines [31–33]. Coffee includes any form of regular or decaffeinated coffee product or coffee substitute (e.g., cereal grain beverage). Tea includes any form of regular or decaffeinated tea product. Alcohol includes beers and ales, cordials and liqueurs, cocktails, wines, and distilled liquors. The definitions on coffee, tea and alcohol are consistent with the USDA FNDDS food/beverage categorization [25]. Beverages in the juice and milk categories were identified based on the Food Patterns Equivalents Database (FPED), which were linked to the NHANES 24-h dietary recall data.

2.6. Added Sugar Consumption

Added sugar is sugar that is not naturally found in a food product but is added during the food production process. The USDA uses ingredient list and total sugar amounts provided to estimate the quantity of added sugar in a food product [34]. We used the FPED which contains the estimated added sugar amounts for each food/beverage consumed by the NHANES 24-h dietary recall participants.

2.7. Onsite Full-Service Restaurant Consumption

The NHANES dietary interviews asked about the source (e.g., restaurant, store, vending machine) of each food/beverage item consumed on a dietary recall day, and also whether the item was consumed at home or away from home. Following An [14] and Powell *et al.* [15], consumption of a food/beverage item qualified for an onsite full-service restaurant consumption if the item was obtained from a "restaurant with waiter/waitress" and consumed away from home.

In the dietary recall data, energy/nutrient derived from each consumed food/beverage item was recorded based on the quantity of food/beverage reported and the corresponding energy/nutrient contents. We calculated daily energy (kcal) and plain water (g), SSBs (g), added sugar (g), saturated fat (g), and sodium (mg) consumed onsite at a full-service restaurant among those NHANES participants who reported any onsite full-service restaurant consumption in the in-person 24-h dietary recall. We further classified full-service restaurant consumers into three mutually-exclusive categories based on their onsite SSB and plain water consumption status—SSB consumption (consumption of any positive grams of SSBs at a full-service restaurant), plain water but no SSB consumption (consumption of any positive grams of plain water but zero grams of SSBs at a full-service restaurant), and no plain water or SSB consumption (consumption of zero grams of plain water and SSBs at a full-service restaurant).

Among a total of 19,245 U.S. adults 18 years of age and above who participated in the in-person 24-h dietary recalls in the NHANES 2005–2012 waves, 934 who were pregnant, lactating, and/or on a special diet to lose weight at the time of interview were excluded. Of the remaining 18,311 participants, 2900 reported onsite full-service restaurant consumption on the dietary recall day. Among full-service restaurant consumers, 523 had SSB consumption, 85 had plain water but no SSB consumption, and the remaining 2292 had no plain water or SSB consumption at the restaurant.

In the analyses, we combined two mutually-exclusive categories, namely SSB but no plain water consumption (consumption of any positive grams of SSBs but zero grams of plain water at a full-service restaurant) and SSB and plain water consumption (consumption of any positive grams of SSBs and plain water at a full-service restaurant), into one category *i.e.*, SSB consumption, because the category of SSB and plain water consumption comprised an insufficient sample size of merely 11. In sensitivity analyses, we regressed each outcome variable (daily energy intake and intake of added sugar, saturated fat, and sodium at a full-service restaurant) on all four categories based on onsite SSB and plain water consumption status (plain water but no SSB consumption, no plain water or SSB consumption, and SSB and plain water consumption, with SSB but no plain water consumption in the reference group). The estimated coefficients were almost identical as those based on the three categories (plain water but no SSB consumption, and no plain water or SSB consumption, with SSB consumption in the reference group). None of the coefficients pertaining to the category of SSB and plain water consumption were statistically significant in the sensitivity analyses.

2.8. Individual Characteristics

The following individual characteristics were adjusted for in regression analyses: a dichotomous variable for sex (female, with male in the reference group); three categorical variables for age groups (18–34 years of age, 35–49 years of age, and 50–64 years of age, with 65 years of age and above in the reference group); three categorical variables for race/ethnicity (non-Hispanic black, non-Hispanic other race or multi-race, and Hispanic, with non-Hispanic white in the reference group); a dichotomous variable for education attainment (college education and above, with high school or lower education in the reference group); two categorical variables for marital status (divorced or separated or widowed, and never married, with married in the reference group); two categorical variables for household income level (130% $\leqslant$ income to poverty ratio [IPR] < 300%, and IPR $\geqslant$ 300%, with IPR < 130% in the reference group; IPR is the ratio of annual household income to poverty level specified in the Department of Health and Human Services' poverty guidelines); a dichotomous variable for body weight status (obesity defined as body mass index [BMI] $\geqslant$ 30 kg/m^2 based on the international classification of adult BMI values [35], with non-obesity in the reference group); a dichotomous variable for smoking status (ever or current smoker, with never smoking in the reference group); a dichotomous variable for self-rated health (good or excellent self-rated health, with poor or fair self-rated health in the reference group); five dichotomous variables for each of the chronic condition diagnoses *i.e.*, diabetes, arthritis, coronary heart disease, stroke, and cancer; a dichotomous variable for day of the week (weekend days including Friday, Saturday, and Sunday, with weekdays including Monday, Tuesday, Wednesday, and Thursday in the reference group) [36]; and three categorical variables for the NHANES waves (2007–2008, 2009–2010, and 2011–2012 waves, with 2005–2006 wave in the reference group).

2.9. Statistical Analyses

We summarized individual characteristics and daily energy/nutrient at full-service restaurants among the 2005–2012 NHANES adult full-service restaurant consumers by onsite SSB and plain water consumption status in descriptive statistics. Linear regressions were performed to estimate the differences in energy/nutrient intake at full-service restaurants by SSB and plain water consumption status, adjusting for individual characteristics. The four outcome variables were daily intake of energy (kcal), added sugar (g), saturated fat (g), and sodium (mg) at a full-service restaurant. Reductions of daily total energy intake and intake of added sugar, saturated fat, and sodium have been the key recommendations of the 2015–2020 Dietary Guidelines for Americans [24]. The key independent variables were two categorical variables for SSB and plain water consumption status at full service restaurant (plain water but no SSB consumption, and no plain water or SSB consumption, with SSB consumption in the reference group).

The dose-response relationship between SSB and plain water consumption and energy/nutrient intake at a full-service restaurant was assessed by regressing the outcome variables on the continuous variables for quantities (g) consumed of SSBs and plain water, adjusting for individual characteristics.

The NHANES 2005–2012 multi-wave sampling design was accounted for in both descriptive statistics and regression analyses. Specifically, we followed the NCHS instructions to construct sampling weights when combining survey waves [37]. We then applied the "svy" commands in Stata to specify sampling weights, sampling strata, and primary sampling units, as well as to conduct regression analyses. All statistical procedures were performed in Stata 14.1 SE version (StataCorp, College Station, TX, USA).

2.10. Human Subjects Protection

The NHANES was approved by the NCHS Research Ethics Review Board. This study used the NHANES de-identified public data and was deemed exempt from human subjects review by the University of Illinois at Urbana-Champaign Institutional Review Board.

3. Results

During 2005–2012, approximately 18.2% of U.S. adults had onsite full-service restaurant consumption on any given day. Among full-service restaurant consumers, 16.7% had SSB consumption, 2.6% had plain water but no SSB consumption, and the remaining 80.7% had no plain water or SSB consumption at the restaurant. Those who had SSB consumption on average consumed 612.0 g of SSB, and those who had plain water but no SSB consumption consumed 639.3 g of plain water at the restaurant. Among those who consumed no plain water or SSB at the restaurant, the prevalence of diet beverage, coffee, tea, alcohol, juice, and milk consumption (mutually-unexclusive) were 9.8%, 13.8%, 21.3%, 14.6%, 17.4%, and 24.1%, respectively.

Table 1 reports individual characteristics of adult full-service restaurant consumers by onsite SSB and plain water consumption status. Compared to women, men were more likely to consume SSBs (63.3%) but less likely to consume plain water (43.1%) in a full-service restaurant. SSB consumers consisted of a larger share of younger adults 18–34 years of age (40.8%) than plain water consumers (24.7%), whereas higher education was less prevalent among SSB consumers (58.6%) than among plain water consumers (67.7%). A smaller proportion of SSB consumers were at the lowest income level (IPR < 130%) but a larger proportion at the middle income level (130% ≤ IPR < 300%) compared to plain water consumers, whereas the prevalence of the highest income level (IPR ≥ 130%) remained similar between these two groups. Obesity rate and the prevalence of poor or fair self-rated health were slightly higher among SSB consumers compared to plain water consumers, and SSB consumers consisted of a larger proportion of former or current smokers.

Table 2 reports daily energy and nutrient intake at a full-service restaurant by onsite SSB and plain water consumption status. Among those three groups, SSB consumers had the highest daily intake of total energy, added sugar, saturated fat, and sodium from a full-service restaurant, whereas plain water consumers had the lowest, with those who consumed neither SSB nor water in between. Daily energy intake at a full-service restaurant totaled 1277.0 kcal among SSB consumers, 527.6 kcal, and 369.8 kcal higher than among plain water consumers and SSB/water nonconsumers, respectively. Daily added sugar intake at a full-service restaurant was 69.3 g among SSB consumers, 60.1 g and 54.5 g higher than among plain water consumers and SSB/water non-consumers, respectively. Daily saturated fat intake at a full-service restaurant was 15.0 g among SSB consumers, 5.7 g and 2.6 g higher than among plain water consumers and SSB/water non-consumers, respectively. Daily sodium intake at a full-service restaurant was 2331.0 mg among SSB consumers, 755.2 mg and 453.1 mg higher than among plain water consumers and SSB/water non-consumers, respectively.

Table 1. Individual characteristics of 2005–2012 NHANES adult full-service restaurant consumers by plain water and sugar-sweetened beverage (SSB) consumption status.

Individual Characteristics (%)	SSB Consumption (95% CI)	Plain Water but No SSB Consumption (95% CI)	No Plain Water or SSB Consumption (95% CI)
Sample size	523	85	2292
Sex			
Male	63.3 (58.2, 68.4)	43.1 (30.2, 56.0)	50.6 (48.5, 52.6)
Female	36.7 (31.6, 41.8)	56.9 (44.0, 69.8)	49.4 (47.4, 51.5)
Age group			
18–34 years of age	40.8 (35.5, 46.1)	24.7 (12.2, 37.1)	25.3 (22.7, 27.9)
35–49 years of age	30.5 (24.7, 36.4)	25.1 (12.9, 37.3)	30.7 (28.4, 33.1)
50–64 years of age	22.7 (17.5, 27.9)	38.6 (25.1, 52.1)	28.1 (25.3, 30.8)
65 years of age and above	6.0 (3.8, 8.1)	11.6 (2.3, 20.9)	15.9 (14.0, 17.8)
Race/ethnicity			
White, non-Hispanic	62.5 (56.2, 68.9)	67.2 (51.7, 82.7)	80.0 (77.2, 82.8)
Black, non-Hispanic	9.5 (6.9, 12.2)	5.2 (1.7, 8.7)	5.6 (4.4, 6.8)
Other race/multi-race, non-Hispanic	6.6 (4.1, 9.0)	8.2 (0.0, 16.9)	5.3 (4.2, 6.4)
Hispanic	21.4 (16.4, 26.4)	19.5 (8.9, 30.0)	9.1 (7.0, 11.2)
Education			
High school and below	41.4 (34.3, 48.5)	32.3 (21.8, 42.9)	31.0 (27.9, 34.1)
College education and above	58.6 (51.5, 65.7)	67.7 (57.1, 78.2)	69.0 (65.9, 72.1)
Marital status			
Married	69.6 (64.3, 74.8)	57.9 (46.2, 69.6)	68.0 (65.4, 70.7)
Divorced, separated, or widowed	10.2 (7.3, 13.0)	21.1 (10.8, 31.5)	15.8 (14.0, 17.7)
Never married	20.3 (15.8, 24.8)	21.0 (10.1, 31.8)	16.2 (13.8, 18.6)
Income to poverty ratio (IPR)			
IPR < 130%	16.6 (11.9, 21.4)	25.90 (11.7, 40.0)	10.5 (8.8, 12.3)
130% ≤ IPR < 300%	27.0 (22.0, 32.1)	17.0 (7.0, 26.9)	24.2 (21.6, 26.9)
IPR ⩾ 300%	56.4 (50.2, 62.5)	57.2 (43.3, 71.1)	65.2 (62.3, 68.1)
Obesity			
Non-obese (BMI < 30)	66.5 (61.5, 71.6)	68.5 (57.4, 79.6)	65.7 (62.8, 68.6)
Obese (BMI ⩾ 30)	33.5 (28.4, 38.6)	31.5 (20.4, 42.6)	34.3 (31.4, 37.2)
Smoking			
Non-smoker	61.2 (55.1, 67.4)	68.6 (53.8, 83.4)	57.4 (54.6, 60.2)
Former or current smoker	38.8 (32.6, 44.9)	31.4 (16.6, 46.2)	42.6 (39.9, 45.4)
Self-rated health			
Good or excellent health	86.4 (82.9, 89.8)	91.8 (86.8, 96.9)	89.0 (87.3, 90.6)
Fair or poor health	13.7 (10.2, 17.1)	8.2 (3.1, 13.2)	11.1 (9.4, 12.7)
Chronic condition			
Diabetes	6.9 (3.4, 10.3)	3.4 (0.6, 6.2)	8.4 (7.0, 9.7)
Arthritis	12.3 (9.0, 15.6)	17.1 (6.8, 27.3)	22.1 (20.0, 24.3)
Coronary artery disease	2.5 (0.5, 4.4)	0.4 (0.0, 1.3)	3.3 (2.4, 4.2)
Stroke	2.2 (0.4, 4.1)	2.7 (0.0, 5.9)	1.5 (0.9, 2.1)
Cancer	4.4 (2.1, 6.7)	12.2 (4.3, 20.0)	9.6 (7.9, 11.3)
Day of the week			
Weekday	27.3 (22.4, 32.2)	34.6 (13.9, 55.4)	33.6 (30.9, 36.2)
Weekend	72.7 (67.8, 77.6)	65.4 (44.7, 86.1)	66.4 (63.8, 69.1)
Survey wave			
2005–2006	28.0 (21.8, 34.2)	21.5 (7.4, 35.5)	25.2 (21.1, 29.3)
2007–2008	25.0 (17.1, 32.9)	22.4 (9.9, 35.0)	25.9 (22.8, 29.1)
2009–2010	20.2 (13.6, 26.9)	23.6 (10.2, 37.0)	23.2 (20.2, 26.2)
2011–2012	26.8 (18.1, 35.5)	32.6 (10.2, 54.9)	25.7 (22.2, 29.1)

Notes: The NHANES multi-wave sampling design was accounted for in estimating the percentages.

Table 2. Daily energy and nutrient intake at full-service restaurant by plain water and sugar-sweetened beverage (SSB) consumption status, 2005–2012 NHANES.

Intake	SSB Consumption (95% CI)	Plain Water but No SSB Consumption (95% CI)	No Plain Water or SSB Consumption (95% CI)
Sample size	523	85	2292
Total energy (kcal)	1277.0 (1184.3, 1369.6)	749.4 (613.5, 885.3)	907.2 (877.2, 937.1)
Added sugar (g)	69.3 (64.3, 74.2)	9.2 (6.2, 12.2)	14.8 (13.6, 16.0)
Saturated fat (g)	15.0 (13.4, 16.5)	9.3 (7.4, 11.2)	12.4 (12.0, 12.9)
Sodium (mg)	2331.0 (2122.0, 2540.1)	1575.8 (1243.4, 1908.2)	1877.9 (1819.8, 1936.1)

Notes: The NHANES multi-wave sampling design was accounted for in estimating the percentages.

Table 3 reports the adjusted differences in daily energy and nutrient intake at a full-service restaurant by onsite SSB and plain water consumption status based on regression estimates. After adjusting for individual characteristics, daily energy intake at a full-service restaurant among SSB consumers was 443.4 (95% confidence interval CI = 297.3, 589.6) kcal and 321.3 (95% CI = 224.0, 418.7) kcal higher than among plain water consumers and SSB/water non-consumers, respectively. Adjusted daily added sugar intake at a full-service restaurant among SSB consumers was 58.2 (95% CI = 52.2, 64.2) g and 53.3 (95% CI = 48.3, 58.4) g higher than among plain water consumers and SSB/water non-consumers, respectively. Adjusted daily saturated fat intake at a full-service restaurant among SSB consumers was 4.4 (95% CI = 2.0, 6.8) g and 2.2 (95% CI = 0.6, 3.8) g higher than among plain water consumers and SSB/water non-consumers, respectively. Adjusted daily sodium intake at a full-service restaurant among SSB consumers was 616.8 (95% CI = 286.8, 946.8) mg and 380.5 (95% CI = 160.8, 600.2) mg higher than among plain water consumers and SSB/water non-consumers, respectively.

Table 3. Adjusted differences in daily energy and nutrient intake at full-service restaurants by plain water and sugar-sweetened beverage (SSB) consumption status, 2005–2012 NHANES.

Independent Variable	Total Energy (kcal) (95% CI)	Added Sugar (g) (95% CI)	Saturated Fat (g) (95% CI)	Sodium (mg) (95% CI)
Sample size	2900	2900	2900	2900
Plain water and SSB intake status				
SSB consumption	Reference	Reference	Reference	Reference
Plain water but no SSB consumption	−443.4 *** (−589.6, −297.3)	−58.2 *** (−64.2, −52.2)	−4.4 ** (−6.8, −2.0)	−616.8 *** (−946.8, −286.8)
No plain water or SSB consumption	−321.3 *** (−418.7, −224.0)	−53.3 *** (−58.4, −48.3)	−2.2 ** (−3.8, −0.6)	−380.5 ** (−600.2, −160.8)
Sex				
Male	Reference	Reference	Reference	Reference
Female	−300.8 *** (−351.0, −250.6)	−6.0 *** (−8.3, −3.7)	−3.9 *** (−4.8, −3.0)	−581.3 *** (−691.0, −471.6)
Age group				
18–34 years of age	Reference	Reference	Reference	Reference
35–49 years of age	46.2 (−34.3, 126.7)	1.4 (−1.8, 4.6)	1.0 (−0.4, 2.3)	254.8 * (55.7, 453.8)
50–64 years of age	−41.2 (−120.8, 38.5)	2.0 (−2.2, 6.1)	−1.0 (−2.4, 0.3)	−6.3 (−171.8, 159.2)
65 years of age and above	−131.8 * (−231.3, −32.2)	−2.6 (−7.0, 1.8)	−2.2 ** (−3.9, −0.6)	−162.5 (−357.8, 32.8)
Race/ethnicity				
White, non-Hispanic	Reference	Reference	Reference	Reference
Black, non-Hispanic	−118.1 ** (−187.2, −49.0)	2.2 (−1.5, 6.0)	−2.5 *** (−3.6, −1.3)	−197.3 * (−350.3, −44.2)
Other race/multi-race, non-Hispanic	−91.6 (−189.7, 6.5)	−7.3 ** (−11.8, −2.8)	−2.3 * (−4.1, −0.5)	258.3 (−5.9, 522.5)
Hispanic	−90.8 * (−176.5, −5.1)	−5.6 * (−10.0, −1.1)	−2.7 *** (−4.1, −1.4)	−129.8 (−302.8, 43.2)

Table 3. Cont.

Independent Variable	Total Energy (kcal) (95% CI)	Added Sugar (g) (95% CI)	Saturated Fat (g) (95% CI)	Sodium (mg) (95% CI)
Education				
High school and below	Reference	Reference	Reference	Reference
College education and above	−11.7 (−77.7, 54.4)	−3.5 * (−6.8, −0.2)	0.00 (−1.1, 1.1)	1.4 (−134.0, 136.9)
Marital status				
Married	Reference	Reference	Reference	Reference
Divorced, separated, or widowed	2.7 (−69.8, 75.2)	−1.5 (−5.7, 2.7)	0.2 (−1.1, 1.5)	47.0 (−128.2, 222.2)
Never married	7.8 (−68.7, 84.2)	−0.3 (−3.9, 3.2)	−0.5 (−1.7, 0.8)	−6.2 (−167.8, 155.3)
Income to poverty ratio (IPR)				
IPR < 130%	Reference	Reference	Reference	Reference
130% ⩽ IPR < 300%	−35.8 (−138.6, 67.0)	−1.0 (−6.9, 4.8)	0.1 (−1.4, 1.6)	−76.3 (−265.1, 112.4)
IPR ⩾ 300%	−14.6 (−114.5, 85.4)	−4.0 (−9.2, 1.2)	0.2 (−1.3, 1.7)	16.5 (−177.7, 210.6)
Obesity				
Non-obese (BMI < 30)	Reference	Reference	Reference	Reference
Obese (BMI ⩾ 30)	27.6 (−29.6, 84.9)	−1.7 (−4.8, 1.4)	0.8 (−0.2, 1.8)	128.6 (−3.1, 260.3)
Smoking				
Non-smoker	Reference	Reference	Reference	Reference
Former or current smoker	49.6 (−9.1, 108.3)	1.2 (−1.6, 4.1)	0.4 (−0.8, 1.5)	88.8 (−32.9, 210.5)
Self-rated health				
Good or excellent health	−25.0 (−106.7, 56.7)	3.0 (−0.2, 6.3)	−1.5 * (−2.9, −0.1)	−90.4 (−325.0, 144.2)
Fair or poor health	Reference	Reference	Reference	Reference
Chronic condition				
Diabetes	−46.1 (−140.2, 48.0)	−1.3 (−6.1, 3.6)	−0.2 (−1.9, 1.5)	−131.7 (−337.8, 74.3)
Arthritis	13.8 (−55.1, 82.8)	1.8 (−0.6, 4.2)	0.5 (−0.7, 1.7)	86.8 (−66.6, 240.1)
Coronary artery disease	−108.0 * (−213.0, −2.9)	2.3 (−5.1, 9.8)	−0.1 (−1.9, 1.8)	−211.6 (−477.0, 53.8)
Stroke	97.1 (−201.2, 395.3)	−3.5 (−9.4, 2.4)	0.9 (−3.6, 5.4)	391.8 (−242.5, 1026.1)
Cancer	−79.1 (−160.7, 2.5)	−1.6 (−6.8, 3.5)	−1.3 (−2.7, 0.1)	−193.9 * (−357.3, −30.6)
Day of the week				
Weekday	Reference	Reference	Reference	Reference
Weekend	88.6 ** (38.2, 139.0)	5.2 *** (3.2, 7.2)	0.8 (−0.2, 1.8)	51.1 (−62.5, 164.6)
Survey wave				
2005–2006	Reference	Reference	Reference	Reference
2007–2008	19.6 (−56.0, 95.2)	−2.7 (−6.6, 1.2)	0.6 (−0.7, 2.0)	62.7 (−81.5, 206.9)
2009–2010	−41.4 (−118.5, 35.7)	−1.4 (−5.7, 3.0)	−0.3 (−1.6, 1.0)	−53.8 (−197.4, 89.8)
2011–2012	1.3 (−81.5, 84.1)	0.7 (−3.6, 5.0)	−0.7 (−2.1, 0.7)	−68.8 (−237.2, 99.7)

Notes: Linear regressions were performed to estimate the adjusted differences in daily energy and nutrient intake at full-service restaurants by plain water and SSB consumption status, accounting for the NHANES multi-wave sampling design. * $0.01 \leqslant p < 0.05$; ** $0.001 \leqslant p < 0.01$; and *** $p < 0.001$.

Women consumed less daily total energy, added sugar, saturated fat, and sodium at a full-service restaurant than men. Compared to those 18–34 years of age, those 35–49 years of age consumed more sodium, whereas those 65 years of age and above consumed less total energy and saturated fat at a full-service restaurant. Compared to non-Hispanic whites, non-Hispanic blacks consumed less total energy, saturated fat, and sodium, Hispanics consumed less total energy, added sugar, and sodium, and non-Hispanic other race/multi-race consumed less added sugar and saturated fat at a full-service restaurant. Those with good or excellent self-rated health consumed less saturated fat at a full-service restaurant than those with poor or fair self-rated health. Those with coronary artery disease consumed less total energy and those with cancer consumed less sodium at a full-service restaurant than those without such chronic conditions. Full-service restaurant consumption during weekend days was associated with higher total energy and added sugar intake than consumption during weekdays. Compared to those with high school or lower education, those with college or higher education consumed less added sugar at a full-service restaurant. Daily total energy, added sugar, saturated fat, and sodium intake at a full-service restaurant were not found to be associated with marital status, income level, obesity, or smoking. No temporal trend in daily total energy, sugar, saturated fat, and sodium intake at a full-service restaurant was identified as none of the coefficients with respect to survey waves were statistically significant at $p < 0.05$.

A dose-response relationship between onsite SSB consumption and energy/nutrient intake at a full-service restaurant was identified, whereas such relationship pertaining to onsite plain water consumption was statistically significant for total energy, added sugar, and saturated fat intake but not for sodium intake. An increase in onsite SSB consumption by 100 g was associated with an increase in daily intake of total energy at a full-service restaurant by 65.1 (95% CI = 50.6, 79.5) kcal, added sugar by 9.3 (95% CI = 8.7, 9.8) g, saturated fat by 0.5 (95% CI = 0.2, 0.8) g, and sodium by 78.9 (95% CI = 44.0, 113.7) mg. An increase in onsite plain water consumption by 100 g was associated with a reduction in daily intake of total energy at a full-service restaurant by 17.8 (95% CI = 0.6, 35.0) kcal, added sugar by 0.5 (95% CI = 0.1, 0.8) g, saturated fat by 0.3 (95% CI = 0.0, 0.6) g, and sodium by 32.0 (95% CI = −6.1, 70.2) mg.

4. Discussion

This study examined plain water and SSB consumption in relation to energy and nutrient intake at full-service restaurants among U.S. adults, using 24-h dietary recall data from a nationally-representative health survey. Over 18% of U.S. adults had onsite full-service restaurant consumption on any given day during 2005–2012. Among full-service restaurant consumers, approximately 16.7% consumed SSBs, 2.6% consumed plain water but no SSBs, and the remaining 80.7% consumed neither beverage at the restaurant. Adjusting for individual characteristics and accounting for sampling design, those consuming SSBs onsite had the highest daily intake of total energy, added sugar, saturated fat, and sodium at a full-service restaurant, whereas those consuming plain water but no SSBs had the lowest, with those consuming neither beverage was in between. Compared to onsite SSB consumption, plain water but no SSB consumption was associated with a reduction in daily total energy intake at a full-service restaurant by 443.4 kcal, added sugar intake by 58.2 g, saturated fat intake by 4.4 g, and sodium intake by 616.8 mg, respectively.

Replacing SSBs with plain water consumption has shown to be associated with reduced daily intake of total energy, added sugar, saturated fat, and sodium in some intervention and epidemiological studies [38–40]. Dining out at a full-service restaurant has been linked to increased energy intake and reduced diet quality [14,15,41]. Findings from this study confirmed the beneficial nutritional implications of plain water consumption at the full-restaurant setting. Drinking plain water in substitution for SSBs could help cut total calories as well as intake of certain nutrients that are of major public health concern, such as added sugar, saturated fat, and sodium when dining at a full-service restaurant.

Despite the nutritional desirability of replacing SSBs with plain water consumption, only a tiny proportion of full-service consumers chose to drink plain water, whereas the prevalence of onsite SSB consumption remained over five-fold larger. The lack of popularity in plain water consumption contrasts the fact that plain water is often easily accessible and made free-of-charge at a full-service restaurants as a "default" service to diners. Compared to eating at a fast-food restaurant, where plain water can be hard to find and a combo meal that includes SSBs is served as the "norm", it could be more convenient and advantageous for full-service restaurant consumers to balance their dietary intake and prevent overconsumption through onsite plain water consumption.

A dose-response relationship between onsite SSB and plain water consumption and energy/nutrient intake at a full-service restaurant was identified (although the associations between plain water consumption and sodium intake were statistically nonsignificant). Higher levels of onsite SSB consumption were associated with increased daily intake of total energy, added sugar, saturated fat, and sodium at a full-service restaurant; whereas higher levels of plain water consumption were associated with reduced intake of total energy and saturated fat. Plain water consumption delivers satiety and reduces the feelings of hunger and desire to eat but adds no calories to one's diet [17]. This study finding indicates that increasing onsite plain water consumption while refraining from SSB consumption could help achieve additional reduction in energy intake at full-service restaurant setting.

We restricted our classification of beverage consumption status at a full-service restaurant to the "dichotomy" of plain water and SSBs. This simplification allows us to examine the key contrasts of interest, which are based upon the accumulating evidence on the health benefits of plain water consumption and the detrimental impacts of SSB consumption on diet quality and obesity [42,43]. Arguably, other types of beverages (e.g., diet drinks, coffee, tea, alcohol, juice, and milk) also play important roles in determining energy and nutrient intake at full-service restaurants. For example, the prevalence of tea consumption is substantial, and if a large proportion of tea is calorically sweetened, it would constitute another large source of added sugar. However, a comprehensive examination of all beverage types is beyond the scope of this study.

A few limitations of this study should be noted. Dietary intake in the NHANES was self-reported and subject to measurement error and social desirability bias [44]. Prevalence of plain water consumption at full-service restaurants was low and this was possibly due to under-reporting of water intake. This study adopted a cross-sectional design. Although we attempted to reduce the influence of potential confounders by including a large set of covariates, it is possible that some unobserved differences in individual characteristics such as taste preferences and/or eating habits that are correlated with both outcomes and water/SSB consumption status at restaurants. A cross-sectional study design would not allow us to completely eliminate the possibility of confounding issue and, thus, the study findings warrant confirmation through controlled interventions. Despite use of multiple waves of data from a large nationally representative survey, only a tiny fraction (2.6%; $N = 85$) of the study sample drank plain water at a full-service restaurant, which compromised estimation precision and precluded further sample stratification and subgroup analyses by individual demographics and/or socioeconomic status. A dose-response relationship between onsite plain water consumption and sodium intake at a full-service restaurant was unidentified, possibly due to the very small sample size of plain water consumers and consequent lack of variations in quantities consumed. The NHANES is a probability sample of the U.S. non-institutionalized population, and patients in penal/mental facilities, institutionalized older adults, and/or military personnel on active duty are not represented.

5. Conclusions

Using 24-h dietary recall data from the 2005–2012 NHANES, this study assessed the relationship between plain water and SSB consumption and energy/nutrient intake at full-service restaurants in U.S. adults. Compared to onsite SSB consumption, plain water, but no SSB consumption, was associated with reduced daily intake of total calories, added sugar, saturate fat, and sodium at full-service restaurants. In comparison to home-prepared meals, dining out is prone to overeating and poorer dietary quality. Given that plain water is mostly available and free-of-charge at full-service restaurants, restricting one's beverage consumption to only plain water when dining out could be a cost-free and easily-adaptable strategy to balance energy and nutrient intake and prevent overconsumption.

Acknowledgments: The author has no funding source to declare.

Author Contributions: Ruopeng An designed the study, conducted statistical analyses, and wrote the manuscript.

Conflicts of Interest: The author declares no conflict of interest.

Abbreviations

The following abbreviations are used in this manuscript:

SSB	sugar-sweetened beverages
NHANES	National Health and Nutrition Examination Survey
NCHS	National Center for Health Statistics
FNDDS	Food and Nutrient Database for Dietary Studies
NCI	National Cancer Institute
CDC	Centers for Disease Control and Prevention (CDC)
FPED	Food Patterns Equivalents Database
IPR	income to poverty ratio
BMI	body mass index
CI	confidence interval

References

1. Guthrie, J.F.; Lin, B.H.; Frazao, E. Role of food prepared away from home in the American diet, 1977–1978 *versus* 1994–1996: Changes and consequences. *J. Nutr. Educ. Behav.* **2002**, *34*, 140–150. [CrossRef]
2. Kant, A.K.; Graubard, B.I. Eating out in America, 1987–2000: Trends and nutritional correlates. *Prev. Med.* **2004**, *38*, 243–249. [CrossRef] [PubMed]
3. Bowman, S.A.; Vinyard, B.T. Fast food consumption of U.S. adults: Impact on energy and nutrient intakes and overweight status. *J. Am. Coll. Nutr.* **2004**, *23*, 163–168. [CrossRef] [PubMed]
4. French, S.A.; Harnack, L.; Jeffery, R.W. Fast food restaurant use among women in the Pound of Prevention study: Dietary, behavioral and demographic correlates. *Int. J. Obes. Relat. Metab. Disord.* **2000**, *24*, 1353–1359. [CrossRef] [PubMed]
5. Paeratakul, S.; Ferdinand, D.P.; Champagne, C.M.; Ryan, D.H.; Bray, G.A. Fast-food consumption among US adults and children: Dietary and nutrient intake profile. *J. Am. Diet. Assoc.* **2003**, *103*, 1332–1338. [CrossRef]
6. Schröder, H.; Fíto, M.; Covas, M.I.; REGICOR investigators. Association of fast food consumption with energy intake, diet quality, body mass index and the risk of obesity in a representative Mediterranean population. *Br. J. Nutr.* **2007**, *98*, 1274–1280.
7. Boutelle, K.N.; Fulkerson, J.A.; Neumark-Sztainer, D.; Story, M.; French, S.A. Fast food for family meals: Relationships with parent and adolescent food intake, home food availability and weight status. *Public Health Nutr.* **2007**, *10*, 16–23. [CrossRef] [PubMed]
8. Bowman, S.A.; Gortmaker, S.L.; Ebbeling, C.B.; Pereira, M.A.; Ludwig, D.S. Effects of fast-food consumption on energy intake and diet quality among children in a national household survey. *Pediatrics* **2004**, *113*, 112–118. [CrossRef] [PubMed]
9. French, S.A.; Story, M.; Neumark-Sztainer, D.; Fulkerson, J.A.; Hannan, P. Fast food restaurant use among adolescents: Associations with nutrient intake, food choices and behavioral and psychosocial variables. *Int. J. Obes. Relat. Metab. Disord.* **2001**, *25*, 1823–1833. [CrossRef] [PubMed]
10. Maddock, J. The relationship between obesity and the prevalence of fast food restaurants: State-level analysis. *Am. J. Health Promot.* **2004**, *19*, 137–143. [CrossRef] [PubMed]
11. Niemeier, H.M.; Raynor, H.A.; Lloyd-Richardson, E.E.; Rogers, M.L.; Wing, R.R. Fast food consumption and breakfast skipping: Predictors of weight gain from adolescence to adulthood in a nationally representative sample. *J. Adolesc. Health* **2006**, *39*, 842–849. [CrossRef] [PubMed]
12. Pereira, M.A.; Kartashov, A.I.; Ebbeling, C.B.; Van Horn, L.; Slattery, M.L.; Jacobs, D.R., Jr.; Ludwig, D.S. Fast-food habits, weight gain, and insulin resistance (the CARDIA study): 15-year prospective analysis. *Lancet* **2005**, *365*, 36–42. [CrossRef]
13. Schmidt, M.; Affenito, S.G.; Striegel-Moore, R.; Khoury, P.R.; Barton, B.; Crawford, P.; Kronsberg, S.; Schreiber, G.; Obarzanek, E.; Daniels, S. Fast-food intake and diet quality in black and white girls: The National Heart, Lung, and Blood Institute Growth and Health Study. *Arch. Pediatrics Adolesc. Med.* **2005**, *159*, 626–631. [CrossRef] [PubMed]
14. An, R. Fast-Food and Full-Service Restaurant Consumption and Daily Energy and Nutrient Intakes in U.S. Adults. *Eur. J. Clin. Nutr.* **2016**, *70*, 97–103. [CrossRef] [PubMed]

15. Powell, L.M.; Nguyen, B.T.; Han, E. Energy intake from restaurants: Demographics and socioeconomics, 2003–2008. *Am. J. Prev. Med.* **2012**, *43*, 498–504. [CrossRef] [PubMed]

16. Popkin, B.M.; D'Anci, K.E.; Rosenberg, I.H. Water, hydration and health. *Nutr. Rev.* **2010**, *68*, 439–458. [CrossRef] [PubMed]

17. Campbell, S.M. Hydration needs throughout the lifespan. *J. Am. Coll. Nutr.* **2007**, *26*, 585S–587S. [CrossRef] [PubMed]

18. Dennis, E.A.; Flack, K.D.; Davy, B.M. Beverage consumption and adult weight management: A review. *Eat. Behav.* **2009**, *10*, 237–246. [CrossRef] [PubMed]

19. Muckelbauer, R.; Sarganas, G.; Grüneis, A.; Müller-Nordhorn, J. Association between water consumption and body weight outcomes: A systematic review. *Am. J. Clin. Nutr.* **2013**, *98*, 282–299. [CrossRef] [PubMed]

20. Stookey, J.D. Drinking water and weight management. *Nutr. Today* **2010**, *45*, S7–S12. [CrossRef]

21. Tate, D.F.; Turner-McGrievy, G.; Lyons, E.; Stevens, J.; Erickson, K.; Polzien, K.; Diamond, M.; Wang, X.; Popkin, B. Replacing caloric beverages with water or diet beverages for weight loss in adults: Main results of the Choose Healthy Options Consciously Everyday (CHOICE) randomized clinical trial. *Am. J. Clin. Nutr.* **2012**, *95*, 555–563. [CrossRef] [PubMed]

22. Hernández-Cordero, S.; Barquera, S.; Rodríguez-Ramírez, S.; Villanueva-Borbolla, M.A.; González de Cossio, T.; Dommarco, J.R.; Popkin, B. Substituting water for sugar-sweetened beverages reduces circulating triglycerides and the prevalence of metabolic syndrome in obese but not in overweight Mexican women in a randomized controlled trial. *J. Nutr.* **2014**, *144*, 1742–1752. [CrossRef] [PubMed]

23. Dennis, E.A.; Dengo, A.L.; Comber, D.L.; Flack, K.D.; Savla, J.; Davy, K.P.; Davy, B.M. Water consumption increases weight loss during a hypocaloric diet intervention in middle-aged and older adults. *Obesity* **2010**, *18*, 300–307. [CrossRef] [PubMed]

24. U.S. Department of Agriculture and U.S. Department of Health and Human Services. Dietary Guidelines for Americans, 2015–2020 (8th Edition). Available online: http://health.gov/dietaryguidelines/2015/guidelines/ (accessed on 25 January 2016).

25. An, R. Beverage consumption in relation to discretionary food intake and diet quality among U.S. Adults, 2003–2012. *J. Acad. Nutr. Diet.* **2016**, *116*, 28–37. [CrossRef] [PubMed]

26. Centers for Disease Control and Prevention. National Health and Nutrition Examination Survey. Available online: http://www.cdc.gov/nchs/nhanes/index.htm (accessed on 19 April 2016).

27. An, R.; McCaffrey, J. Plain water consumption in relation to energy intake and diet quality among US adults, 2005–2012. *J. Hum. Nutr. Diet.* **2016**. [CrossRef] [PubMed]

28. Drewnowski, A.; Rehm, C.D.; Constant, F. Water and beverage consumption among children age 4–13 years in the United States: Analyses of 2005–2010 NHANES data. *Nutr. J.* **2013**, *12*, 85. [CrossRef] [PubMed]

29. Drewnowski, A.; Rehm, C.D.; Constant, F. Water and beverage consumption among adults in the United States: Cross-sectional study using data from NHANES 2005–2010. *BMC Public Health* **2013**, *13*, 1068. [CrossRef] [PubMed]

30. National Cancer Institute. Sources of Beverage Intakes among the US Population, 2005–2006. Available online: http://riskfactor.cancer.gov/diet/foodsources/beverages/ (accessed on 25 November 2016).

31. Ogden, C.L.; Kit, B.K.; Carroll, M.D.; Park, S. Consumption of sugar drinks in the United States, 2005–2008. *NCHS Data Briefs* **2011**, *71*, 1–8.

32. Fakhouri, T.H.; Kit, B.K.; Ogden, C.L. Consumption of diet drinks in the United States, 2009–2010. *NCHS Data Briefs* **2012**, *109*, 1–8.

33. U.S. Food and Drug Administration. Guidance for Industry: A Food Labeling Guide. Available online: http://www.fda.gov/downloads/Food/GuidanceRegulation/UCM265446.pdf (accessed on 25 January 2016).

34. Erickson, J.; Slavin, J. Total, added, and free sugars: Are restrictive guidelines science-based or achievable? *Nutrients* **2015**, *7*, 2866–2878. [CrossRef] [PubMed]

35. World Health Organization. The International Classification of Adult Underweight, Overweight and Obesity According to BMI. Available online: http://apps.who.int/bmi/index.jsp?introPage=intro_3.html (accessed on 25 January 2016).

36. An, R. Weekend-weekday differences in diet among U.S. adults, 2003–2012. *Ann. Epidemiol.* **2016**, *26*, 57–65. [CrossRef] [PubMed]

37. National Center for Health Statistics. When and How to Construct Weights When Combining Survey Cycles. Available online: http://www.cdc.gov/nchs/tutorials/nhanes/SurveyDesign/Weighting/Task2.htm (accessed on 25 January 2016).

38. Akers, J.D.; Cornett, R.A.; Savla, J.S.; Davy, K.P.; Davy, B.M. Daily self-monitoring of body weight, step count, fruit/vegetable intake, and water consumption: A feasible and effective long-term weight loss maintenance approach. *J. Acad. Nutr. Diet.* **2012**, *112*, 685–692. [CrossRef] [PubMed]

39. Stookey, J.D.; Constant, F.; Popkin, B.M.; Gardner, C.D. Drinking water is associated with weight loss in overweight dieting women independent of diet and activity. *Obesity* **2008**, *16*, 2481–2488. [CrossRef] [PubMed]

40. Sichieri, R.; Yokoo, E.M.; Pereira, R.A.; Veiga, G.V. Water and sugar-sweetened beverage consumption and changes in BMI among Brazilian fourth graders after 1-year follow-up. *Public Health Nutr.* **2013**, *16*, 73–77. [CrossRef] [PubMed]

41. An, R.; Liu, J. Fast-food and full-service restaurant consumption in relation to daily energy and nutrient intakes among US adult cancer survivors, 2003–2012. *Nutr. Health* **2013**, *22*, 181–195. [CrossRef] [PubMed]

42. Daniels, M.C.; Popkin, B.M. Impact of water intake on energy intake and weight status: A systematic review. *Nutr. Rev.* **2010**, *68*, 505–521. [CrossRef] [PubMed]

43. Malik, V.S.; Schulze, M.B.; Hu, F.B. Intake of sugar-sweetened beverages and weight gain: A systematic review. *Am. J. Clin. Nutr.* **2006**, *84*, 274–288. [PubMed]

44. Hebert, J.R.; Hurley, T.G.; Peterson, K.E.; Resnicow, K.; Thompson, F.E.; Yaroch, A.L.; Ehlers, M.; Midthune, D.; Williams, G.C.; Greene, G.W.; *et al.* Social desirability trait influences on self-reported dietary measures among diverse participants in a multicenter multiple risk factor trial. *J. Nutr.* **2008**, *138*, 226S–234S. [PubMed]

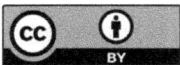

nutrients

MDPI

Article
Physical Activity and Beverage Consumption among Adolescents

Maria del Mar Bibiloni [1,2], Asli Emine Özen [3], Antoni Pons [1,2], Marcela González-Gross [2,4] and Josep A. Tur [1,2,*]

1   Research Group on Community Nutrition and Oxidative Stress, University of Balearic Islands,
    Palma de Mallorca E-07122, Spain; mar.bibiloni@uib.es (M.M.B.); antonipons@uib.es (A.P.)
2   CIBEROBN (Physiopathology of Obesity and Nutrition), Instituto de Salud Carlos III,
    Madrid E-28029, Spain; marcela.gonzalez.gross@upm.es
3   Department of Gastronomy and Culinary Arts, Reha Midilli Foça Faculty of Tourism,
    Dokuz Eylül University, Foça-Izmir 35680, Turkey; asli.ozen@deu.edu.tr
4   ImFINE Research Group, Department of Health and Human Performance,
    Faculty Physical Activity & Sport Sciences-INEF, Technical University of Madrid, Madrid E-28040, Spain
*   Correspondence: pep.tur@uib.es; Tel.: +34-971-173146; Fax: +34-971-173184

Received: 9 April 2016; Accepted: 14 June 2016; Published: 23 June 2016

Abstract: This study assessed the relationship between physical activity and beverage consumption among adolescents with a population based cross-sectional survey was carried out in the Balearic Islands, Spain (n = 1988; 12–17 years old). Body composition, educational and income level, physical activity (PA), and beverage consumption and energy intake were assessed. Sixty-two percent of adolescents engaged in >300 min/week of PA. Boys were more active than girls, younger adolescents were more active than older counterparts, low parental income was associated with physical inactivity, and time spent watching TV (including, TV, Internet or handheld cellular devices) was inversely associated with PA practice. The average beverage intake of the studied adolescents was 0.9 L/day, higher in boys than in girls. Beverage intake was positively associated with PA practice, and the highest amount of energy intake from beverages was observed in active boys and girls. Most of the studied adolescent population met the PA recommendations. Gender, age, parental income, and time spent watching TV were significant determinants of PA. Type and amount of beverages drunk varied according to gender and PA, and general daily total beverage intake was lower than recommended adequate fluid intake. PA behavior should be considered when analyzing beverage consumption in adolescents.

Keywords: beverage consumption; physical activity; adolescents

1. Introduction

Physical activity (PA) is important for a healthy development [1], and adequate levels of PA are currently included in most, if not all, public health guidelines for children and adolescents [2]. As PA increases cell metabolism, it causes an increase in body temperature, and sweating is the main way of maintaining heat balance during PA, especially in hot climates [2–4], increasing the needs of body water to keep adequate thermoregulation functioning, and even though fluid needs will be obviously different in both PA for health and PA as a sport, both show a common physiological basis. Contrary to former statements, current research indicates that young people have similar thermoregulatory ability to adults and that an adequate hydration contributes to a better thermoregulatory ability [5].

Insufficient voluntary fluid intake is common among active young people [6] and if they fail to replace fluid loss during and after exercise, it could lead to more heat storage in the body [7,8]. Hypohydration affects prolonged aerobic exercise more than it affects short, high-intensity anaerobic exercise [9,10]. Adolescents need to consume enough fluid to maintain an appropriate euhydration [7]. Fluid ingested before, during, and after exercise decreases dehydration, core temperature for a given heat production, heart rate, and cardiac strain [11], and then contributes to maintain skin blood flow and to increase exercise performance [12,13].

Beverages are an important source of fluids to maintain appropriate hydration level, but fluid requirements of physically active people are influenced by climate, age, sex, body size, sweat production, and food habits, as well as intensity and duration of PA [14–16]. One study has published beverage consumption in European adolescents [17], but most publications are mainly focused on sugar-sweetened beverages and overweight [18,19].

Therefore, fluid intake is essential for health, but also for a good PA performance, mainly in developing bodies, as in adolescents. However, scarce studies have assessed the relation between physical activity and beverage consumption among adolescents, and then recommendations do not distinguish between physically active and inactive subjects [20]. This study assessed the relationship between physical activity and beverage consumption among an adolescent population.

2. Materials and Methods

2.1. Study Design

The study is a population-based cross-sectional survey carried out in the Balearic Islands (Spain), a Mediterranean region, between 2007 and 2008.

2.2. Study Population

A multicenter study was performed on Balearic Islands' adolescents aged 12–17 years. The population was selected by means of a multiple-step, simple random sampling, taking into account first the location of all the Balearic Islands (Palma de Mallorca 400,578 habitants, Calvià 50,328, Inca 30,651, Manacor 40,170, Maó 28,006, Eivissa 49,975, Llucmajor 34,618, Santa Margalida 11,672, S'Arenal 16,719, and Sant Jordi de Ses Salines 8048) and then by random assignment of the schools within each city. Sample size was stratified by age and gender. The socio-economic variable was considered to be associated to geographical location and type of school. As the selection of schools was done by random selection and fulfilling quota, this variable was also considered to be randomly assigned.

In order to calculate a representative number of adolescents, the variable Body Mass Index (BMI) with the greatest variance for this age group from the data published in the literature at the time the study was selected. The sampling was determined for the distribution of this variable; the confidence interval (CI) was established at 95% with an error ± 0.25. The total number of subjects was uniformly distributed in the cities and proportionally distributed by sex and age. Exclusion criteria were: self-reported type 2 diabetes, pregnancy, alcohol or drug abuse, and non-directly related nutritional medical conditions.

The sample was oversized to prevent loss of information and as necessary to do the fieldwork in complete classrooms. In each school, classrooms were randomly selected among those of the same grade or level, and all the adolescents of one classroom were proposed to participate in the survey. A letter about the nature and purpose of the study informed parents or legal guardians. After receiving their written consent, the adolescents were considered for inclusion in the study. All responses of questionnaires were filled in by adolescents. After finishing the field study, the adolescents who did not fulfill the inclusion criteria were excluded. Finally, the sample was adjusted by a weight factor in order to balance the sample in accordance to the distribution of the Balearic Islands' population and to guarantee the representativeness of each of the groups, already defined by the previously mentioned factors (age and sex). The final number of subjects included in the study was 1988 adolescents (82.8% participation), a representative sample of the Balearic Islands' adolescent population.

The reasons to not participate were: (a) the subject declined to be interviewed; and (b) the parents did not authorize the interview.

This study was conducted according to the guidelines laid down in the Declaration of Helsinki, and all procedures involving human subjects were approved by the Balearic Islands' Ethics Committee (Palma de Mallorca, Spain) No. IB-530/05-PI.

2.3. General Questionnaire

Educational and income level of the parents was determined by means of a questionnaire incorporating the following questions: father's and mother's educational level (grouped according to years and type of education into low, <6 years at school; medium, 6–12 years of education; and high, >12 years of education), father's and mother's income (based on the occupation and classified as low, <12,000 euros/year; medium, 12,000–22,500 euros/year; and high, >22,500 euros/year), according to the methodology described by the Spanish Society of Epidemiology [21].

Information about smoking habits and alcohol intake was collected as described: smoking habit no; yes; occasionally, less than 1 cigarette/day; alcohol consumption no; frequently; occasionally, less than 1 drink/week.

2.4. Body Composition

Height was determined to the nearest millimeter using a mobile anthropometer (Kawe 44444, Kirchner & Wilhelm GmBH Co., KG, Asperg, Germany) with the subject's head in the Frankfurt plane. Body weight was determined to the nearest 100 g using a digital scale (Tefal, sc9210, Groupe SEB, Rumilly, France). The subjects were weighed barefoot wearing light underwear, as previously described [22]. BMI was computed as weight (kg) per height squared (m^2), and study participants were age- and gender-specific categorized using the BMI cut-offs developed and proposed by the International Obesity Task Force [23] and Cole et al. [24] definitions, and categorized as underweight (≤5th percentile), normal-weight (>5th–≤85th percentile), overweight (>85th percentile) and obese (≥95th percentile).

2.5. Physical Activity Assessment

Physical activity was assessed according to the guidelines for data processing and analysis of the short-form International Physical Activity Questionnaire [25], and its specific modification for adolescents (IPAQ-A) [26]. The specific types of activity assessed were: walking, moderate-intensity activities (i.e., PA at school) and vigorous-intensity activities (i.e., sport practice). An additional question about the time spent on a typical day sitting and watching TV (including, TV, Internet or handheld cellular devices), playing computer games, or talking with friends, but also time spent sitting at school and for homework, was used as an indicator variable of time spent at sedentary activities. According to the Patient-centered Assessment & Counseling for Exercise (PACE) + Adolescent Physical Activity Measure and existing guidelines [27,28], adolescents were also asked about the number of days with PA of at least 60 min/day of moderate-vigorous physical activity (≥3 Metabolic Equivalents or METs) during the past 7 days and during a typical week. The number of active days during the past week and during a typical week was averaged. On the basis of their total weekly PA (at least 60 min/day of moderate-vigorous physical activity on at least 5 day/week), the subjects were divided into 2 groups: inactive (<300 min/week) and active (≥300 min/week), according to the current PA recommendations for young people [28,29].

2.6. Assessment of Beverage Consumption and Energy Intake

Beverage consumption and energy intake were assessed using two non-consecutive 24 h diet recalls period, one was administered in the warm season (May–September) and another in the cold season (November–March) to account for the effect of seasonal variations. To bias brought on by day-to-day intake variability, the recalls were administered homogeneously from Monday to

Sunday. Well-trained dieticians administered the recalls and verified and quantified the food records. Recalls were performed face-to-face at the participants' classroom. Volumes and portion sizes were reported in natural units, household measures or with the aid of a manual of sets of photographs [30] Well-trained dieticians administered the recalls and verified and quantified the information obtained from the 24 h recalls.

Beverages were categorized into eleven groups: water (tap water, bottled water, and sparkling water), low-fat milk (low-fat and skimmed milk), whole-fat milk, diet soda (low calorie carbonated soft drinks), coffee/tea (coffee, black tea and herbal tea), fruit juice 100% (all kinds of natural fruit juice), non-diet soda (all kinds of carbonated sugared soft drinks), fruit juice (all kinds of fruit juice sweetened with sugar), alcohol (wine, beer, vodka, and whisky), energy/sports beverages, and others (carrot juice, beer without alcohol, chocolate milkshake, vanilla milkshake, strawberry milkshake, diet milkshake, soy milk, rice milk, oat milk, fermented milk drink with sugar, fermented milk drink, kefir, horchata, and sugar added iced tea).

Total energy intake (TEI) from whole diet and from beverages were calculated using a computer program (ALIMENTA®, NUCOX, Palma, Spain) based on Spanish [31,32] and European Food Composition Tables [33], and complemented with food composition data available for Balearic food items [34]. Identification of misreporters: an energy intake (EI)/basal metabolic rate (BMR) ratio <0.92 (boys) and <0.85 (girls) was considered to represent under-reporters [35], and an EI/BMR $\geqslant$ 2.4 as over-reporters [36].

2.7. Statistical Analyses

Statistical Package for the Social Sciences for Windows version 21.0 (SPSS Inc., Chicago, IL, USA) was used. Absolute numbers and percentages of participants according to physical activity practice were calculated by using a general lineal model adjusted by age, sex, and BMI. Significant differences in mean daily beverage and energy intake were tested by means of ANOVA. Significant differences in percentages were tested by means of χ^2. Crude and adjusted by potential confounders (age and sex), odds ratios (OR) and 95% confidence intervals (CI) were calculated to examine the relationship between the risk of being inactive and socio-demographic and lifestyle characteristics. Linear regression analysis was used to evaluate associations between physical activity and beverage consumption. For all statistical tests, $p < 0.05$ was taken as the significant level.

3. Results

3.1. Socio-Demographic and Lifestyle Characteristics of the Population

Twenty-two percent of the final sample did not report their energy intake accurately (underreporters 20% and overreporters 2%) and were excluded from further analysis. Table 1 shows the socio-demographic and lifestyle characteristics of the study population according to PA level. Sixty-two percent of the adolescents met the recommendations (>300 min/week). Sex, age, parental education level and income, alcohol intake and time spent watching TV, were significant determinants of PA practice. Boys and younger adolescents had lower risk of being inactive. Adolescents whose father had lower income were more likely to be inactive. The length of time spent watching TV was positively associated with PA, and the risk of being inactive was lower among adolescents who watched TV $\leqslant$ 1 h/day.

3.2. Daily Beverage Consumption and Energy Intake

Daily beverage, energy intake and percentage of consumers among adolescents related with PA practice are shown in Table 2. Beverage and energy intake were obtained only from those adolescents who consumed the drinks. Physically active girls had higher mean daily water, total beverage, and beverage TEI, and lower fruit drink intake than inactive girls. Physically active boys showed higher total beverage, dietary TEI, and beverage TEI than inactive boys. Gender differences were also observed: inactive boys showed higher consumption of whole-fat milk, and soda, as well as higher dietary and beverage TEI than inactive girls; and active boys showed higher consumption of whole milk, fruit drinks, and soda consumption, and dietary and beverage TEI, as well as lower low-fat milk than active girls. Percentage of consumers of whole milk, fruit juice and fruit drinks, and energy/sport beverages are higher among active boys; proportion of consumers of low-fat and whole milk, fruit juice, and energy/sport beverages are higher among active girls. Among inactive adolescents, boys showed higher percentage of consumers of low-fat milk, diet soda, and other beverages, whereas girls showed higher proportion of consumers of fruit drinks, soda, coffee/tea, and other beverages than active peers.

Table 1. Socio-demographic and lifestyle characteristics, according to physical activity and multivariable analysis of risk factors for low physical activity versus moderate and high physical activity groups.

	Inactive [1]	Active [2]	χ^2	Risk of Being Inactive
	n (%) [3]	n (%) [3]		OR [4] (95% CI)
Sex			<0.0001	
Male	171 (23.2)	568 (76.8)		0.31 (0.25–0.39) *
Female	415 (51.1)	397 (48.9)		1.00
Age (Years)			0.001	
12–13	112 (30.5)	256 (69.5)		0.59 (0.42–0.82) *
14–15	274 (38.5)	437 (61.5)		0.82 (0.63–1.06)
16–17	220 (46.6)	252 (53.4)		1.00
Father's Education Level [5]			<0.0001	
Low	200 (41.4)	283 (58.6)		0.94 (0.63–1.39)
Medium	257 (39.2)	397 (60.8)		1.08 (0.78–1.49)
High	124 (29.9)	290 (70.1)		1.00
Mother's Education Level [5]			<0.0001	
Low	188 (42.6)	254 (57.4)		1.48 (0.99–2.20)
Medium	270 (38.8)	426 (61.2)		1.27 (0.92–1.75)
High	126 (30.6)	287 (69.4)		1.00
Father's Income			<0.0001	
Low	239 (42.6)	321 (57.4)		1.66 (1.12–2.45) *
Medium	252 (35.7)	452 (64.3)		1.28 (0.90–1.83)
High	87 (30.3)	200 (69.7)		1.00
Mother's Income			0.013	
Low	245 (31.1)	544 (68.9)		0.72 (0.47–1.10)
Medium	206 (34.4)	393 (65.6)		0.68 (0.46–1.01)
High	60 (36.8)	103 (63.2)		1.00
BMI (kg/m^2)			0.870	
Underweight	14 (41.5)	20 (58.5)		1.08 (0.50–2.30)
Normal weight	427 (37.8)	703 (62.2)		0.83 (0.56–1.23)
Overweight	99 (39.7)	148 (60.3)		0.94 (0.60–1.47)
Obese	55 (39.2)	85 (60.8)		1.00
Smoking			0.473	
Yes	40 (43.4)	52 (56.6)		1.09 (0.67–1.77)
Occasionally	149 (37.8)	245 (62.2)		1.01 (0.78–1.30)
No	400 (37.6)	665 (62.4)		1.00
Alcohol Intake			0.032	
Yes	336 (36.1)	595 (63.9)		1.02 (0.80–1.31)
No	254 (41.0)	366 (59.0)		1.00
Time Spent Watching TV			0.001	
<1 h/day	74 (31.0)	165 (69.0)		0.68 (0.48–0.97) *
1–2 h/day	328 (36.7)	565 (63.3)		0.82 (0.64–1.04)
>2 h/day	184 (43.9)	235 (56.1)		1.00

[1] Physical activity < 300 min/week; [2] Physical activity $\geqslant$ 300 min/week; [3] Percentage of population was tested by χ^2; [4] Odds ratios (ORs) and 95% Confidence Interval (95% CI) were adjusted by age and gender; * Odds ratios within a column, for a characteristic, were statistically significant from 1.00 ($p < 0.05$); [5] Educational level of parents: low: <6 years, medium 6–12 years, high: >12 years.

Table 2. Daily beverage (mL), energy intake and percentage of consumers among active and inactive adolescents.

Beverages (mL)	Boys					Girls				
	Inactive (n = 171)		Active (n = 568)			Inactive (n = 415)		Active (n = 397)		
	Mean ± SEM	% Consumers	Mean ± SEM	% Consumers	p Value [1]	Mean ± SEM	% Consumers	Mean ± SEM	% Consumers	p Value [1]
Water	760.9 ± 45.9	73.7	871.3 ± 28.7	73.1	0.058	728.0 ± 28.1	80.7	885.1 ± 33.5	81.9	0.001
Low-Fat Milk	281.4 ± 17.0	27.5	301.5 ± 10.2 *	25.2	0.323	272.3 ± 9.1	32.0	277.1 ± 8.7	37.0	0.701
Whole Milk	298.5 ± 20.3	55.6	301.9 ± 7.9 *	62.9	0.854	276.3 ± 9.9	44.3	265.0 ± 8.0	46.9	0.371
Fruit Juice (100%)	200.0 ± 20.7	4.7	246.3 ± 22.3	7.0	0.363	237.5 ± 26.1	7.7	213.5 ± 8.8	12.1	0.318
Fruit Drinks	370.8 ± 20.9	23.4	338.3 ± 15.9 **	34.3	0.466	312.6 ± 22.0	36.1	269.7 ± 12.4	32.0	0.107
Soda	441.6 ± 31.5	33.9	474.0 ± 20.4 ***	33.6	0.428	400.4 ± 19.7	26.5	365.4 ± 22.1	24.7	0.236
Diet Soda	330.0 ± 30.1	2.3	396.7 ± 36.9	0.5	0.586	266.7 ± 36.7	0.7	410.0 ± 49.3	0.8	0.159
Coffee/Tea	99.6 ± 18.8	7.0	85.0 ± 9.0 *	7.9	0.469	101.2 ± 12.1	10.8	131.3 ± 21.1	7.1	0.188
Alcoholic Beverages	220.0 ± 15.1	0.6	225.0 ± 20.5	0.4	0.983	250.0 ± 23.0	0.2	280.0 ± 35.0	0.3	0.323
Energy/Sport Beverages	495.0 ± 16.5	1.2	337.1 ± 29.8	2.5	0.115	233.3 ± 36.7	0.7	330.0 ± 26.4	1.8	0.133
Others [2]	461.3 ± 46.1	19.3	531.2 ± 64.4	10.9	0.501	501.7 ± 61.2	22.7	573.8 ± 67.2	16.6	0.443
Total Beverage	1004.4 ± 46.5	100.0	1141.7 ± 27.9	100.0	0.015	1003.9 ± 29.0	100.0	1060.3 ± 30.8	100.0	0.012
Dietary TEI (kcal/day)	2254.4 ± 51.3 ***	100.0	2378.7 ± 32.8 ***	100.0	0.042	1952.6 ± 28.5	100.0	1923.8 ± 30.2	100.0	0.486
Beverage TEI (kcal/day)	253.9 ± 44.1 ***	100.0	274.4 ± 23.7 ***	100.0	0.006	238.3 ± 25.9	100.0	230.8 ± 31.4	100.0	0.002

Inactive: <300 min/week. Active: >300 min/week; [1] p value: Active vs. inactive boys, and active vs. inactive girls by ANOVA; Active boys vs. active girls, and inactive boys vs. inactive girls by ANOVA (* $p < 0.05$; ** $p < 0.01$; *** $p < 0.001$); TEI = total energy intake; [2] Others include carrot juice, beer without alcohol, chocolate milkshake, vanilla milkshake, strawberry milkshake, diet milkshake, soy milk, rice milk, oat milk, fermented milk drink, kefir, horchata, and sugar added iced tea.

Table 3. Daily beverage (mL), energy intake and percentage of consumers among active and inactive boys according to the season.

Beverages (mL)	Inactive Boys (n = 171)					Active Boys (n = 568)					
	Cold Season		Warm Season		p Value[1]	Cold Season		Warm Season		p Value[1]	
	Mean ± SEM	% Consumers	Mean ± SEM	% Consumers		Mean ± SEM	% Consumers	Mean ± SEM	% Consumers		
Water	721.6 ± 51.4	65.3	855.4 ± 95.2	76.2	0.007	803.7 ± 30.9 **	63.0	1013.0 ± 59.4 **	78.0	0.001	
Low-Fat Milk	275.9 ± 24.1	17.4	289.5 ± 23.0	36.5	0.700	277.5 ± 12.2	12.0	338.8 ± 16.9 *	30.0	0.003	
Whole Milk	281.0 ± 14.7	67.2	368.4 ± 82.8	46.5	0.086	295.6 ± 8.9	66.0	324.6 ± 17.5 *	46.0	0.131	
Fruit Juice (100%)	200.0 ± 27.2	3.1	280.6 ± 42.0	5.8	0.325	260.4 ± 35.5 *	1.0	225.0 ± 17.1 *	9.0	0.444	
Fruit Drinks	313.3 ± 47.8	16.8	490.0 ± 58.3	26.0	0.018	314.0 ± 17.9	21.0	389.2 ± 30.9 *	36.0	0.026	
Soda	400.0 ± 45.4	25.5	498.8 ± 40.4	37.7	0.400	459.3 ± 22.5	23.0	512.3 ± 44.4	38.0	0.245	
Diet Soda	320.6 ± 27.1	1.9	421.2 ± 38.3	3.9	0.056	330.6 ± 25.3	0.3	430.0 ± 23.0	0.6	0.043	
Coffee/Tea	94.5 ± 19.4	9.2	125.0 ± 75.0	5.8	0.370	88.5 ± 10.6 *	9.0	68.8 ± 13.1 *	4.0	0.409	
Alcoholic Beverages	330.0 ± 18.1	1.0	170.0 ± 20.5	0.4	0.007	330.2 ± 22.5	0.6	120.6 ± 35.8 *	0.3	0.005	
Energy/Sport Beverages	330.9 ± 25.8	0.5	377.8 ± 58.9	1.8	0.779	344.0 ± 33.4	4.0	346.7 ± 55.6	3.0	0.794	
Others[2]	485.0 ± 46.1	29.9	350.3 ± 70.0	9.8	0.002	480.2 ± 58.7	12.0	463.8 ± 63.5	8.0	0.097	
Total Beverage	913.5 ± 47.5	100.0	1281.1 ± 51.2	100.0	0.001	1025.0 ± 29.1	100.0	1454.9 ± 60.5 *	100.0	0.001	
Dietary TEI (kcal/day)	2373.2 ± 95.1	100.0	2213.8 ± 64.5	100.0	0.045	2511.6 ± 40.5 *	100.0	2230.3 ± 53.6	100.0	0.032	
Beverage TEI (kcal/day)	324.1 ± 47.8	100.0	236.8 ± 22.7	100.0	0.009	341.3 ± 52.1	100.0	250.9 ± 19.9	100.0	0.007	

Inactive: <300 min/week. Active: >300 min/week; [1] p value: Warm vs. cold season by ANOVA; Active vs. inactive by ANOVA (* $p < 0.05$; ** $p < 0.01$; *** $p < 0.001$); TEI = total energy intake; [2] Others include carrot juice, beer without alcohol, chocolate milkshake, vanilla milkshake, strawberry milkshake, diet milkshake, soy milk, rice milk, oat milk, fermented milk drink with sugar, fermented milk drink, kefir, horchata, and sugar added iced tea.

Table 4. Daily beverage (mL), energy intake and percentage of consumers among active and inactive girls according to the season.

Beverages (mL)	Inactive Girls (n = 415)					Active Girls (n = 397)				
	Cold Season		Warm Season		p Value [1]	Cold Season		Warm Season		p Value [1]
	Mean ± SEM	% Consumers	Mean ± SEM	% Consumers		Mean ± SEM	% Consumers	Mean ± SEM	% Consumers	
Water	705.8 ± 32.4	78.5	754.1 ± 54.1	83.1	0.003	838.8 ± 43.8	80.1	950.2 ± 51.6 *	83.8	0.006
Low-Fat Milk	273.8 ± 10.7	35.0	268.4 ± 17.3	32.1	0.590	266.3 ± 9.7	36.9	288.4 ± 14.6	39.1	0.206
Whole Milk	272.3 ± 11.6	46.2	280.1 ± 18.3	41.6	0.353	262.7 ± 7.9	48.4	272.1 ± 21.8	43.3	0.318
Fruit Juice (100%)	243.3 ± 53.3	4.2	233.5 ± 16.1	10.6	0.177	193.5 ± 6.5	7.0	282.0 ± 15.0 *	15.0	0.027
Fruit Drinks	331.9 ± 30.7	35.2	268.9 ± 17.1	38.8	0.188	273.8 ± 16.9	29.9	260.5 ± 13.5	33.4	0.223
Soda	403.5 ± 24.5	26.1	393.7 ± 33.2	22.9	0.419	358.9 ± 28.5	24.4	374.3 ± 35.1	24.6	0.534
Diet Soda	246.7 ± 56.7	0.8	266.7 ± 65.7	0.6	0.521	390.0 ± 39.3 *	0.6	430.0 ± 33.3 *	1.8	0.154
Coffee/Tea	106.8 ± 14.9	9.8	92.5 ± 20.4	10.5	0.450	152.4 ± 41.0	5.8	120.0 ± 50.0	5.4	0.550
Alcoholic Beverages	270.0 ± 33.0	0.4	243.2 ± 28.4	0.1	0.005	295.0 ± 33.0	0.2	274.2 ± 43.0	0.3	0.009
Energy/Sport Beverages	332.0 ± 36.5	0.3	185.0 ± 45.2	1.3	0.667	321.0 ± 25.8	0.9	337.0 ± 18.7 *	2.4	0.425
Others [2]	526.2 ± 88.4	23.7	490.3 ± 43.5	21.3	0.361	569.3 ± 41.0	16.0	604.6 ± 34.3	17.4	0.141
Total Beverage	949.9 ± 34.6	100.0	1142.5 ± 50.8	100.0	0.007	925.7 ± 35.4	100.0	1320.2 ± 53.4 *	100.0	0.001
Dietary TEI (kcal/day)	1951.6 ± 35.6	100.0	1954.9 ± 46.9	100.0	0.356	1898.0 ± 36.7	100.0	1942.2 ± 52.8	100.0	0.242
Beverage TEI (kcal/day)	236.1 ± 24.9	100.0	238.5 ± 32.1	100.0	0.754	224.0 ± 15.1	100.0	228.7 ± 25.9	100.0	0.542

Inactive: <300 min/week. Active: >300 min/week; [1] p value: Warm vs. cold season by ANOVA; Active vs. inactive by ANOVA (* p < 0.05; ** p < 0.01; *** p < 0.001); TEI = total energy intake; [2] Others include carrot juice, beer without alcohol, chocolate milkshake, vanilla milkshake, strawberry milkshake, diet milkshake, soy milk, rice milk, oat milk, fermented milk drink with sugar, fermented milk drink, kefir, horchata, and sugar added iced tea.

3.3. Beverage Consumption According to Seasons

Tables 3 and 4 (boys and girls, respectively) show daily beverage, energy intake and percentage of consumers among active and inactive adolescents according to seasons. More water, diet soda, and total beverages are consumed in the warm than in the cold season in both active and inactive boys and girls. Alcoholic beverages as well as dietary and beverage total energy intake are more consumed in the cold season. In boys, activity in the cold season increased water, fruit juice (100%) and dietary TEI and decreased coffee/tea consumption, whereas in the warm season there were increased water, low-fat milk and total beverage consumption, and decreased whole milk, fruit juice (100%), fruit drinks, coffee/tea and alcoholic beverage consumption. In girls, activity in the cold season increased diet soda consumption, whereas in the warm season there were increased water, fruit juice (100%), diet soda, energy/sport beverages, and total beverage consumption.

3.4. Beverage Consumption According to Physical Activity

Proportions of consumers of each beverage according to physical activity level are shown in Figure 1. More than half of the consumers for each beverage were physically active. Highest consumption of energy/sport beverage drinkers was found among active adolescents, whereas the highest proportion of diet soda drinkers was observed among inactive subjects.

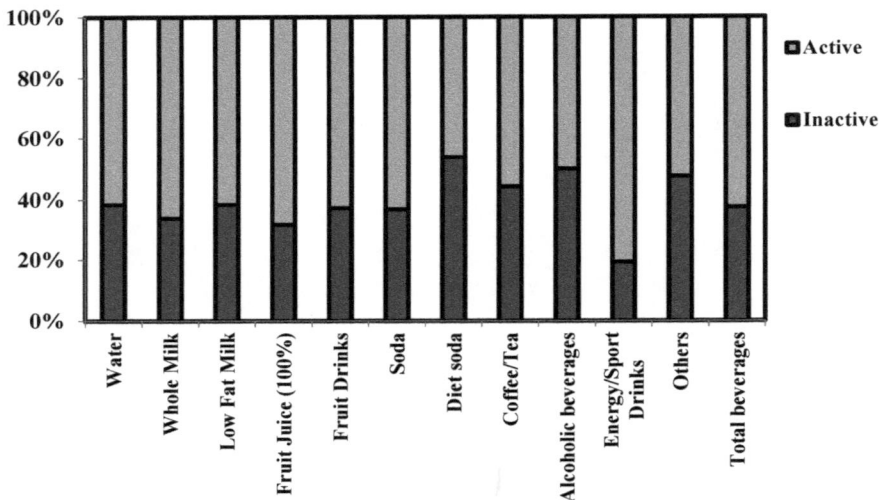

Figure 1. Proportions of consumers of each beverage according to physical activity level (others include carrot juice, beer without alcohol, chocolate milkshake, vanilla milkshake, strawberry milkshake, diet milkshake, soy milk, rice milk, oat milk, fermented milk drink with sugar, fermented milk drink, kefir, horchata, and sugar added iced tea).

Results of the linear regression analysis on the association between PA level and beverage consumption are shown in Table 5. A statistically significant and positive association was observed between PA level and total beverage consumption in model 2 (adjusted data by age, gender, total energy intake and BMI; $p = 0.032$).

Table 5. Association between physical activity and beverage consumption.

Beverages	Physical Activity					
	Model 1 [1]			Model 2 [2]		
	β	SE	p	β	SE	p
Water	0.164	0.130	0.205	0.190	0.137	0.166
Low Fat Milk	−0.021	0.029	0.478	−0.018	0.031	0.566
Whole Milk	0.018	0.037	0.620	0.046	0.038	0.213
Fruit Juice (100%)	0.016	0.014	0.246	0.021	0.015	0.157
Fruit Drinks	−0.023	0.040	0.564	−0.029	0.043	0.493
Soda	0.081	0.047	0.087	0.089	0.050	0.073
Diet Soda	0.011	0.007	0.092	0.010	0.007	0.152
Coffee/Tea	0.006	0.007	0.435	0.008	0.007	0.300
Alcoholic Beverages	0.002	0.005	0.674	0.002	0.006	0.725
Energy/Sport Beverages	0.003	0.009	0.772	0.003	0.010	0.743
Others [3]	−0.010	0.020	0.609	−0.011	0.021	0.611
Total Beverage	0.265	0.147	0.072	0.313	0.146	0.032

[1] Adjusted by age and gender; [2] Adjusted by age, gender, total energy intake and BMI; [3] Others include carrot juice, beer without alcohol, chocolate milkshake, vanilla milkshake, strawberry milkshake, diet milkshake, soy milk, rice milk, oat milk, fermented milk drink with sugar, fermented milk drink, kefir, horchata, and sugar added iced tea.

4. Discussion

Fluid intake either from water, beverages or foods is necessary for physical and mental function [5,14]. However, fluid needs for individuals are variable depending on age, body size, PA level, perspiration, food habits, and environmental conditions [14–16]. Hydration plays an important role in the ability to perform PA, but not in short bout exercise (power or anaerobic activities) [37]. Physical performance is impaired by dehydration, even during relatively short-duration, intermittent exercise, which may provoke changes in cardiovascular, thermoregulatory, metabolic, and central nervous function that become greater as dehydration worsens [38]. Therefore, hydration status should be controlled among people practicing PA, and beverages are an important source of fluids to maintain appropriate levels of hydration.

In addition to normal meals and fluid intake, appropriate prehydrating with beverages is useful to start the PA euhydrated, mainly taking water as the main hydration source. It should be started at least several hours before the activity. During exercise, consuming beverages will allow to prevent dehydration to avert compromised performance. After exercise, beverage consumption will allow to replace any fluid deficit [39].

Participating in regular PA and eating a balanced diet are recognized to be beneficial for health [40], but physical inactivity of adolescents has been usually reported [1,41,42]. In the present analysis most of the studied adolescents were physically active, which is similar to previous results reported in developed countries [43–47], and higher than in developing countries [48,49], measured by means of self-reported instruments of PA assessment similar to the method used in this study. In agreement with previous findings [1,41–51], boys were more active than girls, younger adolescents were physically more active than their older counterparts, low parental income was associated with increased likelihood of being physically inactive, and time spent watching TV was inversely associated with PA. Displacement of PA by TV viewing decreases energy expenditure [41]. In addition, during TV viewing the consumption of beverages, mainly sugar-sweetened beverages, may increase the total energy intake [19,50]. It has been shown among our inactive girls that showed higher total energy intake from beverages than active girls.

Consumption of beverages varied according to sex and PA. The average beverage intake of the studied adolescents was 0.9 L/day, higher in boys than in girls, but these values were lower than the European Food Safety Authority [20] recommended adequate fluid intake (9–13 years: boys

2.1 L/day and girls 1.9 L/day; ≥14 years: boys 2.5 L/day and girls 2.0 L/day), and lower than mean beverage consumption of European adolescents (1.6 L/day in boys and 1.3 L/day in girls) [16]. However, these recommendations of adequate intakes are applied only to conditions of moderate environmental temperature and moderate PA levels.

Accordingly, water, soft drinks and total beverage consumption were higher in the warm than the cold season, whereas alcohol and beverage total energy intake were higher in the cold season. These results are quite different from previous results in Korean school students that showed no differences between winter and summer on amounts of beverage per day and the daily energy intake from beverage consumption [52]. However, Korean girls, similarly to ours, also showed higher consumption of sweetened beverages in the warm season. Furthermore, no evidence that fluid consumption among children was significantly related to the mean temperature in modern conditions [53]. The 1997 Spanish National Household Health Survey showed that Spanish adolescents did not show seasonality of alcohol drinking habits, and they were only weekly drinkers, mainly on weekends [54]. Then, it could be inferred that most consumed beverages to recover fluid loss (i.e., water) are linked to the environmental heat, whereas consumption of hot (i.e., coffee or tea) and alcoholic beverages, with an additional calorific action, are linked to the environmental cold. However, changes in beverage consumption are mainly related to PA practice, and when these differences appeared in seasons, they may be the result of both PA and season, according to loss or need of fluids and nutrients.

As expected, total beverage intake of the studied adolescents was positively associated with PA. The highest amount of beverage TEI was observed in active boys and girls, in spite that it was lower than beverage TEI of European adolescents [16]. Active boys preferred to consume high energy beverages such as whole fat milk, or fruit drinks, whereas active girls preferred to consume low energy beverage such as low-fat milk, which may be related to the girls' preference for a slim body shape [55].

Except diet soda and alcoholic beverage drinkers, more than 50% of all other beverage consumers met the PA recommendations. It is usually recommended to increase the daily PA level to lose weight in conjunction with better diet quality may contribute to better body weight control and prevention of various chronic diseases [56], but PA is also important for disease prevention, weight maintenance and overall health, including optimal growth and development for children and adolescents, and then it is usually recommended both to control dietary intake and also to practice PA. In this way, the highest proportion of diet soda drinkers was found among inactive adolescents. Perhaps adolescents drink diet soda with the recognition that they have not been expending enough energy.

Otherwise, exercise increases the requirement of many electrolytes due to their loss via sweat [57], and isotonic beverages are used for recovery of missing water and electrolytes during or after physical activity [57,58]. The highest proportion of energy/sport drink consumers was found among active adolescents, as previously registered [59], and this behavior might be due to compliment higher energy expenditure but also to imitate what done by elite sportsmen. The consumption of these beverages among adolescents may be recommended only after vigorous and prolonged activity [59].

Strengths and Limitations of the Study

This is the first time that the consumption of any kind of beverage and their relationship with PA has been assessed among adolescents. This study also assessed the percentage of the population consuming the different beverages, avoiding the sometimes misleading mean intake data.

This study has also limitations. Dietary questionnaires have inherent limitations, mainly because they are subjective in nature. The difficulties to assess food and beverage intake in humans are well-known. However, in many cases, self-reporting is the only feasible method of assessing dietary intake in epidemiological studies. Using single 24-h dietary recalls is not the best method to represent typical consumption patterns of individuals, because food and beverage consumption individually vary from day to day and 24-h dietary recalls have limitations related to memory and bias [60].

PA was assessed according to self-reported questionnaire, and may be affected by recall bias because adolescents might not able to accurately remember and capture their activities [61].

5. Conclusions

Most of the studied adolescent population met the PA recommendations. Gender, age, parental income, and time watching TV were significant determinants of PA. Consumption of beverages varied according to gender and PA, and daily total beverage intake was lower than recommended adequate fluid intake. PA behavior should be considered when assessing beverage consumption in adolescents.

Acknowledgments: The study was supported by the Spanish Ministry of Health and Consumption Affairs (Programme of Promotion of Biomedical Research and Health Sciences, Projects 11/01791, 14/00636, Red Predimed-RETIC RD06/0045/1004, and CIBEROBN CB12/03/30038), Grant of support to research groups No. 35/2011 (Balearic Islands Gov.) and EU FEDER funds. The Research Group on Community Nutrition and Oxidative Stress of the University of Balearic Islands and the ImFINE Research Group of the Technical University of Madrid belong to the Exernet Network.

Author Contributions: A.E.O. and J.A.T. conceived, designed and devised the study; M.M.B. collected and supervised the samples; A.E.O., M.M.B., M.G.G. and J.A.T. analyzed the data and wrote the manuscript; A.P. and J.A.T. obtained funding.

Conflicts of Interest: The authors declare no conflict of interest.

References

1. Kristjansdottir, G.; Vilhjalmsson, R. Sociodemographic differences in patterns of sedentary and physically active behavior in older children and adolescents. *Acta Paediatr.* **2001**, *90*, 429–435. [CrossRef] [PubMed]
2. WHO. Global Recommendations on Physical Activity for Health. Geneva, WHO 2010. Available online: http://whqlibdoc.who.int/publications/2010/9789241599979_eng.pdf?ua=1 (accessed on 7 July 2013).
3. Maughan, R.J.; Shirreffs, S.M.; Watson, P. Exercise, heat, hydration and the brain. *J. Am. Coll. Nutr.* **2007**, *26*, 604–612. [CrossRef]
4. Miller, V.S.; Bates, G.P. Hydration, Hydration, Hydration. *Ann. Occup. Hyg.* **2010**, *54*, 134–136. [CrossRef] [PubMed]
5. Popkin, B.M.; D'Anci, K.E.; Rosenberg, I.H. Water, hydration, and health. *Nutr. Rev.* **2010**, *68*, 439–458. [CrossRef] [PubMed]
6. Naughton, G.A.; Carlson, J.S. Reducing the risk of heat-related decrements to physical activity in young people. *J. Sci. Med. Sport* **2008**, *11*, 58–65. [CrossRef] [PubMed]
7. Rivera-Brown, A.M.; Gutiérrez, R.; Gutiérrez, J.C.; Frontera, W.R.; Bar-Or, O. Drink composition, voluntary drinking, and fluid balance in exercising, trained, heat-acclimatized boys. *J. Appl. Physiol.* **1999**, *86*, 78–84. [PubMed]
8. Rowland, T. Thermoregulation during exercise in the heat in children: Old concepts revisited. *J. Appl. Physiol.* **2008**, *105*, 718–724. [CrossRef] [PubMed]
9. Gisolfi, C.V.; Duchman, S.M. Guidelines for optimal replacement beverages for different athletic events. *Med. Sci. Sports Exerc.* **1992**, *24*, 679–687. [CrossRef] [PubMed]
10. American Academy of Pediatrics: Committee on Sports Medicine and Fitness. Promotion of Healthy Weight-Control Practices in Young Athletes. *Pediatrics* **2005**, *116*, 1557–1564.
11. Bar-Or, O. *Nutrition for Child and Adolescent Athletes*; Sports Science Center, Gatorade Sports Science Institute: Chicago, IL, USA, 2000.
12. Montain, S.; Coyle, E.F. Influence of the timing of fluid ingestion on temperature regulation during exercise. *J. Appl. Physiol.* **1993**, *75*, 688–695. [PubMed]
13. Below, P.R.; Mora-Rodriquez, R.; González-Alonso, J.; Coyle, E.F. Fluid and carbohydrate ingestion independently improve performance during 1 h of intense exercise. *Med. Sci. Sports Exerc.* **1995**, *27*, 200–210. [CrossRef] [PubMed]
14. Hargreaves, M.; Dillo, P.; Angus, D.; Febbraio, M. Effect of fluid ingestion on muscle metabolism during prolonged exercise. *J. Appl. Physiol.* **1996**, *80*, 363–366. [PubMed]

15. Lieberman, H.R. Hydration and cognition: A critical review and recommendations for future research. *J. Am. Coll. Nutr.* **2007**, *26*, 555S–561S. [CrossRef] [PubMed]

16. Manz, R. Hydration in children. *J. Am. Coll. Nutr.* **2007**, *26*, 526S–569S. [CrossRef]

17. Duffey, K.J.; Huybrechts, I.; Mouratidou, T.; Libuda, L.; Kersting, M.; DeVriendt, T.; Gottrand, F.; Widhalm, K.; Dallongeville, J.; Hallström, L.; et al. Beverage consumption among European adolescents in the HELENA Study. *Eur. J. Clin. Nutr.* **2012**, *66*, 244–252. [CrossRef] [PubMed]

18. Malik, V.B.; Schulze, M.B.; Hu, F.B. Intake of sugar-sweetened beverages and weight gain: A systematic review. *Am. J. Clin. Nutr.* **2006**, *84*, 274–288. [PubMed]

19. De Craemer, M.; De Decker, E.; De Bourdeaudhuij, I.; Deforche, B.; Vereecken, C.; Duvinage, K.; Grammatikaki, E.; Iotova, V.; Fernández-Alvira, J.M.; Zych, K.; et al. Physical activity and beverage consumption in preschoolers: Focus groups with parents and teachers. *BMC Public Health* **2013**, *13*. [CrossRef] [PubMed]

20. EFSA. Scientific Opinion on Dietary Reference Values for Water. Available online: http://www.efsa.europa.eu/en/scdocs/scdoc/1459.htm (accessed on 25 July 2013).

21. Alvarez-Dardet, C.; Alonso, J.; Domingo, A.; Regidor, E. Grupo de trabajo de la Sociedad española de Epidemiología. In *La Medición de la Clase Social en Ciencias de la Salud*; SG Editores: Barcelona, Spain, 1995.

22. WHO. Physical Status: The use and interpretation of anthropometry. In *Technical Report Series*; World Health Organization: Geneva, Switzerland, 1995.

23. International Association for the Study of Obesity (IASO). 2013. Available online: http://www.iaso.org/resources/aboutobesity/child-obesity/newchildcutoffs/ (accessed on 7 July 2013).

24. Cole, T.J.; Bellizzi, M.C.; Flegal, K.M.; Dietz, W.H. Establishing a standard definition for child overweight and obesity worldwide: International survey. *Br. Med. J.* **2000**, *320*, 1240–1243. [CrossRef]

25. IPAQ International Physical Activity Questionnaire. Guidelines for Data Processing and Analysis of the International Physical Activity Questionnaire (IPAQ). Available online: http://www.ipaq.ki.es/ (accessed on 20 July 2013).

26. Hagströmer, M.; Bergman, P.; De Bourdeaudhuij, I.; Ortega, F.B.; Ruiz, J.R.; Manios, Y.; Rey-López, J.P.; Phillipp, K.; von Berlepsch, J.; Sjöström, M. Concurrent validity of a modified version of the International Physical Activity Questionnaire (IPAQ-A) in European adolescents: The HELENA Study. *Int. J. Obes.* **2008**, *32*, S42–S48. [CrossRef] [PubMed]

27. Prochaska, J.J.; Sallis, J.F.; Long, B. A physical activity screening measure for use with adolescents in primary care. *Arch. Pediatr. Adolesc. Med.* **2001**, *155*, 554–559. [CrossRef] [PubMed]

28. WHO. Global Strategy on Diet, Physical Activity and Health Website, Physical Activity and Young People. 2013. Available online: http://www.who.int/dietphysicalactivity/factsheet_young_people/en/index.html (accessed on 31 July 2013).

29. Andersen, L.B.; Harro, M.; Sardinha, L.B.; Froberg, K.; Ekelund, U.; Brage, S.; Anderssen, S.A. Physical activity and clustered cardiovascular risk in children: A cross-sectional study (The European Youth Heart Study). *Lancet* **2006**, *368*, 299–304. [CrossRef]

30. Gómez, C.; Kohen, V.L.; Nogueira, T.L. *Guía Visual de Alimentos y Raciones*; Editores Médicos S.A. (EDIMSA): Madrid, Spain, 2007.

31. Mataix, J.; Mañas, M.; Llopis, J.; Martínez de Victoria, E.; Juan, J.; Borregón, A. *Tablas de Composición de Alimentos Españoles*; INTA-Universidad de Granada: Granada, Spain, 2004.

32. Ortega, R.M.; López, A.M.; Requejo, A.M.; Andrés, P. *La Composición de los Alimentos. Herramienta Básica Para la Valoración Nutricional*; Complutense: Madrid, Spain, 2004.

33. Feinberg, M.; Favier, J.C.; Ireland-Ripert, J. *Repertoire General des Aliments*; Tec & Doc Lavoisier: Paris, France, 1995.

34. Ripoll, L. *Cocina de las Islas Baleares*, 5th ed.; L. Ripoll Pub. Co.: Palma de Mallorca, Spain, 1992.

35. Livingstone, M.B.E.; Black, A.E. Biomarkers of nutritional exposure and nutritional status. *J. Nutr.* **2005**, *133*, 895S–920S.

36. Johansson, L.; Solvoll, K.; Bjørneboe, G.A.; Drevon, C.A. Under- and overreporting of energy intake related to weight status and lifestyle in a nationwide sample. *Am. J. Clin. Nutr.* **1998**, *68*, 266–274. [PubMed]

37. Kenefick, R.W.; Cheuvront, S.N. Hydration for recreational sport and physical activity. *Nutr. Rev.* **2012**, *70*, S137–S142. [CrossRef] [PubMed]

38. Murray, B. Hydration and physical performance. *J. Am. Coll. Nutr.* **2007**, *26*, 542S–548S. [CrossRef] [PubMed]

39. Sawka, M.N.; Burke, L.M.; Eichner, E.R.; Maughan, R.J.; Montain, S.J.; Stachenfeld, N.S. American College of Sports Medicine position stand. Exercise and fluid replacement. *Med. Sci. Sports Exerc.* **2007**, *39*, 377–390. [PubMed]
40. Platat, C.; Perrin, A.E.; Oujaa, M.; Wagner, A.; Haan, M.C.; Schlienger, J.L.; Simon, C. Diet and physical activity profiles in French preadolescents. *Br. J. Nutr.* **2006**, *96*, 501–507. [PubMed]
41. Gordon-Larsen, P.; McMurray, R.G.; Popkin, B.M. Determinants of adolescent physical activity and inactivity patterns. *Pediatrics* **2000**, *105*. [CrossRef]
42. Ceschini, F.L.; Andrade, D.R.; Oliveira, L.C.; Araujo Junior, J.F.; Matsudo, V.K. Prevalence of physical inactivity and associated factors among high school students from state's public schools. *J. Pediatr.* **2009**, *85*, 301–306. [CrossRef]
43. Gordon-Larsen, P.; Nelson, M.C.; Popkin, B.M. Longitudinal physical activity and sedentary behavior trends: Adolescence to adulthood. *Am. J. Prev. Med.* **2004**, *27*, 277–283. [CrossRef] [PubMed]
44. Koezuka, N.; Koo, M.; Allison, K.R.; Adlaf, E.M.; Dwyer, J.J.; Faulkner, G.; Goodman, J. The relationship between sedentary activities and physical inactivity among adolescents: Results from the Canadian Community Health Survey. *J. Adolesc. Health* **2006**, *39*, 515–522. [CrossRef] [PubMed]
45. Janssen, I. Physical activity guidelines for children and youth. *Can. J. Public Health* **2007**, *98*, S109–S121. [PubMed]
46. De Cocker, K.; Ottevaere, C.; Sjöström, M.; Moreno, L.A.; Wärnberg, J.; Valtueña, J.; Manios, Y.; Dietrich, S.; Mauro, B.; Artero, E.G.; et al. Self-reported physical activity in European adolescents: Results from the HELENA (Healthy Lifestyle in Europe by Nutrition in Adolescence) study. *Public Health Nutr.* **2011**, *14*, 246–254. [CrossRef] [PubMed]
47. Bergier, J.; Kapka-Skrzypczak, L.; Bilinski, P.; Paprzycki, P.; Wojtyla, A. Physical activity of Polish adolescents and young adults according to IPAQ: A population based study. *Ann. Agric. Environ. Med.* **2012**, *19*, 109–115. [PubMed]
48. Sisson, S.B.; Katzmarzyk, P.T. International prevalence of physical activity in youth and adults. *Obes. Rev.* **2008**, *9*, 606–614. [CrossRef] [PubMed]
49. Guthold, R.; Cowan, M.J.; Autenrieth, C.S.; Kann, L.; Riley, L.M. Physical activity and sedentary behavior among schoolchildren: A 34-country comparison. *J. Pediatr.* **2010**, *157*, 43–49. [CrossRef] [PubMed]
50. Seabra, A.F.; Mendonça, D.M.; Thomis, M.A.; Malina, R.M.; Maia, J.A. Correlates of physical activity in Portuguese adolescents from 10 to 18 years. *Scand. J. Med. Sci. Sports* **2011**, *21*, 318–323. [CrossRef] [PubMed]
51. Tudor-Locke, C.; Craig, C.L.; Cameron, C.; Griffiths, J.M. Canadian children's and youth's pedometer-determined steps/day, parent-reported TV watching time, and overweight/obesity: The Canplay Surveillance Study. *Int. J. Behav. Nutr. Phys. Act.* **2011**, *8*. [CrossRef] [PubMed]
52. Kim, S.Y.; Lee, Y.L. Seasonal and gender differences of beverage consumption in elementary school students. *Nutr. Res. Pract.* **2009**, *3*, 234–241. [CrossRef] [PubMed]
53. Rio, M.C.; Prada, C.; Alvarez, F.J. Drinking habits throughout the seasons of the year in the Spanish population. *J. Stud. Alcohol Drugs* **2002**, *63*, 577–580.
54. Sohn, W.; Heller, K.E.; Burt, B.A. Fluid consumption related to climate among children in the United States. *J. Public Health Dent.* **2001**, *61*, 99–106. [CrossRef] [PubMed]
55. Neumark-Sztainer, D.; Paxton, S.J.; Hannan, P.J.; Haines, J.; Story, M. Does body satisfaction matter? Five-year longitudinal associations between body satisfaction and health behaviors in adolescent females and males. *J. Adoles. Health* **2006**, *39*, 244–251.
56. Blair, S.N.; LaMonte, M.J.; Nichaman, M.Z. The evolution of physical activity recommendations: How much is enough? *Am. J. Clin. Nutr.* **2004**, *79*, 913–920.
57. Shirreffs, S.M.; Armstrong, L.E.; Cheuvront, S.N. Fluid and electrolyte needs for preparation and recovery from training and competition. *J. Sports Sci.* **2004**, *22*, 57–63. [CrossRef] [PubMed]
58. Aoi, W.; Naito, Y.; Yoshikawa, T. Exercise and functional foods. *Nutr. J.* **2006**, *5*, 15. [CrossRef] [PubMed]
59. Larsson, N.; Dewolfe, J.; Story, M.; Neumark-Sztainer, D. Adolescent consumption of sports and energy drinks: Linkages to higher physical activity, unhealthy beverage patterns, cigarette smoking, and screen media use. *J. Nutr. Educ. Behav.* **2014**, *46*, 181–187. [CrossRef] [PubMed]

60. Thompson, F.E.; Subar, A.F. Dietary Assessment Methodology. In *Nutrition in the Prevention and Treatment of Disease*, 2nd ed.; Coulston, A.M., Boushey, C.J., Eds.; Academic Press: San Diego, CA, USA, 2008; pp. 5–7.
61. Taber, D.R.; Stevens, J.; Murray, D.M.; Elder, J.P.; Webber, L.S.; Jobe, J.B.; Lytle, L.A. The effect of a physical activity intervention on bias in self-reported activity. *Ann. Epidemiol.* **2009**, *19*, 316–322. [CrossRef] [PubMed]

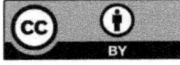

nutrients

MDPI

Article

Beverage Intake Assessment Questionnaire: Relative Validity and Repeatability in a Spanish Population with Metabolic Syndrome from the PREDIMED-PLUS Study

Cíntia Ferreira-Pêgo [1,2], Mariela Nissensohn [2,3], Stavros A. Kavouras [4], Nancy Babio [1,2], Lluís Serra-Majem [2,3], Adys Martín Águila [5], Andy Mauromoustakos [6], Jacqueline Álvarez Pérez [2,3] and Jordi Salas-Salvadó [1,2,*]

[1] Human Nutrition Unit, Biochemistry Biotechnology Department, Faculty of Medicine and Health Sciences, Universitat Rovira i Virgili, IISPV (Institut d'Investigació Sanitària Pere Virgili); Hospital Universitari de Sant Joan de Reus, C/Sant Llorenç, 21, Reus 43201, Spain; cintia.ferreira@iispv.cat (C.F.-P.); nancy.babio@urv.cat (N.B.)

[2] CIBEROBN (Centro de Investigación Biomédica en Red Fisiopatología de la Obesidad y Nutrición), Instituto de Salud Carlos III, Av. Monforte de Lemos, 3-5. Pabellón 11. Planta 0, Madrid 28029, Spain; mnissensohn@acciones.ulpgc.es (M.N.); lluis.serra@ulpgc.es (L.S.-M.); jalvarez@proyinves.ulpgc.es (J.Á.P.)

[3] Research Institute of Biomedical and Health Sciences, University of Las Palmas de Gran Canaria, Paseo Blas Cabrera Felipe "Físico" (s/n), Las Palmas de Gran Canaria 35016, Spain

[4] Hydration Science Lab, 155 Stadium dr-HPER 308Q, University of Arkansas, Fayetteville, AR 72701, USA; kavouras@uark.edu

[5] Clinical Analysis Unit, University Hospital of Gran Canaria Dr. Negrin, Barranco de la Ballena, s/n, Las Palmas de Gran Canaria 35010, Spain; maradys47@gmail.com

[6] Agricultural Statistics Lab, 101 Agricultural Annex Building, University of Arkansas, Fayetteville, AR 72701, USA; amauro@uark.edu

* Correspondence: jordi.salas@urv.cat; Tel.: +34-977-759312; Fax: +34-977-759322

Received: 9 June 2016; Accepted: 27 July 2016; Published: 30 July 2016

Abstract: We assess the repeatability and relative validity of a Spanish beverage intake questionnaire for assessing water intake from beverages. The present analysis was performed within the framework of the PREDIMED-PLUS trial. The study participants were adults (aged 55–75) with a BMI $\geqslant 27$ and <40 kg/m^2, and at least three components of Metabolic Syndrome (MetS). A trained dietitian completed the questionnaire. Participants provided 24-h urine samples, and the volume and urine osmolality were recorded. The repeatability of the baseline measurement at 6 and 1 year was examined by paired Student's *t*-test comparisons. A total of 160 participants were included in the analysis. The Bland–Altman analysis showed relatively good agreement between total daily fluid intake assessed using the fluid-specific questionnaire, and urine osmolality and 24-h volume with parameter estimates of -0.65 and 0.22, respectively ($R^2 = 0.20$; $p < 0.001$). In the repeatability test, no significant differences were found between neither type of beverage nor total daily fluid intake at 6 months and 1-year assessment, compared to baseline. The proposed fluid-specific assessment questionnaire designed to assess the consumption of water and other beverages in Spanish adult individuals was found to be relatively valid with good repeatability.

Keywords: relative validity; repeatability; fluid questionnaire; beverage; PREDIMED-PLUS study; Spain

1. Introduction

Nowadays, estimating the total fluid intake and real beverage pattern of a population may be considered as a real challenge in nutritional epidemiology. The associations between hydration, water, or beverage intake with health or disease has recently become an important area of research [1,2]. Several authors have assessed the relationship between the consumption of beverages and specific outcomes: for example, the intake of sugar-sweetened beverages (SSBs) and metabolic syndrome (MetS) or type 2 diabetes (T2DM) [3], hypertension [4–6] and other cardiometabolic variables [7]; or the intake of drinking water and its relationship to cardiovascular diseases (CVD) [8]. However, the results in some cases are controversial [9–11] and it is probably partially attributable to the difficulties in assessing the real fluid pattern [12]. Water is an essential nutrient for life [13] and the research on its contribution to human health is very important, so it is essential that the technique used to assess the consumption of different types of beverage is sufficiently sensitive.

To evaluate total fluid intake (all drinking water and beverages), it is common to use food frequency questionnaires (FFQ) or 24-h recall [14,15]. However, these questionnaires were mainly designed to evaluate food intake, and not fluid consumption as a whole. In addition, most food records or dietary recalls do not evaluate the consumption of drinking water because they do not provide calories. The assessment of beverage intake in recent years has mostly focused on SSBs and alcoholic drinks [16,17]. For this reason, and also because fluids are often consumed between meals and are not perceived as a food, fluid intake tends to be underestimated by the individual and the interviewer [3,18–20].

In 2010, Hedrick and coworkers published a questionnaire designed to assess the consumption of different types of beverage in the American population [21]. However, to the best of our knowledge, there is no standardized and validated questionnaire in Spanish that has been developed as a research tool for the specific assessment of beverage intake.

For this reason, the main aim of the present study was to assess the repeatability and the relative validity of a new fluid-specific questionnaire designed to measure the habitual consumption of drinking water and different types of beverages in a Spanish population.

2. Material and Methods

2.1. Subjects and Design

The present analysis was performed within the framework of the PREDIMED-PLUS trial, the design of which has been described elsewhere [22]. Briefly, the PREDIMED-PLUS is a large, multicenter, parallel group, randomized and controlled clinical trial designed for evaluating the safety and effectiveness of a multifaceted intervention program for alleviating excessive cardiovascular morbidity and mortality in overweight and obese individuals.

The primary endpoint of the PREDIMED-PLUS trial is to determine the effect on CVD morbidity and mortality of an intensive weight loss intervention program based on an energy-restricted traditional Mediterranean diet (MedDiet), increased physical activity and behavioral therapy in comparison with an intervention based on traditional Mediterranean diet advice (energy-unrestricted MedDiet) and traditional health care for CVD prevention.

All participants provided written informed consent, and the PREDIMED-PLUS protocol and procedures were approved by the Institutional Review Board Comité de Ética de Investigación Clínica del Hospital Universitario de Gran Canaria Dr. Negrín (code 130093, 30 January 2014) and Comité Ètic d'Investigació Clínica del Hospital S. Joan de Reus (code 13-07-25/7proj2, 25 July 2013). The trial is registered at clinicaltrials.gov; identifier: ISRCTN89898870.

The study participants were adult men aged 55–75 and women aged 60–75 with a body mass index (BMI) $\geqslant$27 and <40 kg/m^2 and who met at least three of the following criteria for the MetS: abdominal obesity for European individuals (waist circumferences $\geqslant$88 cm in women and $\geqslant$102 cm in men), hypertriglyceridemia ($\geqslant$150 g/dL) or drug treatment for high plasma triglyceride (TG) concentration, low high-density lipoprotein (HDL)-cholesterol (<50 mg/dL in women and <40 mg/dL in men), high blood pressure (systolic blood pressure $\geqslant$130 mmHg or diastolic blood pressure $\geqslant$85 mmHg) or antihypertensive drug treatment, or high fasting glucose ($\geqslant$100 mg/dL) or drug treatment for T2DM.

MetS was defined in accordance with the updated harmonized criteria of the International Diabetes Federation and the American Heart Association and National Heart, Lung and Blood Institute [23].

The analysis included a total random sample of 160 individuals randomized to the PREDIMED-PLUS trial from the Reus and Las Palmas de Gran Canaria centers.

2.2. Assessment of Fluid Intake

A trained dietician, on behalf of participants at an interview, filled in the fluid-specific questionnaire, recording the daily and weekly consumption of different types of beverage over the previous month (Figure 1 in English and Supplementary materials Figure S1 in Spanish). The average daily fluid intake from beverages was estimated on the basis of servings of each type of beverage. The questionnaire items on beverages included: tap water, bottled water, natural fruit juices, bottled fruit juices, natural vegetable juices, bottled vegetable juices, whole milk, semi-skimmed milk, skimmed milk, drinking yogurt (100 and 200 cc), milkshakes, vegetable drinks, soups, jellies and sorbets, sugar-sweetened beverages (SSBs) (200 and 330 cc), artificially-sweetened beverages (ASBs) (200 and 330 cc), espresso (sweetened and unsweetened), white coffee (sweetened and unsweetened), tea (sweetened and unsweetened), other infusions (sweetened and unsweetened), beer (200 and 330 cc), non-alcoholic beer (200 and 330 cc), wine, sprits, mixed alcoholic drinks, energy drinks, sports drinks (200 and 330 cc), meal replacement shakes and other beverages. Total fluid intake was considered to be the sum of all types of beverage.

The amount of water in each beverage was estimated using the percentage of water values from the United States Department of Agriculture (USDA) online database [24]. All of the analyses were performed taking into account the mL of water content in each beverage.

2.3. Urine Collection

Participants provided a 24-h urine sample, and trained personnel recorded the volume, the day it was provided and the mean environmental temperature of the collection day. Participants were advised that, in the morning, the first urine of the collection day should be discarded, and the first urine sample of the following day included, thus concluding the 24-h cycle. After receiving the urine sample, the trained personnel aliquoted the samples and kept them at $-80\,^\circ$C. Urine osmolality (Uosm) was measured (mOsm/kg) before 31 weeks of freezing using the refractive index method and the osmometer ARKRAY OM6050 (Arkay Global Business, Kyoto, Japan) Osmo Station. Urine osmolality is a measure of the number of dissolved particles per unit of water in urine. Some of these particles can include chloride, glucose, potassium, sodium or urea. In the context of nutrition, the osmolality of a 24-h urine sample reflects the self-regulating activity of renal concentration or dilution mechanisms during a 24-h period. It measures the functional surplus of water and characterizes 24-h hydration status [25].

2.4. Assessment of Other Covariates

At baseline and in each visit during the follow-up, questionnaires were administered about lifestyle variables, educational achievement, history of illness, and medication use. Physical activity was assessed using a validated Spanish version of the Minnesota Leisure-Time Physical Activity questionnaire [26]. Trained personnel took the anthropometric measurements. Weight and height were measured with light clothing, and no shoes with calibrated scales and a wall-mounted stadiometer (Certified scale BARYS with stadiometer T2), respectively. Trained dietitians completed a 137-item semi-quantitative and validated [27] FFQ in a face-to-face interview with the participant. Energy and protein intake were estimated using a Spanish food composition table [28,29]. In addition, dietitians administered a 17-item MedDiet screener, adapted from the 14-item questionnaire validated for the PREDIMED study [30], to assess the degree of adherence to the traditional MedDiet.

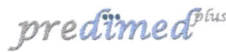

SPANISH BEVERAGE INTAKE ASSESSMENT QUESTIONNAIRE

predïmed*plus*

Centre | Participant | Visit | Date

Instructions:
Please indicate your answer for your consumption last month.
For each type of beverage consumed, indicate the number of times per day or per week, and with an "X" the moment of the day that you consumed it.
For example, if you drank 2 glasses of wine per week with lunch, mark "lunch" in the "moment of the day" column and put a 2 in "per week" column. If a drink is consumed every day, for example water, indicate how many times "per day" you consumed it. For example: 6 times a day.
Do not take into account the liquids used in the kitchen or in other culinary preparations, such as sauce or homemade dessert.
If you drink coffee with milk, mark it in the category "coffee with milk" and not in the dairy categories.

TYPE OF BEVERAGE		FREQUENCY OF CONSUMPTION										
		TIMES		MOMENT OF THE DAY								
		RARELY OR NEVER	PER WEEK	PER DAY	BEFORE BREAKFAST	BREAKFAST	BETWEEN BREAKFAST AND LUNCH	LUNCH	BTEWEEN LUNCH AND DINNER	DINNER	AFTER DINNER	DURING NIGHT
Tap water	200 cc											
Bottled water (sparkling/ still)	200 cc											
Natural fruit juices	200 cc											
Bottled fruit juices	200 cc											
Natural vegetable juices (gazpacho, tomato, etc.)	200 cc											
Bottled vegetable juices (gazpacho, tomato, etc.)	200 cc											
Whole milk	200 cc											
Semi-skimmed milk	200 cc											
Skimmed milk	200 cc											
Drinking yogurt	100 cc											
	200 cc											
Milkshakes	200 cc											
Vegetable drinks (soy, oat, almond, etc.)	200 cc											
Soups	200 cc											
Jellies and sorbets	120 cc											
Sugar sweetened beverages	200 cc											
	330 cc											
Artificially sweetened beverages	330 cc											
	200 cc											
Espresso (sweetened)	30-50 cc											
Espresso (unsweetened or sugar-free)	30-50 cc											
White coffee (sweetened)	125 cc											
White coffee (unsweetened or sugar-free)	125 cc											
Tea (sweetened)	200 cc											
Tea (unsweetened or sugar-free)	200 cc											
Other infusions (sweetened)	200 cc											
Other infusions (unsweetened or sugar-free)	200 cc											
Beer	200 cc											
	330 cc											
Non-alcoholic beer	330 cc											
	200 cc											
Wine, champagne	120 cc											
High alcoholic content beverages (whisky, rum, vodka, gin)	50 cc											
Mixed alcoholic drinks (cocktails, gin tonic, piña colada, etc.)	200 cc											
Energy drinks (Red Bull, Burn, etc.)	200 cc											
Sport/ Isotonic drinks	200 cc											
	330 cc											
Meal replacement shakes	200 cc											
Other drinks:												

Figure 1. The beverage intake assessment questionnaire in English (translated version and not validated tool).

2.5. Statistical Analysis

Beverages and total fluid intake (mL/day) and demographic characteristics are presented as a means (SD) for continuous variables or percentages (numbers) for dichotomous variables. Student's *t*-test or Pearson's χ^2 tests were used to compare the quantitative or categorical general characteristics of the participants.

To assess relative validity, the total daily fluid intake assessed by the fluid-specific questionnaire was compared to the urine osmolality and the 24-h urine volume values. Associations among these variables were assessed using the correlational analysis Bland–Altman agreement method. A total of 160 participants were included in the validity analysis. A stepwise method was used to select only the significant predictors for urine osmolality. The list of covariates that were not kept in the final model (i.e., did not contribute significantly) to the model urine osmolality were: sex, height, weight, center of recruitment, intervention group, total protein intake, MedDiet adherence, leisure-time physical activity, mean environmental temperature, urine albumin and urine creatinine. The covariates that were kept in the model included age, BMI and total energy consumption. The model for the 24-h urine volume analysis included age and total energy intake. No predictor interactions were found with any of the aforementioned variables. Quintiles of total water intake, osmolality and 24-h urine volume were calculated. The osmolality and 24-h urine volume values were adjusted by the same covariates as were used in the validity analysis. The degree of gross misclassification in the fluid-specific questionnaire with respect to the adjusted osmolality and adjusted 24-h urine volume values was evaluated using contingency tables. The proportions of correctly categorized subjects in the same or adjacent quintiles, and also the individuals classified in extreme quintiles were calculated.

The repeatability of the fluid-specific questionnaire was examined by comparing baseline, and six-month and 12-month values (in 45 and 34 individuals, respectively) with paired Student's *t*-tests. For a comparison between repeatedly measured variables of consumption of each type of beverage and total fluid intake during time (baseline, six month and one year), a linear mixed-effect model for repeated measures was used. In order to avoid the effect of the intervention on beverage and total-water intake, only individuals from the control group were included in the repeatability analysis.

The level of significance for all the statistical tests was set at $p < 0.05$ for bilateral contrast. Analyses were performed using JMP version 12.1.0 (SAS Institute Inc., Cary, NC, USA) and with SPSS software, version 22.0 (SPSS Inc., Chicago, IL, USA).

3. Results

A total of 160 participants (68 men and 92 women) with a mean age of 65.3 years (range 55 to 75 years) were included in the present analysis. Height and weight, but not BMI, were significantly different between men and women. Such lifestyle variables as leisure-time physical activity, MedDiet adherence and total energy consumed were different between genders. Levels of urine osmolality, urine creatinine and urine albumin were higher in men. Women took significantly more pain relief pills and tranquilizers than men. The general characteristics of the study participants are summarized in Table 1.

Table 1. General characteristics of the study population.

Variables	All Population (*n* = 160)	Men (*n* = 68)	Women (*n* = 92)	*p*-Value [a]
Age, years	65.3 (4.9)	64.5 (5.9)	65.9 (3.9)	0.097
Height, m	1.62 (0.09)	1.69 (0.06)	1.56 (0.06)	<0.001
Weight, kg	86.7 (14.3)	94.3 (12.5)	81.9 (12.9)	<0.001
BMI, kg/m^2	33.0 (4.3)	32.9 (3.6)	33.1 (4.7)	0.328
Leisure-time physical activity, METs/week	3123 (2804)	4006 (2945)	2471 (2518)	<0.001
Mediterranean diet score, (0–17 points)	9.2 (2.5)	8.5 (2.6)	9.8 (2.3)	<0.005
Total energy intake, kcal/day	2229 (551)	2330 (606)	2155 (497)	<0.005
Total protein intake, g/day	134 (357)	189 (545)	93 (22)	0.276
Urine volume, mL/day	1722 (651)	1762 (698)	1693 (616)	0.506
Urine osmolality, mOsm/kg	551 (211)	631 (204)	492 (196)	<0.001
Urine albumin, mg/dL	13.8 (31.8)	20.0 (39.5)	9.0 (23.4)	0.047
Urine creatinine, μmol/dL	7718 (3760)	9440 (4204)	6431 (2783)	<0.001
Urine albumin to creatinine ratio, mg/g	17.1 (43.4)	22.2 (53.2)	13.2 (33.9)	0.228
Use of medications, % (*n*)				
Aspirin	24.4 (39)	26.5 (18)	22.8 (21)	0.596
Pain relief	33.7 (54)	17.6 (12)	45.6 (42)	<0.005
Tranquilizers	27.5 (44)	17.6 (12)	34.8 (32)	0.016
Vitamin/minerals	6.9 (11)	2.9 (2)	9.8 (9)	0.091
Heart problems	4.4 (7)	5.9 (4)	3.3 (3)	0.423
Antihypertensive agents	79.4 (127)	82.3 (56)	77.2 (71)	0.423
Statins	56.9 (91)	50.0 (34)	62.0 (57)	0.131
Insulin	6.2 (10)	5.9 (4)	6.5 (6)	0.869
Oral anti-diabetic drugs	30.0 (48)	30.9 (21)	29.3 (27)	0.834
Others	68.1 (109)	63.2 (43)	71.7 (66)	0.254

Data expressed as means (SD) or percentages (*n*). Abbreviations: BMI, body mass index. [a] *p*-Values for comparisons between groups were tested by Student's *t*-test or χ^2 as appropriate.

3.1. Relative Validity of the Questionnaire

Total daily fluid intake from beverages assessed by the specific questionnaire was negatively associated with age and urine osmolality, and positively associated with BMI and total energy intake (R^2: 0.20; $p < 0.001$). The Bland–Altman analysis showed relatively good agreement between total daily fluid intake assessed using the fluid-specific questionnaire, and urine osmolality and 24-h volume with parameter estimates of −0.65 and 0.22, respectively. The validity results for the total daily fluid intake assessed with the specific questionnaire are presented in Table 2. The Bland–Altman plot showing the relationship between total daily fluid intake and 24-h urine volume is shown in a supplementary file (Figure S2).

Table 2. Parameter estimates for two candidate models (osmolality and urine volume) with similar predictive ability of total daily beverage intake.

Term	Parameter Estimate	Standardized β *	Standard Error	*p*-Value	R^2
Intercept	2278				
Osmolality	−0.65	−0.26	0.18	0.0005	0.20
Age	−25.13	−0.23	7.94	0.0019	
BMI	23.86	0.15	11.38	0.0376	
Total energy	0.27	0.25	0.08	0.0007	
Intercept	2455				
Urine volume	0.22	0.27	0.06	0.0003	0.20
Age	−26.03	−0.24	7.93	0.0013	
Total energy	0.24	0.23	0.07	0.0019	

* Standardized beta weights are indicative of effect size.

The percentage of gross misclassification (both over-and underestimation by the fluid-specific questionnaire) as indices of validity of the fluid-specific questionnaire in categorizing individuals was performed (Supplementary Materials Table S1). Osmolality analysis classified 66% of the individuals into the same or the adjacent quintile (±1 quintile) with both methods. A total of 4.4% of the individuals were classified into quintiles at opposite ends of the scale (highest quintile of total water from beverage intake and lowest quintile of osmolality). A total of 6.9% of the population was classified into the lowest quintile of total water intake and the highest quintile of osmolality, suggesting that the total water intake from fluids may have been underestimated. In the 24-h urine volume analysis, 65.7% of the individuals were categorized in the same or the adjacent quintile (± 1 quintile) by both methods. A total of 4.4% and 1.3% of the population studied were misclassified in extreme quintiles (the highest quintile of total water intake and the lowest 24-h urine volume quintile, and the lowest of the total water intake and the highest 24-h urine volume quintiles, respectively).

3.2. Repeatability of the Questionnaire

Table 3 shows the repeatability of the fluid-specific questionnaire measurements for each type of beverage analyzed (baseline vs. six months and baseline vs. one year). The consumption in mL/day of each type of beverage and total daily fluid intake at baseline, six months and one year is described. The differences in the consumption (mL/day) between baseline and six months and baseline and one year, and differences in the consumption during all the visits are also shown in the table. No significant differences were found in the fluid consumption from beverages between the baseline and six months or one-year assessments.

Table 3. Repeatability of the beverage intake assessment questionnaire.

Beverage Category	Baseline (mL/day) (n = 67)	Baseline vs. 6 Months				Baseline vs. 1 Year			
		6 Months (mL/day) (n = 45)	Mean (SD) Differences from Baseline	p-Value [a]	1 Year (mL/day) (n = 34)	Mean (SD) Differences from Baseline	p-Value [a]	p-Value [b]
Tap water	289 (571)	449 (657)	62 (413)	0.32	360 (577)	−23 (502)	0.79	0.389
Bottled water	755 (539)	773 (714)	80 (505)	0.29	813 (612)	125 (577)	0.22	0.905
Natural fruit juices	39 (69)	27 (54)	1 (79)	0.92	28 (61)	16 (75)	0.21	0.537
Bottled fruit juices	26 (93)	22 (52)	7 (46)	0.33	19 (44)	7 (29)	0.16	0.880
Natural vegetable juices	6 (28)	16 (36)	9 (29)	0.05	1 (9)	−1 (16)	0.79	0.073
Bottled vegetable juices	14 (69)	4 (14)	−5 (32)	0.25	4 (18)	−7 (41)	0.35	0.451
Whole milk	24 (92)	3 (17)	−16 (89)	0.22	25 (74)	4 (125)	0.86	0.284
Semi-skimmed milk	43 (81)	67 (126)	8 (125)	0.67	63 (123)	9 (131)	0.69	0.467
Skimmed milk	95 (146)	59 (107)	−19 (145)	0.38	54 (102)	−36 (151)	0.17	0.192
Drinking yogurt (100 cc)	13 (32)	10 (32)	−6 (32)	0.23	8 (23)	−6 (25)	0.18	0.765
Drinking yogurt (200 cc)	6 (31)	13 (46)	5 (61)	0.58	10 (42)	4 (54)	0.56	0.562
Milkshakes	0 (2)	0 (0)	0 (3)	0.32	2 (10)	1 (11)	0.53	0.289
Vegetable drinks	21 (80)	9 (39)	5 (49)	0.47	38 (128)	33 (133)	0.16	0.330
Soups	36 (30)	34 (35)	0 (45)	0.93	50 (56)	17 (52)	0.07	0.144
Jellies and sorbets	2 (11)	1 (5)	−1 (9)	0.61	1 (4)	−1 (7)	0.64	0.594
SSBs (200 cc)	11 (34)	11 (38)	3 (31)	0.53	7 (32)	−3 (18)	0.32	0.862
SSBs (330 cc)	8 (39)	18 (90)	6 (92)	0.68	10 (51)	5 (54)	0.59	0.707
ASBs (200 cc)	7 (48)	21 (118)	11 (134)	0.57	39 (158)	37 (157)	0.18	0.363
ASBs (330 cc)	42 (164)	8 (32)	−54 (200)	0.08	18 (45)	−61 (215)	0.11	0.292
Espresso sweetened	16 (31)	9 (20)	−4 (31)	0.33	9 (18)	−4 (20)	0.25	0.287
Espresso unsweetened	24 (35)	36 (38)	7 (36)	0.22	31 (37)	2 (23)	0.62	0.223
White coffee sweetened	23 (63)	5 (25)	−3 (40)	0.66	4 (21)	−2 (36)	0.69	0.063
White coffee unsweetened	9 (31)	3 (18)	−5 (35)	0.32	7 (28)	3 (36)	0.57	0.492

Table 3. Cont.

Beverage Category	Baseline (mL/day) (n = 67)	Baseline vs. 6 Months			Baseline vs. 1 Year			
		6 Months (mL/day) (n = 45)	Differences from Baseline Mean (SD)	p-Value [a]	1 Year (mL/day) (n = 34)	Differences from Baseline Mean (SD)	p-Value [a]	p-Value [b]
Tea sweetened	7 (29)	2 (13)	−7 (26)	0.09	14 (48)	2 (65)	0.82	0.246
Tea unsweetened	25 (87)	34 (105)	17 (79)	0.15	19 (51)	−2 (54)	0.82	0.718
Other infusions sweetened	27 (96)	13 (66)	12 (67)	0.23	17 (55)	15 (56)	0.13	0.646
Other infusions unsweetened	34 (91)	51 (107)	14 (90)	0.30	54 (139)	12 (106)	0.51	0.613
Beer (200 cc)	18 (67)	10 (32)	−12 (68)	0.24	1 (4)	−18 (71)	0.13	0.266
Beer (330 cc)	32 (91)	47 (119)	2 (131)	0.92	26 (66)	6 (69)	0.63	0.580
Non-alcoholic beer (200 cc)	5 (25)	11 (39)	−8 (45)	0.21	5 (24)	−4 (20)	0.28	0.581
Non-alcoholic beer (330 cc)	13 (54)	3 (14)	4 (22)	0.25	2 (15)	−11 (58)	0.25	0.283
Wine	35 (63)	41 (68)	−7 (60)	0.46	60 (85)	9 (55)	0.35	0.257
High alcoholic content beverages	1 (3)	1 (4)	0 (3)	0.66	1 (2)	0 (3)	0.26	0.988
Mixed alcoholic beverages	1 (6)	0 (3)	0 (0)	-	0 (0)	0 (3)	0.32	0.388
Energy drinks	0 (0)	0 (0)	0 (4)	0.32	0 (0)	0 (0)	-	-
Sports drinks (200 cc)	0 (3)	0 (0)	0 (4)	0.32	0 (0)	0 (0)	-	0.558
Sports drinks (330 cc)	0 (0)	2 (13)	2 (13)	0.32	0 (0)	0 (0)	-	0.328
Meal replacement shakes	0 (0)	0 (0)	0 (0)	-	0 (0)	0 (0)	-	-
Other drinks	0 (0)	0 (0)	0 (0)	-	0 (0)	0 (0)	-	-
Total water intake	1711 (64)	1816 (498)	106 (475)	0.14	1804 (435)	128 (559)	0.19	0.477

Data expressed as means (SD). [a] p-values for comparisons between groups were tested by Student's t-test; [b] p-Values for comparisons between repeated measures were tested by linear mixed models test.

4. Discussion

The main objective of the present analysis was to assess the relative validity and repeatability of a fluid-specific questionnaire designed to measure the habitual consumption of drinking water and different types of beverage. We report for the first time that the use of a fluid-specific questionnaire in Spanish and designed for the Spanish population seems to be highly repeatable, and relatively valid for estimating the daily intake of water from beverages. This tool may be useful for clinicians and researchers interested in assessing habitual water-drinking and beverage-consumption patterns, particularly in large-scale investigations, in which other resource-intensive dietary intake assessment techniques are not so accurate [31].

Although the present fluid-specific questionnaire is the only one to have been validated in Spanish, other questionnaires designed to evaluate beverage intake have been published and validated by a variety of different methods [17,21,31,32]. In 2009, Neuhouser and coworkers developed a questionnaire for assessing the consumption of snacks and beverages, mainly sweetened beverages, by young adolescents [31]. The participants filled in the self-reported beverage questionnaire and also a four-day dietary record. This second method was compared with the beverage questionnaire to assess its validity. The same method was used by Hedrick in 2010 to validate a questionnaire designed to assess the intake of water and caloric beverages [21]. This study used the energy intake from the four-day food record as a method for validating the fluid questionnaire. Although urine samples were collected, they were used to objectively determine total fluid intake and to encourage accurate self-reporting, not for purposes of validation. To date, and to the best of our knowledge, only one questionnaire has been validated using hydration indices with 24-h urine samples [32]. In 2012, Malisova and colleagues developed a "water balance questionnaire", designed to evaluate water drinking and also water intake from solids and other beverages [32]. For validation purposes, urine was collected from 40 healthy adults and osmolality, 24-h volume, specific gravity, pH and color were evaluated. Although all of these indices have been demonstrated to be biomarkers of hydration, nowadays there is still no biomarker universally accepted as the "gold standard" [33,34]. Nevertheless, in the Malisova study, urine osmolality was proposed as the most promising urine biomarker of all the ones used [32,35]. In the present analysis, the 24-h urine samples were frozen for a few weeks, and the freezing-point depression method could not be used for assessing osmolality. Even though the method used in our study was not the same as the one used in the previously mentioned paper, the validation results were very similar in both studies. The results were also similar for the 24-h urine volume as a biomarker of hydration status. Urine volume in both of our studies and Malisova's was found to be significantly related to hydration, but not as strongly as to urine osmolality.

In our study, only 1% to 7% of the subjects were misclassified into extreme quintiles. We found that total water intake was considerably underestimated with the fluid-specific questionnaire in comparison with adjusted-osmolality values. This may be because beverages, mainly drinking water, are consumed during the day and often between meals, so they are not perceived as an important food by the participants and tend to be underestimated [18,19].

The second important outcome of the present study is that the repeatability of the Spanish fluid-specific questionnaire was tested. No differences were found for any of the beverages or in the total daily fluid intake at the different times of evaluation (baseline versus six months or one year), either during all the visits as repeated measures. Therefore, beverage intake and patterns can be compared over time.

The test–retest interval between the three evaluation times of the questionnaire is a factor that has an important influence on repeatability [27]. If the interval is too short, the following evaluations can be influenced by the memory of the first answers, and repeatability will be overestimated. On the other hand, if the interval is too long, the drinking patterns may have changed, which could lead to an underestimation of repeatability [36]. According to a comprehensive review, the time intervals in reports using FFQs range between 2 h and 15 years [37]. In the present analysis, we chose time intervals of six months and one year to prevent the types of bias mentioned above.

This study has several strengths. The ability to accurately assess the validity and repeatability of a questionnaire relies on having a large sample [38] and using multiple statistical methods, which has been achieved in this present study. The second strength is the use of hydration biomarkers instead of dietary intake methods to determine the validity of the analysis. Biomarkers make it possible to improve validation, as they avoid bias caused by measurement errors (memory of the interviewers, errors in estimating food intake), which impact on the statistical power of the study. Another important strength of the present analysis is that the questionnaire was completed by trained dietitians. By avoiding the use of self-reported data we significantly reduced the risk of underreporting errors. However, the study also has several limitations. The present questionnaire may underestimate certain beverage categories because of the serving sizes established (for example, water intake (tap and bottled)). However, estimated mean daily water intake and also total daily fluid intake are very similar to those reported in 2014 in a Spanish population [39], and the present findings did not indicate a ceiling effect. Due to the fact that our population was middle-aged and elderly rather than healthy individuals, future studies should focus on healthy adults and children and other minorities to determine if the fluid-specific questionnaire is a valid tool across other population groups. Another limitation was the lack of a measure to assure the completeness of the 24 h urine samples. However, at the moment the urine was brought in, we asked the participants whether they had followed the instructions and whether they had had any problem with the collection. A final limitation was the use of frozen samples. It has been suggested that freezing urine samples generates urinary sediments that consist predominantly of endogenous calcium oxalate dehydrate and amorphous calcium crystals [40] and that this may account for the changes in osmolality observed after freezing. However, several studies have shown that the changes in frozen urine osmolality are trivial and physiologically irrelevant, especially because daily variations in urine osmolality are considerably larger than these changes [41,42]. The long-term stability and measurement validity for frozen urine were found to be good without the addition of a preservative. The prospective storage of frozen urine aliquots, even exceeding 10 years, appears to be an acceptable and valid tool in epidemiological settings for subsequent urine analysis [43]. Nevertheless, in the present study, we measured osmolality levels in a subsample of urine just after the collection (n = 59), without freezing, and no significant differences were found (data not shown).

5. Conclusions

The present fluid-specific questionnaire appears to be a relatively valid and a highly reliable tool for assessing intake of water and other types of beverages in Spanish adults. The Spanish beverage intake assessment questionnaire may help nutrition researchers and clinicians to evaluate beverages, patterns and changes in consumption and their influence on health or disease.

Supplementary Materials: The following are available online at http://www.mdpi.com/2072-6643/8/8/475/s1, Figure S1: The beverage intake assessment questionnaire in Spanish (validated tool); Figure S2: Bland–Altman plots showing the relationship between total daily water intake (mL/day) and 24-h urine volume (mL/day); Table S1: Contingency tables for the gross misclassification between quintiles of total daily water intake and (A) osmolality adjusted or (B) 24-h urine volume adjusted.

Acknowledgments: The present study was conducted according to the guidelines laid down in the Declaration of Helsinki and the Institutional Review Board of each participating center approved all the procedures of the study protocol. Written informed consent was obtained from all subjects. Sources of Funding: This study was supported, in part, by the official funding agency for biomedical research of the Spanish Ministry of Health Instituto de Salud Carlos III (ISCIII) through grants provided to research networks specifically developed for the trial (PI13/00462); and by RecerCaixa (2013ACUP00194). None of the funding sources played a role in the design, collection, analysis, or interpretation of the data or in the decision to submit the manuscript for publication. Centro de Investigación Biomédica En Red - fisiopatología de la OBesidad y Nutrición (CIBEROBN) is an initiative of ISCIII, Spain.

Author Contributions: L.S.-M. and J.S.-S. designed the PREDIMED-PLUS study and were the coordinators of subject recruitment and follow-up at the outpatient clinics; C.F.-P., M.N., N.B., L.S.-M., J.Á.-P. and J.S.-S. conducted the research; C.F.-P., S.A.K., A.M. and J.S.-S. analysed the data; C.F.-P., N.B. and J.S.-S. wrote the manuscript; A.M.Á. performed the urine laboratory analysis; N.B. and J.S.-S. had full access to all of the data in the study and

Nutrients **2016**, *8*, 475

takes responsibility for the integrity of the data and the accuracy of the data analysis. All authors have read and approved the final manuscript.

Conflicts of Interest: Cíntia Ferreira-Pêgo declares no conflict of interests. Stavros A. Kavouras is member of the scientific advisory board on fluid intake of Danone Research and has received research grants from Danone Research. Nancy Babio has received travel support and grant support through her institution from Danone. Lluís Serra-Majem is member of the Scientific Advisory Board and has received consulting fees and grant support from the European Hydratation Institute; and he has received lecture fees from the International Nut Council and travel support for conferences from Nestle. Jordi Salas-Salvadó reports serving on the board of Instituto Danone España, and receiving grant support through his institution from Danone, Eroski and Nestlé.

Abbreviations

SSBs, sugar-sweetened beverages; ASBs, artificially-sweetened beverages; FFQ, food frequency questionnaire; CVD, cardiovascular diseases; MetS, metabolic syndrome; MedDiet, Mediterranean diet; USDA, United States Department of Agriculture; SD, Standard Deviation; ANOVA, analysis of variance; BMI, body mass index.

References

1. Johnson, E.C.; Muñoz, C.X.; Le Bellego, L.; Klein, A.; Casa, D.J.; Maresh, C.M.; Armstrong, L.E. Markers of the hydration process during fluid volume modification in women with habitual high or low daily fluid intakes. *Eur. J. Appl. Physiol.* **2015**, *115*, 1067–1074. [CrossRef] [PubMed]
2. Lafontan, M. H4H—Hydration for health. *Obes. Facts* **2014**, *7* (Suppl. S2), 1–5. [CrossRef] [PubMed]
3. Malik, V.S.; Popkin, B.M.; Bray, G.A.; Despres, J.-P.; Willett, W.C.; Hu, F.B. Sugar-Sweetened Beverages and Risk of Metabolic Syndrome and Type 2 Diabetes: A meta-analysis. *Diabetes Care* **2010**, *33*, 2477–2483. [CrossRef] [PubMed]
4. Cohen, L.; Curhan, G.; Forman, J. Association of sweetened beverage intake with incident hypertension. *J. Gen. Intern. Med.* **2012**, *27*, 1127–1134. [CrossRef] [PubMed]
5. Sonestedt, E. Artificial and sugar-sweetened beverages are associated with increased incidence of hypertension. *Evid.-Based Med.* **2013**, *18*, e38. [CrossRef] [PubMed]
6. Sayon-Orea, C.; Martinez-Gonzalez, M.A.; Gea, A.; Alonso, A.; Pimenta, A.M.; Bes-Rastrollo, M. Baseline consumption and changes in sugar-sweetened beverage consumption and the incidence of hypertension: The SUN project. *Clin. Nutr.* **2014**, *34*, 1133–1140. [CrossRef] [PubMed]
7. Malik, V.S.; Hu, F.B. Fructose and Cardiometabolic Health: What the Evidence from Sugar-Sweetened Beverages Tells Us. *J. Am. Coll. Cardiol.* **2015**, *66*, 1615–1624. [CrossRef] [PubMed]
8. Sauvant, M.P.; Pepin, D. Drinking water and cardiovascular disease. *Food Chem. Toxicol.* **2002**, *40*, 1311–1325. [CrossRef]
9. Khosravi-Boroujeni, H.; Sarrafzadegan, N.; Mohammadifard, N.; Alikhasi, H.; Sajjadi, F.; Asgari, S.; Esmaillzadeh, A. Consumption of sugar-sweetened beverages in relation to the metabolic syndrome among Iranian adults. *Obes. Facts* **2012**, *5*, 527–537. [CrossRef] [PubMed]
10. Odegaard, A.O.; Koh, W.-P.; Yuan, J.-M.; Pereira, M.A. Beverage habits and mortality in Chinese adults. *J. Nutr.* **2015**, *145*, 595–604. [CrossRef] [PubMed]
11. Rippe, J.M. The Metabolic and Endocrine Response and Health Implications of Consuming Sugar-Sweetened Beverages: Findings from Recent Randomized Controlled Trials. *Adv. Nutr.* **2013**, *4*, 677–686. [CrossRef] [PubMed]
12. Armstrong, L.E. Challenges of linking chronic dehydration and fluid consumption to health outcomes. *Nutr. Rev.* **2012**, *70* (Suppl. S2), S121–S127. [CrossRef] [PubMed]
13. Popkin, B.B.M.; D'Anci, K.K.E.; Rosenberg, I.I.H. Water, hydration, and health. *Nutr. Rev.* **2010**, *68*, 439–458. [CrossRef] [PubMed]
14. Manz, F.; Johner, S.A.; Wentz, A.; Boeing, H.; Remer, T. Water balance throughout the adult life span in a German population. *Br. J. Nutr.* **2012**, *107*, 1673–1681. [CrossRef] [PubMed]
15. Riebl, S.K.; MacDougal, C.; Hill, C.; Estabrooks, P.A.; Dunsmore, J.C.; Savla, J.; Frisard, M.I.; Dietrich, A.M.; Davy, B.M. Beverage Choices of Adolescents and Their Parents Using the Theory of Planned Behavior: A Mixed Methods Analysis. *J. Acad. Nutr. Diet.* **2016**, *116*, 226–239. [CrossRef] [PubMed]

16. Serra-Majem, L.; Santana-Armas, J.F.; Ribas, L.; Salmona, E.; Ramon, J.M.; Colom, J.; Salleras, L. A comparison of five questionnaires to assess alcohol consumption in a Mediterranean population. *Public Health Nutr.* **2002**, *5*, 589–594. [CrossRef] [PubMed]

17. Hedrick, V.E.; Savla, J.; Comber, D.L.; Flack, K.D.; Estabrooks, P.A.; Nsiah-Kumi, P.A.; Ortmeier, S.; Davy, B.M. Development of a brief questionnaire to assess habitual beverage intake (BEVQ-15): Sugar-Sweetened beverages and total beverage energy intake. *J. Acad. Nutr. Diet.* **2012**, *112*, 840–849. [CrossRef] [PubMed]

18. Le Bellego, L.; Jean, C.; Jiménez, L.; Magnani, C.; Tang, W.; Boutrolle, I. Understanding Fluid Consumption Patterns to Improve Healthy Hydration. *Nutr. Today* **2010**, *45*, S22–S26. [CrossRef]

19. Popkin, B.B.M.; Armstrong, L.L.E.; Bray, G.M.; Caballero, B.; Frei, B.; Willett, W.C. A new proposed guidance system for beverage consumption in the United States. *Am. J. Clin. Nutr.* **2006**, *83*, 529–542. [PubMed]

20. Han, E.; Powell, L.M. Consumption patterns of sugar-sweetened beverages in the United States. *J. Acad. Nutr. Diet.* **2013**, *113*, 43–53. [CrossRef] [PubMed]

21. Hedrick, V.E.; Comber, D.L.; Estabrooks, P.A.; Savla, J.; Davy, B.M. The beverage intake questionnaire: Determining initial validity and reliability. *J. Am. Diet. Assoc.* **2010**, *110*, 1227–1232. [CrossRef] [PubMed]

22. PREDIMED-PLUS. Available online: http://predimedplus.com/ (accessed on 8 June 2016).

23. Alberti, K.G.M.M.; Eckel, R.H.; Grundy, S.M.; Zimmet, P.Z.; Cleeman, J.I.; Donato, K.A.; Fruchart, J.-C.; James, W.P.T.; Loria, C.M.; Smith, S.C. Harmonizing the metabolic syndrome: a joint interim statement of the International Diabetes Federation Task Force on Epidemiology and Prevention; National Heart, Lung, and Blood Institute; American Heart Association; World Heart Federation; International Atherosclerosis Society; and International Association for the Study of Obesity. *Circulation* **2009**, *120*, 1640–1645. [PubMed]

24. United States Department of Agriculture USD. A Online Database. Available online: https://ndb.nal.usda.gov/ (accessed on 8 June 2016).

25. Manz, F.; Wentz, A.; Sichert-Hellert, W. The most essential nutrient: defining the adequate intake of water. *J. Pediatr.* **2002**, *141*, 587–592. [CrossRef] [PubMed]

26. Elosua, R.; Marrugat, J.; Molina, L.; Pons, S.; Pujol, E. Validation of the Minnesota Leisure Time Physical Activity Questionnaire in Spanish men. The MARATHOM Investigators. *Am. J. Epidemiol.* **1994**, *139*, 1197–1209. [PubMed]

27. Fernández-Ballart, J.D.; Piñol, J.L.; Zazpe, I.; Corella, D.; Carrasco, P.; Toledo, E.; Perez-Bauer, M.; Martínez-González, M.A.; Salas-Salvadó, J.; Martín-Moreno, J.M. Relative validity of a semi-quantitative food-frequency questionnaire in an elderly Mediterranean population of Spain. *Br. J. Nutr.* **2010**, *103*, 1808–1816. [CrossRef] [PubMed]

28. Mataix, V. *Tabla de Composición de Alimentos [Food Composition Table]*, 4th ed.; Universidad de Granada: Granada, Spain, 2003. (In Spanish)

29. Moreiras, O.; Cabrera, L. *Tabla de Composición de Alimentos [Food Composition Table]*; Ediciones Pirámide: Madrid, Spain, 2005.

30. Schröder, H.; Fitó, M.; Estruch, R.; Martínez-González, M.A.; Corella, D.; Salas-Salvadó, J.; Lamuela-Raventós, R.; Ros, E.; Salaverría, I.; Fiol, M.; et al. A short screener is valid for assessing Mediterranean diet adherence among older Spanish men and women. *J. Nutr.* **2011**, *141*, 1140–1145. [CrossRef] [PubMed]

31. Neuhouser, M.L.; Lilley, S.; Lund, A.; Johnson, D.B. Development and validation of a beverage and snack questionnaire for use in evaluation of school nutrition policies. *J. Am. Diet. Assoc.* **2009**, *109*, 1587–1592. [CrossRef] [PubMed]

32. Malisova, O.; Bountziouka, V.; Panagiotakos, D.B.; Zampelas, A.; Kapsokefalou, M. The water balance questionnaire: Design, reliability and validity of a questionnaire to evaluate water balance in the general population. *Int. J. Food Sci. Nutr.* **2012**, *63*, 138–144. [CrossRef] [PubMed]

33. Nissensohn, M.; Ruano, C.; Serra-Majem, L. Validation of beverage intake methods vs. hydration biomarker; a short review. *Nutr. Hosp.* **2013**, *28*, 1815–1819. [PubMed]

34. Armstrong, L.E. Assessing hydration status: the elusive gold standard. *J. Am. Coll. Nutr.* **2007**, *26*, 575S–584S. [CrossRef] [PubMed]

35. Shirreffs, S.M. Markers of hydration status. *Eur. J. Clin. Nutr.* **2003**, *57* (Suppl. S2), S6–S9. [CrossRef] [PubMed]

36. Tsubono, Y.; Nishino, Y.; Fukao, A.; Hisamichi, S.; Tsugane, S. Temporal change in the reproducibility of a self-administered food frequency questionnaire. *Am. J. Epidemiol.* **1995**, *142*, 1231–1235. [PubMed]

37. Cade, J.; Thompson, R.; Burley, V.; Warm, D. Development, validation and utilisation of food-frequency questionnaires—A review. *Public Health Nutr.* **2002**, *5*, 567–587. [CrossRef] [PubMed]

38. Willett, W.; Lenart, E. *Nutritional Epidemiology*, 2nd ed.; Oxford University Press: New York, NY, USA, 1998.

39. Ferreira-pêgo, C.; Babio, N.; Fenández-alvira, J.M.; Iglesia, I.; Moreno, L.A. Fluid intake from beverages in Spanish adults: Cross-Sectional study. *Nutr. Hosp.* **2014**, *29*, 1171–1178. [PubMed]

40. Saetun, P.; Semangoen, T.; Thongboonkerd, V. Characterizations of urinary sediments precipitated after freezing and their effects on urinary protein and chemical analyses. *Am. J. Physiol. Ren. Physiol.* **2009**, *296*, F1346–F1354. [CrossRef] [PubMed]

41. Cheuvront, S.N.; Ely, B.R.; Kenefick, R.W.; Sawka, M.N. Biological variation and diagnostic accuracy of dehydration assessment markers. *Am. J. Clin. Nutr.* **2010**, *92*, 565–573. [CrossRef] [PubMed]

42. Sparks, S.A.; Close, G.L. Validity of a portable urine refractometer: The effects of sample freezing. *J. Sports Sci.* **2013**, *31*, 745–749. [CrossRef] [PubMed]

43. Remer, T.; Montenegro-Bethancourt, G.; Shi, L. Long-Term urine biobanking: Storage stability of clinical chemical parameters under moderate freezing conditions without use of preservatives. *Clin. Biochem.* **2014**, *47*, 307–311. [CrossRef] [PubMed]

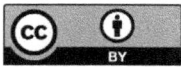

nutrients

MDPI

Article

Water and Beverage Consumption among Children Aged 4–13 Years in Lebanon: Findings from a National Cross-Sectional Study

Lamis Jomaa [1], Nahla Hwalla [1], Florence Constant [2], Farah Naja [1,*,†] and Lara Nasreddine [1,*,†]

1   Department of Nutrition and Food Sciences, Faculty of Agricultural and Food Sciences,
    American University of Beirut, P.O. Box 11-0.236, Riad El Solh, Beirut 11072020, Lebanon;
    lj18@aub.edu.lb (L.J.); nahla@aub.edu.lb (N.H.)
2   Nestle Waters, 12 boulevard Garibaldi, Issy-les-Moulineaux, Paris 92130, France;
    Florence.Constant@waters.nestle.com
*   Correspondence: fn14@aub.edu.lb (F.N.); ln10@aub.edu.lb (L.N.);
    Tel.: +961-1-35000 (ext. 4504) (F.N.); +961-1-35000 (ext. 4547) (L.N.); Fax: +961-1-744460 (L.N. & F.N.)
†   These authors contributed equally to this work.

Received: 29 July 2016; Accepted: 30 August 2016; Published: 8 September 2016

Abstract: This study evaluates total water intake (TWI) from plain water, beverages and foods among Lebanese children and compares TWI to dietary reference intakes (DRIs). In a national cross-sectional survey, data on demographic, socioeconomic, anthropometric, and physical activity characteristics were obtained from 4 to 13-year-old children ($n = 752$). Food and beverage consumption patterns were assessed using a validated food-frequency questionnaire. TWI was estimated at 1651 mL/day, with beverages contributing 72% of the TWI compared to 28% from foods. Beverages with the highest contribution to TWI included plain water, fruit juice and soda. A significantly higher proportion of 9–13-year-old children failed to meet the DRIs compared to 4–8 years old (92%–98% vs. 74%). Gender differentials were observed with a significantly higher proportion of boys meeting the DRIs compared to girls. The water to energy ratio ranged between 0.84 and 0.87, which fell short of meeting the desirable recommendations. In addition, children from higher socioeconomic status had higher intakes of water from milk and bottled water, coupled with lower water intakes from sodas. The study findings show an alarming high proportion of Lebanese children failing to meet TWI recommendations, and call for culture-specific interventions to instill healthy fluid consumption patterns early in life.

Keywords: water intake; beverage consumption; water adequacy; hydration; children; Lebanon

1. Introduction

Water is quantitatively the most important nutrient, playing a critical role in maintaining adequate hydration status [1]. Hypohydration is recognized as a precipitating factor in a number of acute medical conditions [2]. Even short periods of fluid restriction, characterized by a loss of body mass of 1%–2%, may lead to increases in self-reported tiredness and headache and to reductions in the subjective perception of alertness and ability to concentrate [2]. In addition, recent studies suggest that changes of hydration status may affect cognitive performance in children, whereby improved hydration was associated with enhanced performance on cognitive tests such as the digit-span and pair-cancellation tasks and with improved short-term memory [3,4].

Children are amongst the population groups that are at particular risk of hypohydration and inadequate water intakes [2,5,6]. Despite its critical importance in health and nutrition, the array of available research that serves as a basis for assessing the adequacy of water intake, remains limited in comparison with most other nutrients [1]. Adequate intakes for water are defined based on: (1) observed water intakes in various population groups; (2) desirable water volumes per 1000 kcal; and (3) desirable osmolality values in urine. The Dietary Reference Intakes (DRIs) for Water and Electrolytes reported by the Institute of Medicine (IOM) have set the Adequate Intake (AI) for total daily water intake at 1.7 L/day in 4–8-year-old children, 2.1 L/day in 9–13-year-old girls and 2.4 L/day in 9–13-year-old boys [7]. The European Food Safety Authority (EFSA) established total water AI levels at slightly lower levels: 1.6 L/day for boys and girls aged 4–8 years, and at 1.9 L/day for girls and 2.1 L/day for boys aged 9–13 years [8]. The water-to-energy ratio is another proposed index of adequate hydration; an index that incorporates to some degree, body size or surface area, and activity [1,9]. Accordingly, the desirable total water intake (TWI) is estimated to range between 1.0 and 1.5 L per 1000 kcal in children, depending on activity levels and water losses [8,10].

The established DRI values are based on water obtained from plain drinking water (bottled or tap), water from other beverages, and water from foods (both intrinsic water in foods and water added during food preparations) [8,10,11]. The DRIs were set mostly to prevent the adverse effects of dehydration, but beyond issues of hydration, there is increasing interest in characterizing consumption patterns of plain water vs. water arising from other sources. Some epidemiological data suggest that water may have different metabolic effects when consumed alone rather than as a component of flavored, sweetened or caffeinated beverages, but available evidence remains inconclusive [12,13]. Drinking plain water instead of caloric beverages helps to reduce dietary energy density, and may contribute to the regulation of body weight [1,9,14]. Some studies have also suggested that consumption of plain water is associated with better diets and better health behaviors in youth [15]. Based on the 2010 National Youth Physical Activity and Nutrition Study, Park et al. showed that low water intake was associated with poor diet quality and physical inactivity amongst US adolescents [16].

Although beverage consumption patterns and their contribution to energy intake (EI) have been well documented in children, few studies have explored the consumption of plain water and the adequacy of TWI in this age group [9,11,17,18]. A study conducted on a national sample of 4–13-year-old children in the US, showed that plain water, tap and bottled, contributed 25%–30% of total dietary water and that more than 75% of children did not meet the DRIs for TWI [9]. The study by Vieux et al. (2016), on 4–13-year-old French children and the study by Piernas et al. (2014), on Mexican children have also shown that the contribution of plain water to TWI did not exceed 34% and that a high proportion of children did not meet the recommendations (71%–90%) [11,17]. With the exception of few studies reporting on the contribution of various beverages to EI or on the volume of ingested fluids [19,20], no studies have investigated TWI and its adequacy amongst children in the Middle-East and North Africa (MENA), a region that is characterized by a hot climate, a high prevalence of dietary inadequacies in children [21,22] and one of the highest burdens of pediatric overweight and obesity worldwide [22]. Based on a nationally representative survey conducted in 2015, the present study aims at: (1) assessing total dietary water intakes (from foods and beverages) amongst 4–13-year-old children in Lebanon, in comparison with the IOM and EFSA recommendations by gender and age (4–8 years and 9–13 years); (2) investigating the association of water intakes from various sources with demographic, socioeconomic, anthropometric, and physical activity characteristics; (3) estimating EI from beverage and food sources and determining the water per calorie ratio (L/1000 kcal), in relation to desirable values by gender and age; and (4) comparing water intake data presented in this study to those reported from other countries, on the same age group.

2. Methods

2.1. Study Population and Sampling Framework

Data for this study were drawn from a national cross-sectional study conducted among a representative sample of children (4–18 years) and their mothers in Lebanon. A stratified cluster sampling strategy was followed, whereby the strata were the six Lebanese governorates and the clusters were selected further at the level of districts. Each district was divided into clusters comprised of 100–150 households. Households constituted the primary sampling unit within this national study. Within the cluster, households were selected by systematic sampling, based on probability proportional to size technique using the Lebanese Central Administration of Statistics as a reference [23]. For a household to be eligible, children and their mothers had to be present at the time of the interview. Inclusion criteria for children included: (1) Lebanese nationality; (2) child's age between 4 and 18 years; (2) not suffering from any chronic disease; and (3) not taking any medications that may interfere with his/her dietary intake or body weight. Of the 4076 households that were contacted, 3147 accepted to participate in the study (response rate = 77%). Of these, 3147 households, 1221 met the eligibility criteria and 1209 completed the study. The main reasons for refusing to participate in the study were time constraints and lack of interest.

For the purpose of the present study, data for children aged 4–13 years were considered (*n* = 752). Since the evaluation of the TWI amongst 4–13-year-old children and the identification of the proportion of children meeting (or failing to meet) the water intake recommendations were among the main objectives of the national study, sample size calculations were conducted as follows: a minimum of 638 participants were needed to provide 95% confidence interval to estimate a prevalence of water adequacy of 30% with ±3.5% variation in this age group. The estimate of children with adequate water intake levels (30%) for the 4–13-year-old age group used in the sample size calculations was based on results from previously conducted studies reporting water and beverage consumption patterns among a similar age group of children and adolescents in Mexico [11] and the United States [9].

Ethical approval for the study was obtained from the Institutional Review Board at the American University of Beirut. Written informed consents were obtained from all mothers prior to participation in the study. Written assents were also obtained from children aged 6 years and above.

2.2. Data Collection

The survey was conducted over approximately one calendar year, between December 2014 and November 2015, covering weekdays and weekends. Face-to-face interviews with children and their mothers were conducted within their household setting by trained dietitians using a multi-component questionnaire. The questionnaire included information on demographic and socioeconomic characteristics, anthropometric measurements, dietary intake, and physical activity levels of participating children. Mothers served as proxy respondents for children under the age of 10 years and the interviews lasted on average 45 min per household.

Demographic characteristics included sex and age of the child. Indicators of the household's socioeconomic status (SES) included parents' highest educational level (intermediate level or less, high school or technical diploma, university degree or more), employment status (employed or unemployed) and household's income (reported as <1 million Lebanese pounds (LBP)—662 US dollars equivalent, 1–1,999,999 million LBP, and ≥2 million LBP). Additionally, the crowding index, a commonly used criterion to assess the socio-economic status of households, was calculated by dividing the number of persons living in the household over the number of rooms in the households (excluding bathrooms, kitchens and balconies) [24,25]. The questionnaire was designed by a panel of experts including scientists in the fields of epidemiology and nutrition. The questionnaire was used in previous studies conducted in Lebanon [26,27] and was pilot tested on 25 households at the start of the present study to ensure clarity of questions.

Anthropometric measurements were obtained from study participants by trained dietitians using standard techniques and equipment. Children were weighed on a digital scale to the nearest 0.1 kg wearing light clothing, while height was measured to the nearest 0.1 cm, without shoes. Waist circumference (WC) was measured to the nearest 0.1 cm using a calibrated plastic measuring tape at the level of the umbilicus to the nearest 0.1 cm, after normal expiration. All measurements were taken twice and the average of the 2 values was reported. Body Mass Index (BMI) was calculated by dividing the weight in kilograms over the height in meters squared. Using WHO growth charts and criteria (WHO Growth reference 2015), BMI-for-age z-scores were used to classify children as normal weight, overweight, or obese. For children under 5 years, normal weight was classified as BMI between −2 and +2 SD of the WHO growth standard median, overweight as BMI > +2 SD, and obese as BMI > +3 SD. For children 5–13 years in the study sample, normal weight was defined between −2 SD and +1 SD, overweight > +1 SD, and obese > +2 SD above the WHO growth standard median. The Waist to height ratio (WHtR) for abdominal obesity was calculated by dividing WC by height, both measured in centimeters [28]. The suggested cut-off point of ≥0.5 was used to identify children with elevated WHtR [28,29].

Physical activity level of children was assessed using a modified version of the Children and Youth Physical Activity Questionnaire [30]. Children were asked to recall activities that they participated in and their duration during the past week, including weekdays and weekends, and activities within the school as well extra-curricular activities. For the purpose of this study, children engaging in more than 420 minutes per week of moderate to vigorous activities were considered active and those below this cut-off were categorized as inactive [31,32].

2.3. Dietary Intake Assessment and Interpretation

Dietary intake data was collected by trained interviewers using a 187-item food frequency questionnaire (FFQ) that was previously validated among Lebanese children to assess habitual dietary intake over the past year [33]. The FFQ included foods and beverages commonly consumed in Lebanon with a particular focus on a variety of beverages, such as bottled and tap water, milk, sodas, diet drinks, fruit and vegetable juices, hot beverages (coffee and tea), alcoholic beverages, and sports and energy drinks.

For children < 10 years old, mothers as the main meal planners were the proxy respondents to complete the FFQ. Children aged 10–14 years were the main respondents, and their mothers were present at the time of the interview to assist in providing detailed description of foods consumed at home including recipes and portion sizes consumed by children. To assist children and their mothers when estimating the portions and amounts of food and beverages consumed and reported in the FFQs, household measures and two-dimensional portion size posters were used (Millen and Morgan, Nutrition Consulting Enterprises, Framingham, MA, United States). These previously validated visuals [34] have been well-accepted and commonly used in previous national studies conducted in Lebanon [21,35].

2.4. Water and Energy Intake and Beverage Classifications

Daily water and EI from all foods and beverages reported in the FFQ were computed using the food composition database of the Nutritionist Pro software (version 5.1.0, 2014, SR 24, First Data Bank, Nutritionist Pro, Axxya Systems, San Bruno, CA, USA). The food composition database within this software is based on the USDA nutrient database [36]; however it was further expanded by adding analyses of traditional Lebanese foods and recipes reported among participating children using local food composition databases [37].

The present study focused on TWI from all foods and beverages. Results were reported as mL of water content from all foods and beverages, foods only, beverages only, and from specific beverages. Beverages were classified into 8 main groups with subcategories as follows: (1) plain water (bottled and tap); (2) milk and milk alternatives (milk shakes, yoghurt—plain or flavored—and hot chocolate prepared with milk); (3) sodas (regular and diet); (4) fruit juices (fresh fruit juice—100% natural, bottled fruit juice (without sugar), and bottled fruit juice with sugar (fruit drink); (5) vegetable juice; (6) hot beverages (coffee and tea); (7) sports and energy drinks; and (8) alcoholic beverages. EI from beverages were evaluated for the same beverage categories.

TWI from all food and beverages (mL/day) were compared to the Institute of Medicine (IOM) and EFSA water intake recommendations for each age and gender group to assess the shortfall in water consumption and the proportion of children who met or failed to meet the adequate water intake levels [7]. Using the same calculated daily TWI, in conjunction with total EI; water per calorie ratio was calculated and presented as mean (L/1000 kcal) by age and gender.

Water intake data estimated by the present study were compared to those reported by studies conducted in other countries, on similar age groups. Dietary assessment methods varied across countries, with the 24-hour recall data being adopted in Mexico and the US [9,11], and the 7-day food record being used in France [17]. These studies reported on plain water (tap and bottled) and similar beverage groups, while also sharing similar definitions for the assessment of TWIs, water and energy intakes from foods and beverages and their contribution to TWI and EI [9,11,17]. The estimated TWIs were compared to the IOM water intake recommendations in Mexico and the US [9,11], whereas the study conducted in France [17] used the EFSA recommendations [17].

2.5. Statistical Analysis

Continuous variables were presented as means and standard errors (SE), whereas categorical variables were reported as proportions with percentages.

Mean TWI from different beverage groups and from moisture in foods were presented by age group (4–8 years and 9–13 years), gender, socioeconomic, anthropometric and physical activity characteristics. The contribution of water from each beverage type was calculated at the individual level by dividing the water intake from that specific beverage type by the daily TWI. Comparisons of mean daily TWIs and mean % of TWI from each beverage type were conducted by age group (4–8 vs. 9–13 years old) using student t-tests. Associations of water intakes (from foods and beverages; plain water, and beverages (excluding plain water) with demographic, socioeconomic, anthropometric, and physical activity characteristics, were examined using student t-tests and analysis of variance (ANOVAs) with Bonferroni corrections.

In addition, the mean daily intake of energy (kcal) from all foods and beverages, from caloric beverages, and from each beverage type were calculated and presented as means $\pm$ SE and as proportions (percent of total EI). Differences between 4–8- and 9–13-year-old children in terms of mean EI from each beverage type and the contribution of beverages to total EI were conducted using student t-tests. Using the IOM age and gender-specific water recommendations, the proportion of children who met or did not meet the DRIs for water intake, the total shortfall in water consumption, and mean ratio of water per calorie (L/1000 kcal) were calculated. Similar calculations were conducted to compare the average TWI of children in the study sample with EFSA water intake recommendations by age and gender.

All data analyses were conducted using the Statistical Package for the Social and Sciences statistical software package (SPSS) version 22 with p-values of < 0.05 considered statistically significant.

3. Results

3.1. Total Water Intakes among Study Sample in Relation to Recommended Intakes

Average TWI for all children (aged 4–13 years old) in the study sample was assessed to be 1651 mL/day. As shown in Table 1, average TWI was estimated at 1601 mL/day amongst 4–8-year-old children and 1698 mL/day amongst 9–13 years old. Overall, intakes of water from all foods and beverages, plain water and from beverages (excluding plain water) were significantly higher among boys than girls and among older (9–13 years) compared to younger children (4–8 years).

Table 1. Total Water Intakes (mL/day) from foods and beverages by sociodemographic, anthropometric and physical activity characteristics in a representative sample of Lebanese children aged 4–13 years (n = 752).

	Total Mean ± SE or n (%)	TWI from Foods and Beverages (mL/Day)	Water Intakes from All Beverages (mL/Day)	
			Plain Water (Bottled and Tap) (mL/Day)	Beverages (Excluding Plain Water) (mL/Day)
			Mean ± SE	
Age	9.07 ± 0.10			
4–8 years	358 (47.6)	1600.63 ± 12.93 [a]	767.32 ± 11.22 [a]	376.21 ± 7.95 [a]
9–13 years	394 (52.4)	1697.68 ± 16.55 [b]	840.49 ± 13.39 [b]	401.13 ± 9.24 [b]
Gender				
Boys	397 (52.8)	1738.77 ± 17.72 [a]	841.58 ± 13.50 [a]	440.54 ± 9.91 [a]
Girls	355 (47.2)	1553.87 ± 8.81 [b]	765.48 ± 10.97 [b]	331.92 ± 5.47 [b]
Father's educational level				
Intermediate or less	435 (58.2)	1646.44 ± 13.60 [a]	804.73 ± 11.53 [a]	396.18 ± 7.49 [a]
High school/technical diploma	203 (27.2)	1660.32 ± 22.73 [a]	812.81 ± 18.60 [a]	378.70 ± 14.37 [a]
University Degree or more	109 (14.6)	1645.37 ± 27.34 [a]	793.63 ± 21.15 [a]	372.21 ± 12.91 [a]
Mother's educational level				
Intermediate or less	363 (48.3)	1632.03 ± 14.98 [a]	790.21 ± 12.32 [a]	391.70 ± 9.36 [a]
High school/technical diploma	227 (30.2)	1674.59 ± 20.87 [a]	830.57 ± 17.45 [a]	393.16 ± 10.89 [a]
University Degree or more	162 (21.5)	1662.68 ± 22.69 [a]	805.37 ± 18.64 [a]	378.35 ± 12.04 [a]
Father's employment status				
Unemployed	32 (4.3)	1669.58 ± 62.48 [a]	794.76 ± 60.61 [a]	436.67 ± 33.85 [a]
Employed	711 (95.7)	1651.28 ± 11.01 [a]	807.07 ± 8.99 [a]	386.36 ± 6.28 [a]
Mother's employment status	743 (100)			
Unemployed	556 (74.0)	1644.78 ± 12.56 [a]	802.36 ± 10.43 [a]	388.29 ± 7.22 [a]
Employed	195 (26.0)	1669.90 ± 21.04 [a]	814.06 ± 17.21 [a]	391.98 ± 11.88 [a]
Monthly family income (LBP)				
<1,000,000	310 (41.8)	1636.68 ± 16.11 [a]	807.52 ± 14.25 [a]	391.02 ± 8.91 [a]
1,000,000–1,999,999	279 (37.6)	1643.13 ± 16.75 [a]	790.03 ± 14.02 [a]	386.28 ± 9.05 [a]
≥2,000,000	153 (20.6)	1701.01 ± 27.93 [a]	835.94 ± 20.22 [a]	391.31 ± 17.74 [a]

Table 1. *Cont.*

	Total Mean ± SE or *n* (%)	TWI from Foods and Beverages (mL/Day)	Water Intakes from All Beverages (mL/Day)	
			Plain Water (Bottled and Tap) (mL/Day)	Beverages (Excluding Plain Water) (mL/Day)
		Mean ± SE		
Crowding index (person/room)	1.62 ± 0.03			
<2	534 (71.2)	1654.31 ± 13.01 [a]	808.22 ± 10.58 [a]	388.52 ± 7.50 [a]
≥2	216 (28.8)	1644.11 ± 19.30 [a]	799.48 ± 16.74 [a]	390.62 ± 10.72 [a]
BMI z-score	0.92 ± 0.06			
BMI status				
Normal weight	443 (58.9)	1640.08 ± 13.96 [a]	787.19 ± 10.82 [a]	390.21 ± 8.49 [a]
Overweight	152 (20.2)	1657.23 ± 23.68 [a]	824.72 ± 20.89 [a]	376.22 ± 12.41 [a]
Obese	157 (20.9)	1678.07 ± 24.21 [a]	839.29 ± 21.70 [a]	399.24 ± 12.33 [a]
Waist Circumference (cm)	64.11 ± 0.46			
Waist to height ratio (WHtR)	0.48 ± 0.00			
<0.5	489 (65.4)	1660.89 ± 14.08 [a]	807.59 ± 242.03 [a]	392.54 ± 8.17 [a]
≥0.5	259 (34.6)	1631.77 ± 260.18 [a]	803.33 ± 250.37 [a]	382.24 ± 144.39 [a]
Level of physical activity				
Active	434 (57.7)	1676.47 ± 13.94 [a]	817.52 ± 12.16 [a]	404.27 ± 7.39 [a]
Inactive	318 (42.3)	1617.37 ± 16.78 [b]	789.46 ± 12.95 [a]	368.80 ± 10.41 [b]

[a,b] Statistical comparisons were conducted within each sociodemographic group and within anthropometric and physical activity levels based on independent samples *t*-test or ANOVA test. Mean estimates with different superscript letters are significantly different at $p \leq 0.05$.

Total daily water intakes amongst 4–13-year-old Lebanese children were compared to the age and gender-specific water intake recommendations of the IOM (Figure 1). Compared to the AI values, the shortfall in water intake was observed to be higher amongst 9–13-year-old children (592 mL/day in boys and 533 mL/day in girls) compared to their younger counterparts (99 mL/day). Overall, only 15% (*n* = 114) of the study sample met the recommendations for daily TWI, among whom the mean TWI was estimated at 2047 mL/day (SE = 32.2) on average. In addition, a significantly higher proportion of 4–8-year-old children met the AI values compared to 9–13 years old (26% vs. 5%, *p* < 0.001). Amongst the older age group, a higher proportion of boys met the water intake recommendations compared to girls (7.9% vs. 2.2% *p* = 0.012). Similarly, a significantly higher proportion of boys had adequate levels of TWI compared to girls within the 4–8-year-old children group (41.5% vs. 9.7%), *p* < 0.001 (data not shown).

Additional analyses were conducted based on EFSA recommendations for adequate water intakes. Accordingly, 26.5% of 4–13-year-old children were found to meet the AI values. Similar to the observations seen with the IOM DRIs, a higher proportion of younger children met the EFSA water intake recommendations compared to older children (40.5% vs. 13.7%, *p* < 0.001) and a higher proportion of boys had adequate levels of TWI compared to girls, in both age groups (*p* < 0.001).

As for the water-to-energy ratio, the observed water volume per 1000 kcal ranged between 0.84 in 4–8-year-old children and 0.87 in 9–13 years old, with 96%–99% of the children not meeting the desirable IOM recommendations for this indicator.

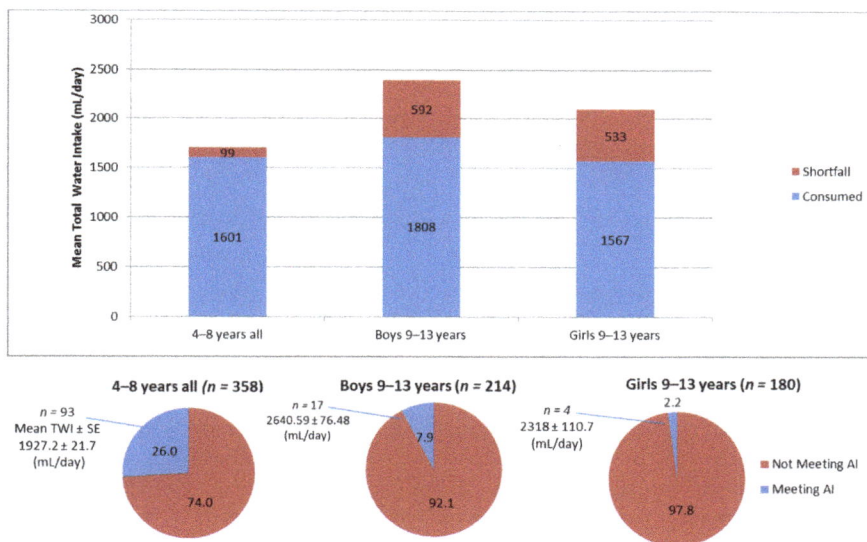

Figure 1. Shortfalls in total water intakes amongst 4–13-year-old Lebanese children as compared to the IOM adequate intake (AI) and proportion of children meeting the age and gender-specific AIs. Total daily water intake from all foods and beverages (consumed) by age group and gender compared to Institute of Medicine Recommendations (IOM) (shortfall). Proportions of children meeting and not meeting needs compared to IOM are displayed in the corresponding pie charts.

3.2. Water Consumption According to Socioeconomic, Physical Activity and Anthropometric Characteristics

Water intakes were not found to be significantly different according to socioeconomic indicators (household income, crowding index, mother and father's educational level or employment status) (Table 1). However, results showed that children reporting active physical activity levels had significantly higher TWI from foods and beverages and higher water consumption from beverages compared to inactive children. No significant associations were observed between various anthropometric measures (such as BMI and WHtR) with water consumption from total foods and beverages, plain water, and beverages (excluding plain water).

3.3. Patterns of Water Intake from Food and Various Beverage Types by Age and Gender

Table 2 presents the intakes of water from foods and from different beverage types by age group. Overall, water from beverages contributed close to 72% of total daily water intake amongst 4–13-year-old children, compared to 28% from food moisture. Amongst 4–8-year-old children, the three main sources of water included plain water (47.6%), moisture in foods (28.5%), and fruit juice (10.3%). For older children (9–13 years), the main contributors to TWI included plain water (49%), moisture in food (27.7%), and sodas (10.3%). Older children (9–13 years) were found to have significantly higher water intakes from plain water (bottle and tap water), sodas, particularly regular/caloric sodas, hot beverages, energy drinks and alcoholic beverages compared to younger ones (4–8 years). In addition, the contribution of water intake from plain water, sodas, and alcoholic beverages to TWI was significantly higher amongst 9–13-year-old children compared to their younger counterparts. On the other hand, the contribution of water intake from foods, milk and milk alternatives, and fruit juice (fresh and bottled with sugar) were significantly higher amongst 4-8-year-old children compared to the older ones.

Gender differentials in water intakes from foods and from different beverage sources are shown in Figure 2. For the 4–8-year-old children, water intakes from solid foods and from hot beverages (tea/coffee) were found to be significantly higher amongst girls compared to boys. On the other hand, 4–8-year-old boys had significantly higher intakes of water from sodas and fruit drinks (bottled fruit juices with sugar) compared to girls of the same age. Among 9–13-year-old children, significantly higher water intakes from sodas, fruit drinks, and fruit juices (fresh and no sugar added) were noted in boys compared to girls, whereas significantly higher water intakes from milk and milk alternatives were observed in girls compared to boys.

3.4. Water Intake from Specific Beverages by Socioeconomic, Anthropometric and Physical Activity Characteristics

Table 3 presents the intakes of water from specific beverages by socioeconomic, anthropometric, and physical activity characteristics amongst 4–13-year-old Lebanese children. A higher paternal education level (university degree or more) was found to be associated with higher water intakes from bottled water, coupled to lower intakes from tap water and regular soft drinks. As for maternal educational level, it was found to be associated with higher intakes of bottled water, milk and milk alternatives yet with lower intakes of tap water, regular soft drinks and energy drinks. Monthly family income and crowding index, two indicators of socioeconomic status, were also found to be associated with water intakes from specific beverages: Children from households with higher socioeconomic status had higher intakes of water from bottled water, milk and milk alternatives, fresh fruit juice and vegetable juice, yet lower intakes of water from tap water and caloric soft drinks. With respect to physical activity, overall active children had higher intakes of water from beverages compared to inactive ones, with the difference reaching statistical significance for soft drinks and fresh fruit juice. No significant associations were observed between anthropometric measures, such as BMI status and WHtR, with water intakes from plain or bottled water, milk, soft drinks, and juices (data not shown).

Table 2. Intakes of water (mL/day) from different beverage groups and from foods and their contribution to total water intake by age group; children aged 4–13 years, Lebanon (n = 752).

	Total 752		4–8 Years 183 (46.1%)		9–13 Years 214 (53.9%)		p-Value
	Mean ± SE	% of TWI	Mean ± SE	% of TWI	Mean ± SE	% of TWI †	
Total water intake from all food and beverages	1651.48 ± 10.77	100	1600.63 ± 12.93 a	100	1697.68 ± 16.55 b	100	p < 0.001
Water intake from food only	455.79 ± 1.87	28.09	450.69 ± 2.33 a	28.54	460.41 ± 2.86 b	27.68 **	p = 0.009
Plain Water	805.66 ± 8.91	48.36	767.32 ± 11.22 a	47.61	840.49 ± 13.39 b	49.05 *	p < 0.001
Bottled water	685.54 ± 6.98	41.75	671.51 ± 8.67 a	42.15	698.29 ± 10.72 b	41.39	p = 0.053
Tap water	96.36 ± 6.75	5.62	81.26 ± 8.67 a	4.89	110.08 ± 10.15 b	6.29	p = 0.031
Water intake from all beverages (excluding plain water)	1194.92 ± 8.91	71.60	1143.53 ± 14.17 a	70.85	1241.62 ± 17.47 b	72.28	p < 0.001
Milk and milk alternatives	57.72 ± 0.90	3.54	59.59 ± 1.32 a	3.75	56.02 ± 1.22 b	3.34 **	p = 0.048
Milk	25.62 ± 0.81	1.56	26.75 ± 1.20 a	1.67	24.59 ± 1.09 a	1.45 *	p = 0.182
Milk Alternatives ≠	32.10 ± 0.32	1.98	32.84 ± 0.44 a	2.08	31.43 ± 0.45 b	1.89 **	p = 0.026
Sodas	155.68 ± 5.35	9.25	132.14 ± 7.15 a	8.09	177.06 ± 7.74 b	10.31 **	p < 0.001
Regular	142.61 ± 4.81	8.50	114.04 ± 5.15 a	7.06	168.68 ± 7.66 b	9.80 **	p < 0.001
Diet	13.01 ± 2.83	0.75	18.10 ± 5.50 a	1.03	8.38 ± 2.05 a	0.50	p = 0.098
Fruit Juice	160.77 ± 1.39	9.91	163.20 ± 2.21 a	10.33	158.55 ± 1.72 a	9.53 **	p = 0.094
Fresh Fruit Juice (100% Natural)	69.15 ± 0.20	4.29	69.02 ± 0.28 a	4.39	69.23 ± 0.28 a	4.19 **	p = 0.603
Bottled Fruit Juice (with sugar)/Fruit Drink	85.18 ± 0.78	5.25	85.90 ± 1.11 a	5.43	84.52 ± 1.09 a	5.08 **	p = 0.379
Bottled Fruit Juice (without sugar)	6.46 ± 1.18	0.38	8.28 ± 2.07 a	0.51	4.80 ± 1.25 a	0.27	p = 0.152
Vegetable Juice	2.89 ± 0.91	0.17	4.33 ± 1.80 a	0.27	1.58 ± 0.60 a	0.09	p = 0.149
Fresh Vegetable Juice	1.26 ± 0.31	0.07	1.65 ± 0.52 a	0.10	0.91 ± 0.35 a	0.05	p = 0.232
Bottled Vegetable Juice	1.63 ± 0.86	0.10	2.67 ± 1.73 a	0.16	0.68 ± 0.50 a	0.04	p = 0.268
Hot Beverages	57.06 ± 2.04	3.44	52.14 ± 2.80 a	3.26	61.53 ± 2.93 b	3.61	p = 0.021
Sports and Energy Drinks	1.84 ± 0.62	0.10	0.81 ± 0.53 a	0.05	2.77 ± 1.07 a	0.14	p = 0.103
Sports Drinks	0.85 ± 0.49	0.05	0.47 ± 0.47 a	0.03	1.20 ± 0.84 a	0.06	p = 0.463
Energy Drinks	0.99 ± 0.32	0.05	0.34 ± 0.24 a	0.02	1.58 ± 0.57 b	0.08	p = 0.047
Alcoholic beverages	0.51 ± 0.21	0.03	0.02 ± 0.02 a	0.00	0.95 ± 0.40 b	0.06 *	p = 0.019

[a,b] Statistical comparisons were conducted between age groups for the means of water intake from each beverage type using independent samples t-test. Mean estimates within a row with different superscript letters were significantly different at p < 0.05. ≠ Milk alternatives include milk-shakes, yoghurts (plain and flavored), and hot chocolate. † Statistical comparisons were conducted between age groups for the means of contribution of different beverages to total water intake (% TWI) using independent samples T-test; * p ≤ 0.05; ** p ≤ 0.001.

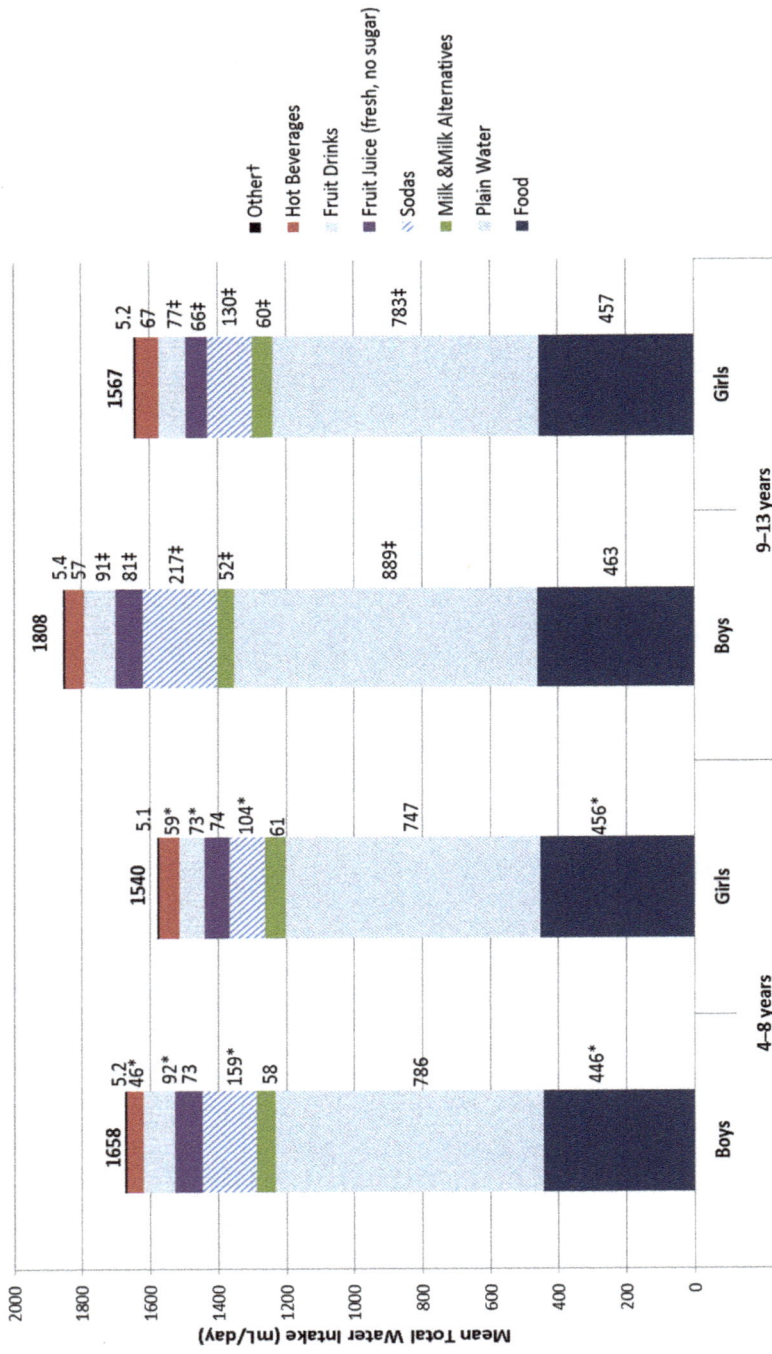

Figure 2. Total daily water intake (mL/day) from all sources by gender, in a national sample of 4–13-year-old children. * Statistical comparisons are made between genders within the 4–8 years age group, derived from independent samples *t*-test, results are significant at *p* < 0.05. ‡ Statistical comparisons are made between genders within the 9–13 years age group, derived from independent samples *t*-test, results are significant at *p* < 0.05. † Other category includes: vegetable juices, sports and energy drinks, and alcoholic beverages.

Table 3. Intakes (mL/day) of water from specific beverages * by socioeconomic ** and physical activity characteristics in a representative sample of Lebanese children aged 4–13 years † (n = 752).

	Bottled Water	Tap Water	Milk and Milk Alternatives	Regular Soft Drinks	Fresh Fruit Juice	Fresh Veg. Juice	Energy Drinks
	685.54 ± 6.98	96.36 ± 6.75	57.72 ± 0.90	142.67 ± 4.81	69.13 ± 0.20	1.26 ± 0.31	0.99 ± 0.32
Father's educational level							
Intermediate or less	670.04 ± 9.09 [a]	115.67 ± 9.65 [a]	56.48 ± 1.18 [a]	155.95 ± 6.20 [a]	69.10 ± 0.26 [a]	1.41 ± 0.47 [a]	0.92 ± 0.40 [a]
High school/technical diploma	699.88 ± 14.23 [a,b]	82.80 ± 12.37 [a,b]	58.98 ± 1.68 [a]	125.42 ± 9.16 [b]	68.95 ± 0.42 [a]	1.25 ± 0.48 [a]	1.63 ± 0.83 [a]
University Degree or more	722.11 ± 16.45 [b]	41.01 ± 9.12 [b]	60.30 ± 2.53 [a]	106.77 ± 9.95 [b,c]	69.53 ± 0.50 [a]	0.76 ± 0.44 [a]	0.11 ± 0.08 [a]
Mother's educational level							
Intermediate or less	653.90 ± 9.453 [a]	122.48 ± 10.76 [a]	53.28 ± 1.00 [a]	168.61 ± 8.00 [a]	68.87 ± 0.30 [a]	0.92 ± 0.33 [a]	1.95 ± 0.66 [a]
High school/technical diploma	714.72 ± 13.68 [b]	82.44 ± 11.64 [b]	62.03 ± 1.95 [b]	125.89 ± 7.36 [b]	69.31 ± 0.34 [a]	1.06 ± 0.47 [a]	0.04 ± 0.03 [b]
University Degree or more	715.57 ± 14.52 [b,c]	57.33 ± 10.77 [b,c]	61.64 ± 2.14 [b,c]	108.04 ± 7.19 [b,c]	69.48 ± 0.44 [a]	2.30 ± 1.02 [a]	0.13 ± 0.10 [a,b]
Monthly family income (LBP)							
≤1,000,000	647.53 ± 10.90 [a]	144.24 ± 12.73 [a]	54.55 ± 1.21 [a]	162.71 ± 8.15 [a]	68.80 ± 0.31 [a]	0.87 ± 0.47 [a]	0.79 ± 0.34 [a]
1,000,000–1,999,999	698.20 ± 10.88 [b]	69.43 ± 9.15 [b]	59.39 ± 1.65 [b]	135.02 ± 6.56 [b]	69.41 ± 0.31 [a]	1.32 ± 0.43 [a]	0.76 ± 0.42 [a]
≥2,000,000	743.9447 ± 15.53 [c]	48.09 ± 9.49 [b,c]	59.72 ± 1.92 [a,b]	116.72 ± 11.21 [b,c]	69.48 ± 0.52 [a]	2.04 ± 0.87 [a]	1.86 ± 1.20 [a]
Crowding index (person/room)							
<2	696.62 ± 8.40 [a]	85.66 ± 7.30 [a]	58.71 ± 1.09 [a]	137.07 ± 5.79 [a]	69.52 ± 0.24 [a]	1.55 ± 0.42 [a]	0.87 ± 0.37 [a]
≥2	657.64 ± 12.49 [b]	123.56 ± 14.89 [b]	54.91 ± 1.55 [a]	156.28 ± 8.56 [a]	68.20 ± 0.35 [b]	0.56 ± 0.23 [b]	1.29 ± 0.63 [a]
Level of physical activity							
Active	691.14 ± 9.42 [a]	99.56 ± 8.82 [a]	58.13 ± 1.21 [a]	155.08 ± 6.43 [a]	69.85 ± 0.25 [a]	1.41 ± 0.46 [a]	1.44 ± 0.53 [a]
Inactive	677.91 ± 10.37 [a]	91.98 ± 10.48 [a]	57.16 ± 1.35 [a]	125.72 ± 7.14 [b]	68.15 ± 0.32 [b]	1.10 ± 0.36 [a]	0.37 ± 0.23 [a]

* Analyses were carried for the remaining beverages (fruit drinks), fruit juice without sugar (fruit drinks), fruit juice without sugar, bottled vegetable juice, diet soft drinks, sports drinks, alcoholic beverages, and hot beverages) but the results were not presented in this table given the lack of significant associations with physical activity or any SES variable. ** Analyses were conducted for father and mother's employment status but the results were not included in this table since these variables were not significantly associated with water intakes from any beverage. † Analyses were carried for anthropometric variables (including BMI status, and WHtR) in relation to water intakes from beverage sources, but the results were not included in the table due to lack of significant associations. [a,b,c] Statistical comparisons are made within each socioeconomic group and within physical activity levels based on independent samples t-test or ANOVA test with Bonferroni-adjustment. Mean estimates with different superscript letters were significantly different at $p < 0.05$.

Table 4. Energy Intake (kcal/day) from different beverage groups and from all solid foods and their contribution to total energy intake by age group; children aged 4–13 years, Lebanon (n = 752).

	Number of Consumers n (%)	Total		4–8 Years 183 (46.1%)		9–13 Years 214 (53.9%)		p-Value
		Mean ± SE	% of Total EI	Mean ± SE	% of Total EI	Mean ± SE	% of Total EI †	
Total energy intake from all foods and beverages	752 (100)	1924.66 ± 7.45	100	1899.34 ± 8.80 a	100	1947.67 ± 11.66 b	100	0.001
Energy intake from foods only	752 (100)	1741.56 ± 6.34	90.54	1720.68 ± 7.71 a	90.62	1760.54 ± 9.77 b	90.47	0.001
Energy intake from caloric beverages	752 (100)	181.16 ± 1.49	9.36	176.76 ± 1.76 a	9.27	185.17 ± 2.33 b	9.44	0.004
Milk and milk alternatives	752 (100)	56.15 ± 1.24	2.92	58.28 ± 1.94 a	3.07	54.20 ± 1.57 a	2.79 *	0.080
Milk	752 (100)	32.25 ± 1.18	1.67	34.45 ± 1.88 a	1.80	30.25 ± 1.46 a	1.55 *	0.079
Milk alternatives	752 (100)	23.90 ± 0.23	1.25	23.84 ± 0.29 a	1.26	23.95 ± 0.35 a	1.24	0.972
Sodas	752 (100)	60.22 ± 1.98	3.06	48.54 ± 2.12 a	2.51	70.83 ± 3.16 b	3.56 **	<0.001
Regular	752 (100)	59.96 ± 1.98	3.05	48.18 ± 2.13 a	2.49	70.67 ± 3.16 b	3.55 **	<0.001
Diet	68 (9.04)	0.26 ± 0.06	0.01	0.36 ± 0.11 a	0.02	0.17 ± 0.04 a	0.01	0.098
Fruit Juice	752 (100)	71.34 ± 0.82	3.71	73.01 ± 1.30 a	3.85	69.82 ± 1.02 a	3.58 **	0.052
Fresh fruit juice (100% natural)	752 (100)	15.24 ± 0.14	0.80	15.48 ± 0.22 a	0.82	15.02 ± 0.18 a	0.78 *	0.096
Bottled fruit juice (with sugar)/fruit drink	752 (100)	52.51 ± 0.48	2.72	52.92 ± 0.68 a	2.78	52.13 ± 0.67 a	2.67 *	0.406
Bottled fruit juice (without sugar)	41 (5.45)	3.59 ± 0.66	0.18	4.61 ± 1.15 a	0.24	2.67 ± 0.69 a	0.13	0.152
Vegetable juice	50 (6.65)	0.56 ± 0.18	0.03	0.84 ± 0.36 a	0.05	0.30 ± 0.12 a	0.02	0.157
Fresh vegetable juice	42 (5.59)	0.23 ± 0.06	0.01	0.30 ± 0.09 a	0.02	0.16 ± 0.06 a	0.01	0.232
Bottled vegetable juice	8 (1.06)	0.33 ± 0.18	0.02	0.54 ± 0.35 a	0.03	0.14 ± 0.10 a	0.01	0.268
Hot Beverages	752 (100)	0.70 ± 0.01	0.037	0.67 ± 0.01 a	0.03	0.72 ± 0.01 b	0.04 *	0.001
Sports and energy drinks	21 (2.79)	0.75 ± 0.23	0.04	0.31 ± 0.18 a	0.02	1.15 ± 0.40 a	0.06	0.059
Sports drinks	6 (0.80)	0.25 ± 0.14	0.01	0.14 ± 0.14 a	0.01	0.35 ± 0.24 a	0.02	0.463
Energy drinks	18 (2.39)	0.50 ± 0.16	0.02	0.17 ± 0.12 a	0.01	0.80 ± 0.29 b	0.04 *	0.047
Alcoholic beverages	13 (1.73)	0.48 ± 0.25	0.02	0.01 ± 0.01 a	0.00	0.90 ± 0.48 a	0.04 *	0.064

a,b Statistical comparisons were carried out between age groups for the means of energy intake from each beverage type using independent samples t-test. Mean estimates within a row with different superscript letters were significantly different at $p < 0.05$. † Statistical comparisons were conducted between age groups for the means of contribution of different beverages to total energy intake (% EI) using independent samples T-test. * $p \leq 0.05$; ** $p \leq 0.001$.

Nutrients **2016**, 8, 554

Table 5. Patterns of water and beverage consumption amongst 4–13-year-old Lebanese children as compared to data reported by other studies on the same age group.

Present Study (Lebanon)	France [a]		USA [b]		Mexico [c]		Present Study (Lebanon)	
	4–8 years	9–13 years	4–8 years	9–13 years	4–8 years	9–13 years	4–8 years	9–13 years
Total water intake (TWI) (mL/day)	1233	1416	1447	1711	1426.8	1658.4	1600.63	1697.68
Plain water intake (mL/day)	407.6	498.2	364.9	496.1	350.2	426.9	767.32	840.49
Contribution of plain water to TWI (%)	33	35	25.2	29	24.5	25.7	47.61	49.05
Water intake from foods (mL/day)	492.3	555.5	431.4	457.5	504.8	597.2	450.69	460.41
Contribution of foods to TWI (%)	40	39.2%	29.8	26.7	35.4	36.0	28.5	27.7
Water intake from all beverages (mL/day)	740.7	860.6	1015.4	1254	922.1	1061.2	1143.53	1241.62
Contribution of all beverages to TWI (%)	60.1	60.7	70.2	73.3	64.6	64.0	70.85	72.28
Water intake from all beverages (excluding plain water) (mL/day)	333.3	362.4	M: 678 [d] F: 621 [d]	M: 814 [d] F: 702 [d]	571.9 [d]	634.3 [d]	376.2	401.1
Contribution of all beverages (excluding plain water) to TWI (%)	27.0	25.6	M: 46.9 F: 43.0	M: 47.6 F: 41.0	40.1	38.2	23.5	23.6
Beverages with the highest contribution to TWI	4–13 years: Plain water (33%–35%); Milk (13.2%); Fruit juice (5.5%)		Plain Water: 25.2% Milk (20.4%) Fruit drink (7.9%)	Plain Water (29%) Milk (15.7%) Soda (12%)	Plain water: (24.5%) Fruit water (8.8%) Milk (5.5%)	Plain water (25.7%) Fruit water (8.6%) Soda (7%)	Plain water (47.6%) Fruit juice (10.3%) Soda (8.1%)	Plain water (49.05%) Soda: 10.3% Fruit juice (9.5%)
Proportion of children not meeting AI *	89	Boys: 90 Girls: 93	75	Boys: 85 Girls: 83	71	Boys: 83 Girls: 81	74.0	Boys: 92.1 Girls: 97.8
Shortfall compared to AI (mL/day) *	367	Boys: 594 Girls: 587	253	Boys: 633 Girls: 444	273	Boys: 668 Girls: 516	99	Boys: 592 Girls: 533
Water to energy ratio	4–13 years: Boys: 0.75; Girls: 0.77		0.85	Boys: 0.88 Girls: 0.95	0.84	Boys: 0.82 Girls: 0.84	0.84	0.87
Contribution of caloric beverages to total EI (%)	11.5	10.1	19.5	18	19.8	17.5	9.27	9.44

EI: Energy Intake; * USA and Mexico: the AI is based on the IOM; France: the AI is based on EFSA; [a] Vieux et al., 2016 [17]; [b] Drewnowski et al., 2013 [9]; [c] Piernas, C, Barquera, S, and Popkin, BM, 2014 [11]; [d] Calculated from data reported by the studies [9,11].

3.5. Contribution of Various Beverage Sources to Total Daily Energy Intake

As shown in Table 4, on average, older children (9–13 years) had a significantly higher EI from all foods and beverages, foods only, and caloric beverages compared to younger ones (4–8 years old). Foods were found to be the main contributors to EI in both age groups (90.5%–90.6% EI), whereas beverages contributed close to 9% of the daily caloric intake. Overall, beverages with the highest contribution to EI of children aged 4–13 years old included fruit juices (mainly fruit drinks), sodas (regular), and milk and milk alternatives. Compared to their younger counterparts, older children (9–13 years) had significantly higher EIs and higher contribution of specific beverages to total daily EI, including regular sodas, hot beverages, and energy drinks. On the other hand, we observed that the contribution of milk and milk alternatives and fruit juices to total daily EI was significantly higher amongst younger compared to older children ($p < 0.05$).

3.6. Comparison of Water Intakes amongst Children in Lebanon with Other Countries

Table 5 compares the results of this study to those reported from other countries, on the same age group [11,17,38]. Accordingly, TWI amongst 4–8-year-old Lebanese children (1600 mL/day) exceeded that reported for French, American and Mexican children (1233–1447 mL/day), while the intake amongst 9–13 years old was within the range reported from other countries. Water intakes from food sources in Lebanon (450–460 mL/day) were inferior to those reported from Mexico (505–597 mL/day) and France (492–555 mL/day), while the consumption of plain water was the highest in Lebanon (767–840 mL/day), exceeding intake levels reported by other studies (350–498 mL/day). Milk's contribution to TWI was low in Lebanon (3.4%), compared to estimates reported by France and the USA (13%–20%). Conversely, soda was identified as one of the three main contributors to water intake in Lebanese children (8%–10%).

4. Discussion

Based on a nationally representative survey, this study explored total water intake amongst 4–13-year-old children in Lebanon, in comparison to international recommendations, making it the first to report on the intake of this critical nutrient among children from the MENA region. Studies of beverage consumption amongst children have mostly focused on caloric beverages such as milk [39,40], fruit juices [41,42], sweetened beverages [40,42–45], and the amount of dietary energy provided in liquid form [17]. Few studies have investigated patterns of water consumption by age group, sex and socioeconomic status, and even fewer studies have compared water intakes amongst children with the existing recommendations and across various countries [9,11,17,18].

This study showed, in agreement with findings reported by other studies [9,11,17], that total daily water intakes amongst 4–13-year-old Lebanese children were below the existing recommendations. When comparing age groups, the study results indicated that a higher proportion of older children failed to meet the IOM DRI values compared to their younger counterparts (4–8 years old). The shortfalls in total daily water intakes, based on the IOM DRI values, were the highest amongst 9–13-year-old children partly because the AI for water increases with age [46]. Data were reanalyzed using the EFSA AI values and the same observations were noted. When comparing our results to those derived by other studies, Lebanon had the highest proportion of 9–13 years old who did not meet the water intake recommendations, followed by France (90%–93%), USA (83%–85%) and Mexico (81%–83%) [9,11,17]. Gender differentials in water intake were also documented in the present study, with a significantly higher TWI observed amongst boys and a significantly higher proportion of boys meeting the AI values compared to girls. The observed gender differentials in water intakes may be a reflection of the significantly higher proportion of boys engaging in physical activity compared to girls in our study sample (66% vs. 49%, $p < 0.001$, data not shown), and therefore of their higher water needs. As for the water to energy ratio, another indicator of hydration, the study findings showed that the water volume per 1000 kcal ranged between 0.84 and 0.87, which fell short of meeting the desirable IOM recommendations of at least 1 L/1000 kcal. Taken together, the study's findings highlight a substantial gap between existing recommendations and actual water intakes in Lebanese children. This is of concern given the vulnerability of this age group to dehydration and its adverse effects. Children have a higher proportion of body water compared to adults; they are also less heat tolerant and more susceptible to dehydration, especially in hot climates and when engaging in physical activity [1,47]. Available studies suggest that low to moderate levels of dehydration may increase fatigue, decrease alertness and impair cognitive function, which may carry implications on school performance [1,3,4,48,49].

The high proportion of children not meeting the international water intake recommendations in Lebanon as well as in other countries may be at least partly explained by the fact that water consumption tends to be underreported, particularly among children [11,38]. This highlights the need for rigorous investigations on probing methods to collect better water recall data and reduce measurement errors, mainly amongst the pediatric population [1]. It is also important to underscore the scarcity of available research serving as evidence for setting adequate water intake levels, despite the critical importance of water in health and nutrition. While this scarcity may be partially explained by the sophisticated set of neurophysiological adaptations and adjustments that occur over a large range of fluid intake to protect body hydration and osmolality, it remains a challenge for nutrition and public health professionals [1]. In addition, given the extreme inter-individual variability in water needs that are not only determined by differences in metabolism, but also by environmental conditions and physical activities, there may not be a single level of water intake that would assure adequate hydration [1]. Water needs may in fact be influenced by the individual's health status, physical activity, dietary intake, including sodium and protein intake, and environmental factors such as temperature and humidity [38].

In order to better contextualize the observed water intake data, the results of this study were compared to those reported from other countries, for the same age group [9,11,17]. The consumption of plain water was found to be the highest in Lebanon exceeding intake levels reported by other studies and contributing to almost half of TWI. Even though milk appeared as one of the main contributors to TWI in France and the USA (13%–20%), milk's contribution to TWI was low in Lebanon, being estimated at 3.5% in the study sample. On the other hand, soda was identified as one of the three main contributors to water intake in Lebanese children, even amongst the younger age group. Water intakes from food sources were lower than those reported from Mexico and France [11,17], suggesting a lower consumption of low-energy-density foods, such as fruits and vegetables, amongst Lebanese children. For instance, the intake of fruits and vegetables was previously estimated at 87 g/d amongst Lebanese children aged 6–11 years [22], compared to estimates ranging between 141–152 g/day amongst 3–14-year-old French children [50].

The present study has also investigated the association between water intakes and SES. Interestingly, and in contrast to data reported from the USA and Mexico [9,11,38], this study's findings showed that total and plain water intakes were not associated with the household's income. When examining the association between SES and water intakes from specific beverage sources, a higher SES was found to be associated with a healthier pattern of beverage consumption. Several SES indicators, including paternal and maternal education levels, family income and crowding index, converged in showing that water intakes from bottled water increased with increasing SES, while the opposite was observed for sodas and tap water. Available evidence suggests that in Lebanon, tap water may not be safe for consumption as its quality tends to deteriorate during distribution, namely due to cross-contamination by wastewater networks and rusting water conduits [51]. This may explain the observed association between higher SES and bottled water consumption, as households who can afford it will naturally opt for safer sources of water. Higher maternal education was associated with a healthier drinking pattern amongst Lebanese children, characterized by higher water intakes from milk, and lower intakes from soft drinks and energy drinks. These findings are in line with those reported by other studies, where soft drink consumption, dairy product intakes and dietary adequacy amongst children were found to be directly related to maternal education levels [52–54]. This highlights the role of the mother's education and awareness in modulating the family environment, which can have a direct influence on the child's lifestyle and dietary behavior, including fluid consumption [52–54].

In this study, physically active children had higher intakes of total water, which is expected given that their hydration needs are higher. Physically active children were also found to have lower intakes of sodas and higher intakes of fresh fruit juice (no added sugar). These findings are aligned with those reported amongst a national sample of Lebanese adolescents aged 13–19 years, where physically active children were found to follow a healthier dietary pattern compared to those with low levels of physical activity. These observations may suggest that the clustering of behavioral risk factors, including physical inactivity and unbalanced diet, which has been repeatedly described among adults [55], is already apparent as early as the childhood and adolescent years [21]. Even though the present study's findings did not document a protective association of TWI or plain water intake against overweight and obesity, other studies have suggested that higher water intakes may be associated with healthier weight in children [1,14]. This may be of direct relevance to the MENA region that harbors one of the highest rates of childhood obesity in the world. In Lebanon, pediatric obesity is following an alarming escalating trend over time, with the prevalence of obesity increasing from 7.3% to 10.9% in 6–19-year-old children and adolescents, over the past decade [56].

The present study showed that the contribution of beverages to daily dietary EI was close to 9% amongst Lebanese children, which is lower than estimates observed in other countries (10%–20%) [9,11,17]. However, unlike data reported from other studies where milk appeared as the beverage with the highest contribution to EI (7%–11%), Lebanese children's milk intake contributed less than 3% to daily EI. At the same time, soda was identified as the beverage with the second most important contribution to EI in both age groups in Lebanon. These findings suggest that soda consumption may be displacing milk drinking in Lebanese children, which could result in decreased calcium intakes, suboptimal bone health [57], disrupted calcium-phosphorus ratio [58,59], overweight and obesity [60,61].

The strengths of this study include the national representativeness of the sample, the use of a validated FFQ in dietary assessment, and the measurements of anthropometric characteristics by trained dietitians instead of self-reporting. The age cut-off points that were selected for this study (4–8 years and 9–13 years) were intentionally similar to those adopted by the IOM and by EFSA when setting DRIs for children, allowing for direct comparisons with the AI values. The results of the present study should, however, be considered in light of the following limitations. Dietary intake data were collected by means of a FFQ that may be subject to respondent and recall bias. Proxy recall for younger children may represent an additional source of bias. Recall bias may be particularly challenging when exploring water intake among children, who may consume it unconsciously during their regular day (within the school meal, when playing in public playgrounds, during social events, and other venues) [9,11]. In addition, there was no measurement of hydration status validating reported TWI in the present study. Another limitation is the lack of data on the time and occasions of water and beverage consumption throughout the regular day (breakfast vs. lunch vs. dinner and snacking patterns). Future studies need to explore potential differences in water and beverage consumption patterns across various occasions, days of the week, and time of day. Finally, the cross-sectional design of the study allowed us to test associations rather than to assess any causal relationships.

5. Conclusions

In conclusion, even though the intakes of plain water in Lebanon were higher than those reported by other countries, and the contribution of caloric beverages to EI were lower than that observed in other countries, the results of this study showed that an alarming high proportion of Lebanese children failed to meet water intake recommendations. In addition, older children aged 9–13 years, and girls were identified by this study as being at particular risk of water intake inadequacies. These findings raise a public health concern, given the vulnerability of children to dehydration and its potential adverse effects [1]. The study's findings have also shown that, compared to children from high SES, children from a lower socioeconomic background had higher water intakes from soda, energy drinks and tap water coupled with lower water intakes from milk, fresh fruit juice, vegetable juice and bottled water. This socioeconomic gradient should be taken into consideration when planning for intervention strategies aiming at instilling healthy drinking habits at an early age in Lebanon. Future dietary guidelines and policy interventions should promote drinking plain water for daily hydration and nutrient-dense beverages, such as low-fat milk, to contribute further to adequate fluid intake and nutrient adequacy amongst children. This is of particular importance given the magnitude of the shortfall between observed TWI and DRIs. A particular challenge would be the safety of tap water in Lebanon, given that surveillance measures and water quality monitoring are lagging behind in the country. Schools should be encouraged to make safe potable water available to all students, by installing fresh water fountains and providing children with easy access to a non-caloric beverage at no charge [9,17]. Along with improving the availability of safe water, it is crucial to decrease students' access to caloric beverages in the school setting, by limiting the sale and marketing of sugar-sweetened beverages. Supportive educational programs targeting students and parents, as agents of change, are needed to foster healthy drinking patterns early in life [62].

Acknowledgments: The authors express their sincere gratitude to all participating children and their mothers and acknowledge the efforts exerted by field workers for their assistance with data collection. In addition, authors acknowledge Hikma Shoaib and Massar Dabbous for their assistance with data cleaning and statistical analyses as part of this study. The national cross-sectional survey was funded by the Lebanese National Council for Scientific Research, the University Research Board at the American University of Beirut, and Nestle Waters (SEML).

Author Contributions: L.J., N.H., F.N., and L.N. conceptualized the national research study. L.J. coordinated data collection and entry, and conducted data analysis. L.N., L.J., and F.N. drafted the manuscript and contributed to data interpretation. F.C. contributed significantly to the review of the manuscript. All authors read and approved the final manuscript.

Conflicts of Interest: FC is employed by Nestle Waters, France. The funding sponsors had no role in the design of the study; in the collection, analyses, or interpretation of data.

References

1. Popkin, B.M.; D'Anci, K.E.; Rosenberg, I.H. Water, hydration, and health. *Nutr. Rev.* **2010**, *68*, 439–458. [CrossRef] [PubMed]
2. Maughan, R. Impact of mild dehydration on wellness and on exercise performance. *Eur. J. Clin. Nutr.* **2003**, *57*, S19–S23. [CrossRef] [PubMed]
3. Fadda, R.; Rapinett, G.; Grathwohl, D.; Parisi, M.; Fanari, R.; Calò, C.M.; Schmitt, J. Effects of drinking supplementary water at school on cognitive performance in children. *Appetite* **2012**, *59*, 730–737. [CrossRef] [PubMed]
4. Perry, C.S.; Rapinett, G.; Glaser, N.S.; Ghetti, S. Hydration status moderates the effects of drinking water on children's cognitive performance. *Appetite* **2015**, *95*, 520–527. [CrossRef] [PubMed]
5. Manz, F. Hydration in children. *J. Am. Coll. Nutr.* **2007**, *26*, 562S–569S. [CrossRef] [PubMed]
6. Manz, F.; Wentz, A.; Sichert-Hellert, W. The most essential nutrient: Defining the adequate intake of water. *J. Pediatr.* **2002**, *141*, 587–592. [CrossRef] [PubMed]
7. Institute of Medicine (IOM). Dietary Reference Intakes Tables and Applications. Available online: http://www.nationalacademies.org/hmd/Activities/Nutrition/SummaryDRIs/DRI-Tables.aspx (accessed on 8 July 2016).
8. European Food Safety Authority (EFSA). Scientific opinion on dietary reference values for water. Efsa panel on dietetic products, nutrition, and allergies. *ESFA J.* **2010**, *8*. [CrossRef]
9. Drewnowski, A.; Rehm, C.D.; Constant, F. Water and beverage consumption among children age 4–13 years in the united states: Analyses of 2005–2010 nhanes data. *Nutr. J.* **2013**, *12*. [CrossRef] [PubMed]
10. Institute of Medicine. *Dietary Reference Intakes for Water, Potassium, Sodium, Chloride, and Sulfate*; National Academies Press: Washington, DC, USA, 2004.

11. Piernas, C.; Barquera, S.; Popkin, B.M. Current patterns of water and beverage consumption among mexican children and adolescents aged 1–18 years: Analysis of the mexican national health and nutrition survey 2012. *Public Health Nutr.* **2014**, *17*, 2166–2175. [CrossRef] [PubMed]

12. Stookey, J.D.; Constant, F.; Gardner, C.D.; Popkin, B.M. Replacing sweetened caloric beverages with drinking water is associated with lower energy intake. *Obesity* **2007**, *15*, 3013–3022. [CrossRef] [PubMed]

13. Stookey, J.D.; Constant, F.; Popkin, B.M.; Gardner, C.D. Drinking water is associated with weight loss in overweight dieting women independent of diet and activity. *Obesity* **2008**, *16*, 2481–2488. [CrossRef] [PubMed]

14. Daniels, M.C.; Popkin, B.M. Impact of water intake on energy intake and weight status: A systematic review. *Nutr. Rev.* **2010**, *68*, 505–521. [CrossRef] [PubMed]

15. Stookey, J.D. Drinking water and weight management. *Nutr. Today* **2010**, *45*, S7–S12. [CrossRef]

16. Park, S.; Blanck, H.M.; Sherry, B.; Brener, N.; O'Toole, T. Factors associated with low water intake among us high school students—National youth physical activity and nutrition study, 2010. *J. Am. Diet. Assoc.* **2012**, *112*, 1421–1427. [CrossRef] [PubMed]

17. Vieux, F.; Maillot, M.; Constant, F.; Drewnowski, A. Water and beverage consumption among children aged 4–13 years in France: Analyses of INCA 2 (etude individuelle nationale des consommations alimentaires 2006–2007) data. *Public Health Nutr.* **2016**, *19*, 2305–2314. [CrossRef] [PubMed]

18. Iglesia, I.; Santaliestra-Pasías, A.; Bel-Serrat, S.; Sadalla-Collese, T.; Miguel-Berges, M.; Moreno, L. Fluid consumption, total water intake and first morning urine osmolality in spanish adolescents from zaragoza: Data from the HELENA study. *Eur. J. Clin. Nutr.* **2015**, *70*, 541–547. [CrossRef] [PubMed]

19. Akpata, E.S.; Behbehani, J.; Akbar, J.; Thalib, L.; Mojiminiyi, O. Fluoride intake from fluids and urinary fluoride excretion by young children in kuwait: A non-fluoridated community. *Community Dent. Oral. Epidemiol.* **2014**, *42*, 224–233. [CrossRef] [PubMed]

20. Bello, L.; Al-hammad, N. Pattern of fluid consumption in a sample of saudi arabian adolescents aged 12–13 years. *Int. J. Paediat. Dent.* **2006**, *16*, 168–173. [CrossRef] [PubMed]

21. Naja, F.; Hwalla, N.; Itani, L.; Karam, S.; Sibai, A.M.; Nasreddine, L. A western dietary pattern is associated with overweight and obesity in a national sample of lebanese adolescents (13–19 years): A cross-sectional study. *Br. J. Nutr.* **2015**, *114*, 1909–1919. [CrossRef] [PubMed]

22. Nasreddine, L.; Naja, F.; Akl, C.; Chamieh, M.C.; Karam, S.; Sibai, A.-M.; Hwalla, N. Dietary, lifestyle and socio-economic correlates of overweight, obesity and central adiposity in lebanese children and adolescents. *Nutrients* **2014**, *6*, 1038–1062. [CrossRef] [PubMed]

23. Central Administration of Statistics (CAS) Lebanon. Population Characteristics in 2007. Available online: http://www.cas.gov.lb/index.php/demographic-and-social-en/population-en (accessed on 11 July 2016).

24. Melki, I.S. Household crowding index: A correlate of socioeconomic status and inter-pregnancy spacing in an urban setting. *J. Epidemiol. Community Health* **2004**, *58*, 476–480. [CrossRef] [PubMed]

25. Goodyear, R.F.A.; Hay, J. Finding the crowding index that works best for new zealand: Applying different crowding indexes to census of population and dwellings data for 1986–2006. *Statistics N. Zeal.* **2012**, *4*, 1–50.

26. Naja, F.; Nasreddine, L.; Itani, L.; Chamieh, M.C.; Adra, N.; Sibai, A.M.; Hwalla, N. Dietary patterns and their association with obesity and sociodemographic factors in a national sample of lebanese adults. *Public Health Nutr.* **2011**, *14*, 1570–1578. [CrossRef] [PubMed]

27. Naja, F.; Nasreddine, L.; Itani, L.; Dimassi, H.; Sibai, A.M.; Hwalla, N. Dietary patterns in cardiovascular diseases prevention and management: Review of the evidence and recommendations for primary care physicians in Lebanon. *J. Med. Liban* **2014**, *62*, 92–99. [CrossRef] [PubMed]

28. Maffeis, C.; Banzato, C.; Talamini, G.; Obesity Study Group of the Italian. Waist-to-height ratio, a useful index to identify high metabolic risk in overweight children. *J. Pediatr.* **2008**, *152*, 207–213. [CrossRef] [PubMed]

29. McCarthy, H.D.; Ashwell, M. A study of central fatness using waist-to-height ratios in UK children and adolescents over two decades supports the simple message—'Keep your waist circumference to less than half your height'. *Int. J. Obes.* **2006**, *30*, 988–992. [CrossRef] [PubMed]

30. Corder, K.; van Sluijs, E.M.; Wright, A.; Whincup, P.; Wareham, N.J.; Ekelund, U. Is it possible to assess free-living physical activity and energy expenditure in young people by self-report? *Am. J. Clin. Nutr.* **2009**, *89*, 862–870. [CrossRef] [PubMed]

31. Coledam, D.H.C.; Ferraiol, P.F.; Júnior, R.P.; Ribeiro, E.A.G.; Ferreira, M.A.C.; de Oliveira, A.R. Agreement between two cutoff points for physical activity and associated factors in young individuals. *Rev. Paul. Pediatr. (Engl. Ed.)* **2014**, *32*, 215–222.

32. United States Department of Health and Human Services. 2008 Physical Activity Guidelines for Americans. Available online: https://health.gov/paguidelines/pdf/paguide.pdf (accessed on 11 July 2016).

33. Moghames, P.; Hammami, N.; Hwalla, N.; Yazbeck, N.; Shoaib, H.; Nasreddine, L.; Naja, F. Validity and reliability of a food frequency questionnaire to estimate dietary intake among Lebanese children. *Nutr. J.* **2016**, *15*. [CrossRef] [PubMed]

34. Posner, B.M.; Smigelski, C.; Duggal, A.; Morgan, J.; Cobb, J.; Cupples, L. Validation of two-dimensional models for estimation of portion size in nutrition research. *J. Am. Diet. Assoc.* **1992**, *92*, 738–741. [PubMed]

35. Naja, F.; Hwalla, N.; Itani, L.; Salem, M.; Azar, S.T.; Zeidan, M.N.; Nasreddine, L. Dietary patterns and odds of type 2 diabetes in Beirut, Lebanon: A case–control study. *Nutr. Metab.* **2012**, *9*. [CrossRef] [PubMed]

36. United States Department of Agriculture (USDA). Usda Food Composition Database. Available online: https://ndb.nal.usda.gov/ (accessed on 11 July 2016).

37. Pellett, P.L.; Shadarevian, S. *Food Composition Tables for Use in the Middle East*; American University of Beirut: Beirut, Lebanon, 1970.

38. Drewnowski, A.; Rehm, C.D.; Constant, F. Water and beverage consumption among adults in the United States: Cross-sectional study using data from NHANES 2005–2010. *BMC Public Health* **2013**, *13*. [CrossRef] [PubMed]

39. Fulgoni, V.L.; Quann, E.E. National trends in beverage consumption in children from birth to 5 years: Analysis of NHANES across three decades. *Nutr. J.* **2012**, *11*. [CrossRef] [PubMed]

40. Collison, K.S.; Zaidi, M.Z.; Subhani, S.N.; Al-Rubeaan, K.; Shoukri, M.; Al-Mohanna, F.A. Sugar-sweetened carbonated beverage consumption correlates with BMI, waist circumference, and poor dietary choices in school children. *BMC Public Health* **2010**, *10*. [CrossRef] [PubMed]

41. Drewnowski, A.; Rehm, C.D. Socioeconomic gradient in consumption of whole fruit and 100% fruit juice among US children and adults. *Nutr. J.* **2015**, *14*. [CrossRef] [PubMed]

42. Sayegh, A.; Dini, E.; Holt, R.; Bedi, R. Food and drink consumption, sociodemographic factors and dental caries in 4–5-year-old children in Amman, Jordan. *Br. Dent. J.* **2002**, *193*, 37–42. [CrossRef] [PubMed]

43. O'Connor, T.M.; Yang, S.-J.; Nicklas, T.A. Beverage intake among preschool children and its effect on weight status. *Pediatrics* **2006**, *118*, e1010–e1018. [CrossRef] [PubMed]

44. Oza-Frank, R.; Zavodny, M.; Cunningham, S.A. Beverage displacement between elementary and middle school, 2004–2007. *J. Am. Diet. Assoc.* **2012**, *112*, 1390–1396. [CrossRef] [PubMed]

45. Ali, H.I.; Ng, S.W.; Zaghloul, S.; Harrison, G.G.; Qazaq, H.S.; El Sadig, M.; Yeatts, K. High proportion of 6 to 18-year-old children and adolescents in the United Arab Emirates are not meeting dietary recommendations. *Nutr. Res.* **2013**, *33*, 447–456. [CrossRef] [PubMed]

46. Senterre, C.; Dramaix, M.; Thiébaut, I. Fluid intake survey among schoolchildren in Belgium. *BMC Public Health* **2014**, *14*. [CrossRef] [PubMed]

47. British Nutrition Foundation. Hydration for Children. Available online: https://www.nutrition.org.uk/healthyliving/hydration/hydration-forchildren.html (accessed on 20 July 2016).

48. Bar-Or, O.; Dotan, R.; Inbar, O.; Rotshtein, A.; Zonder, H. Voluntary hypohydration in 10- to 12-year-old boys. *J. Appl. Physiol.* **1980**, *48*, 104–108. [PubMed]

49. Benton, D.; Braun, H.; Cobo, J.; Edmonds, C.; Elmadfa, I.; El-Sharkawy, A.; Feehally, J.; Gellert, R.; Holdsworth, J.; Kapsokefalou, M. Executive summary and conclusions from the European hydration institute expert conference on human hydration, health, and performance. *Nutr. Rev.* **2015**, *73*, 148–150. [CrossRef] [PubMed]

50. Lioret, S.; Dubuisson, C.; Dufour, A.; Touvier, M.; Calamassi-Tran, G.; Maire, B.; Volatier, J.-L.; Lafay, L. Trends in food intake in French children from 1999 to 2007: Results from the INCA (étude individuelle nationale des consommations alimentaires) dietary surveys. *Br. J. Nutr.* **2010**, *103*, 585–601. [CrossRef] [PubMed]

51. Ministry of Environment/LEDO. *Lebanon State of the Environment Report*; 2001; pp. 109–129. Available online: http://www.moe.gov.lb/ledo/soer2001pdf/preface.pdf (accessed on 22 July 2016).

52. Vereecken, C.; Maes, L. Young children's dietary habits and associations with the mothers' nutritional knowledge and attitudes. *Appetite* **2010**, *54*, 44–51. [CrossRef] [PubMed]

53. Patrick, H.; Nicklas, T.A. A review of family and social determinants of children's eating patterns and diet quality. *J. Am. Coll. Nutr.* **2005**, *24*, 83–92. [CrossRef] [PubMed]

54. De Coen, V.; Vansteelandt, S.; Maes, L.; Huybrechts, I.; De Bourdeaudhuij, I.; Vereecken, C. Parental socioeconomic status and soft drink consumption of the child. The mediating proportion of parenting practices. *Appetite* **2012**, *59*, 76–80. [CrossRef] [PubMed]

55. Naja, F.; Hwalla, N.; Itani, L.; Baalbaki, S.; Sibai, A.; Nasreddine, L. A novel mediterranean diet index from lebanon: Comparison with Europe. *Eur. J. Nutr.* **2015**, *54*, 1229–1243. [CrossRef] [PubMed]

56. Nasreddine, L.; Naja, F.; Chamieh, M.C.; Adra, N.; Sibai, A.-M.; Hwalla, N. Trends in overweight and obesity in Lebanon: Evidence from two national cross-sectional surveys (1997 and 2009). *BMC Public Health* **2012**, *12*. [CrossRef] [PubMed]

57. NIH Consensus Panel. Nih consensus development on optimal calcium intake. *J. Am. Med. Assoc.* **1994**, *272*, 1942–1948.

58. Rampersaud, G.C.; Bailey, L.B.; Kauwell, G.P. National survey beverage consumption data for children and adolescents indicate the need to encourage a shift toward more nutritive beverages. *J. Am. Diet. Assoc.* **2003**, *103*, 97–100. [CrossRef] [PubMed]

59. Nielsen, S.J.; Popkin, B.M. Changes in beverage intake between 1977 and 2001. *Am. J. Prev. Med.* **2004**, *27*, 205–210. [CrossRef] [PubMed]

60. Tam, C.S.; Garnett, S.P.; Cowell, C.T.; Campbell, K.; Cabrera, G.; Baur, L.A. Soft drink consumption and excess weight gain in australian school students: Results from the nepean study. *Int. J. Obes.* **2006**, *30*, 1091–1093. [CrossRef] [PubMed]

61. Must, A.; Barish, E.; Bandini, L. Modifiable risk factors in relation to changes in BMI and fatness: What have we learned from prospective studies of school-aged children&quest. *Int. J. Obes.* **2009**, *33*, 705–715.

62. Abi, H.G.; Lahham, S.N.; Afifi, R. Jarrib Baleha—A pilot nutrition intervention to increase water intake and decrease soft drink consumption among school children in Beirut. *J. Med. Liban* **2010**, *59*, 55–64.

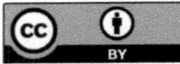

nutrients

MDPI

Article

Water Intake in a Sample of Greek Adults Evaluated with the Water Balance Questionnaire (WBQ) and a Seven-Day Diary

Adelais Athanasatou, Olga Malisova, Aikaterini Kandyliari and Maria Kapsokefalou *

Unit of Human Nutrition, Department of Food Science and Human Nutrition, Agricultural University of Athens, 75 Iera Odos Str., Athens 11855, Greece; dathanasatou@gmail.com (A.A.); olgamalisova@yahoo.gr (O.M.); katerinakand@hotmail.com (A.K.)
* Correspondence: kapsok@aua.gr; Tel.: +30-210-529-4708

Received: 28 July 2016; Accepted: 5 September 2016; Published: 10 September 2016

Abstract: Awareness on the importance of hydration in health has created an unequivocal need to enrich knowledge on water intake of the general population and on the contribution of beverages to total water intake. We evaluated in the past water intake in a sample of Greek adults using two approaches. In study A, volunteers completed the Water Balance Questionnaire (WBQ), a food frequency questionnaire, designed to evaluate water intake (n = 1092; 48.1% males; 43 ± 18 years). In study B, a different population of volunteers recorded water, beverage, and food intake in seven-day diaries (n = 178; 51.1% males; 37 ± 12 years). Herein, data were reanalyzed with the objective to reveal the contribution of beverages in total water intake with these different methodologies. Beverage recording was grouped in the following categories: Hot beverages; milk; fruit and vegetable juices; caloric soft drinks; diet soft drinks; alcoholic drinks; other beverages; and water. Total water intake and water intake from beverages was 3254 (SE 43) mL/day and 2551 (SE 39) mL/day in study A; and 2349 (SE 59) mL/day and 1832 (SE 56) mL/day in study B. In both studies water had the highest contribution to total water intake, approximately 50% of total water intake, followed by hot beverages (10% of total water intake) and milk (5% of total water intake). These two approaches contribute information on water intake in Greece and highlight the contribution of different beverages; moreover, they point out differences in results obtained from different methodologies attributed to limitations in their use.

Keywords: total water intake; beverages consumption; seven-day diary record; water balance questionnaire

---

1. Introduction

Reports that linked hydration with the maintenance of normal physical and cognitive functions [1] engendered the need for data on hydration of the general population and for public health advice on water intake.

Hydration reflects balance between water intake and loss. Water intake consists of water from a variety of sources; namely, drinking water, beverages, and fluid and solid foods. In most studies, drinking water and beverages contribute approximately 80%, and solid and fluid foods approximately 20% to water intake [2–4]. Water loss consists mainly from excretion of water in urine, respiratory water, feces, and sweat [2].

New studies focus on evaluating water intake in the general population in different countries using either new data or retrospective analyses of older studies, thus building information on water intake worldwide [4–8]. For example, total water intake is 1307 mL/day in adults aged 20–54 years, and 1198 mL/day in senior adults in France [6,9], and 3563 mL/day in the USA [10].

Overall, these differences are expected to some extent because water intake reflects environmental conditions and physical activity levels [11] that vary in different countries or population groups. Moreover, water intake is influenced by diverse dietary habits, the availability of a variety of beverages in local markets, and the adoption of drinking-friendly policies in public and private spaces (schools, working environments, hospitals, etc.). In this context, the recording of information on the contribution of different beverages in total water intake deserves attention. For example, in many countries drinking water is the most popular beverage [9,10] but in others, such as in the UK, hot beverages [5] are preferable.

Apart from differences amongst countries, the methodological tools used for evaluating water intake in these studies are inconsistent, some use seven-day diaries, 24 h recalls, or food frequency questionnaires [12]. Moreover, most of these studies used tools that were not specifically designed to evaluate water intake. Therefore, they may not fully capture the consumption of water or of other beverages [13].

Limited information on fluid intake is available for the Greek population [3,8,14]. Cohort studies conducted in Greece do not include the evaluation of water intake [15–17]. We have conducted two studies in the past with the objective to evaluate water intake in a sample of the Greek population. In these studies we analyzed total water intake without specific reference to the variety of beverages consumed. There is a need to obtain this important information because a higher variety has been linked to a higher total water intake [5]. Moreover, these studies used different methodologies; the study of Malisova et al. [8] used the WBQ [18], a semi-quantified food frequency questionnaire and the study of Malisova et al. [3] used a 7-day diary record. There is a need to carefully observe and comment on the use of different tools in the evaluation of water intake.

The objectives of the present study were to reanalyze the existing databases in order: (a) to report water intake and the type of beverages consumed in a sample of Greek adults using a food frequency questionnaire and a seven-day diary; and (b) to compare the water intake recorded from these two approaches, i.e., a semi-quantified food and fluids frequency questionnaire or a seven-day diary record.

2. Materials and Methods

We reanalyzed data from two existing databases; data were obtained from a semi-quantified food frequency questionnaire (study A), and from seven-day diaries (study B). The sample of studies A and B is composed of different subjects. A total of 1270 subjects from the metropolitan area of Athens (Greece) were included in these analyses.

In Study A [8] we used the Water Balance Questionnaire (WBQ) [18], a self-administrated semi-quantified food frequency questionnaire specially designed and validated with urine hydration biomarkers and three-day diaries to estimate water intake from all sources. The exclusion criteria were disease in relation to water balance, including urinary tract infection, kidney disease, and diabetes. All volunteers were informed on the objectives of the study and the procedures involved, and signed an informed consent. In 1092 healthy subjects 18–75 years (age: 43 ± 18 years; males 48.1%) water intake was estimated from the consumption of fifty-eight foods and from drinking water or beverages recorded in detail as glasses, bottles, or cups consumed per day. Employment status, education level, and levels of physical activity estimated from the International Physical Activity Questionnaire (IPAQ) questionnaire [19] were also considered. Height and weight of subjects was measured. Water from solid and fluid foods, recorded from the WBQ, was calculated using data from the USDA National Nutrient Database by multiplying the content in water given from the USDA of any food or beverage (in g or mL) with the portion size (in g or mL) and the number of times that the portion was consumed in the last month.

In study B [3] we used a seven-day diary to record detailed information on foods, and beverages intake. The study protocol had a 24 h urine collection for the same seven days in order to assess hydration status. Exclusion criteria were disease (diabetes insipidus, renal, liver, gastrointestinal, cardiac, pulmonary, or muscle-skeletal diseases), pregnancy, lactation, hypertension, taking diuretic drugs, and following a high-protein or hypocaloric diet. Written informed consent was obtained from all subjects. The recruitment strategy included invitations sent by email to the non-academic and academic personnel; uploaded on social media and published in local newspapers; uploaded on internet sites related to nutrition; and sent by email to other academic and social work institutions. A total of 178 healthy subjects 18–65 years (age: 37 ± 12 years; males 51.1%) recorded the type and amount of food and/or fluid consumption, time, and place immediately after it happened in order to avoid misreporting. Employment status, education level, tobacco use, and levels of physical activity estimated from the International Physical Activity Questionnaire (IPAQ) questionnaire [19] were also considered. Height and weight of subjects was measured. Water from solid and fluid foods, recorded from the seven-day diaries was calculated using the data from the Diet Analysis plus version 6.1 software (ESHA Research, Wadsworth Publishing Co. Inc., Salem, OR, USA).

2.1. Data Analysis

(a) Subjects from studies A and B with anomalous values of energy intake [20] were excluded from the analyses; below 500 calories for females and 800 calories for males, above 3500 calories for females and 4000 calories for males.

(b) Beverage consumption was combined in the eight following categories: (1) hot beverages (including tea and coffee); (2) milk (including regular, light, and chocolate milk); (3) fruit and vegetable juices (including nectar, fresh, and mix juices); (4) caloric soft drinks; (5) diet soft drinks; (6) alcoholic drinks; (7) water (including tap and bottled); and (8) other beverages (i.e., non-alcoholic beer). Total water intake was calculated from the moisture content in foods and the total beverages intake. Beverage intake was the sum of the amounts of these eight categories.

(c) The variety score was calculated as the sum of the beverages consumed from the eight different categories with a minimum value of "0" and a maximum value of "8".

(d) Daily water intake of males and females was compared to the European Food Safety Authority (EFSA) Dietary Reference Values for Adequate Intake of water for males and females (2.5 L and 2.0 L, respectively) [2]. Nordic and German-speaking countries take the approach of inadequate water intake when it is less than 1 g per kilocalorie of energy requirement [2]. Therefore, we used three approaches to define adequate water intake in order to estimate the proportion of subjects that have a low total water intake. A classification based on the adequate intake value, defined by the EFSA, was considered as Criterion 1. Criterion 2 was considered as a ratio of total water intake and energy intake higher than 1. The combination of both (Criterion 1 and 2) was considered as the final criterion (Criterion 3).

2.2. Statistics

Continuous variables are expressed as the mean (standard error) for variables following normal distribution. Normal distribution of all continuous variables was tested with the Shapiro–Wilk parametric test or graphically assessed by histograms. All variables were found to be normal. Correlations were evaluated using Pearson's correlation coefficient. Partial correlations between water intake, energy intake, and beverage consumption adjusted for age, gender, body weight, and physical activity were calculated by the use of a variety score. Differences between genders and age groups were observed using Student's *t*-test. We deemed statistical significance at $\alpha = 0.05$. Statistical analysis was performed by SPSS package, version 18 (SPSS Inc., Chicago, IL, USA).

3. Results

The age, gender distribution, and characteristics in details of subjects of study A are presented in Table 1.

Table 1. Descriptive characteristics of subjects that completed the WBQ (*n* = 1092).

			Total	%	Male	%	Female	%
		Total	1092	100	532	48.1	575	51.9
Age (years)	18–39	Count	488	44.7	230	44.1	258	45.3
	40–64	Count	390	35.7	187	35.8	203	35.6
	65–75	Count	214	19.6	105	20.1	109	19.1
Unemployed		Count	139	13.2	61	12.0	78	14.1
Level of physical activity	Inactive	Count	71	6.4	37	7.0	34	5.9
	Active	Count	1036	93.6	495	93.0	541	94.1
Level of education	Primary or less	Count	129	14.1	47	10.8	82	17.2
	Secondary	Count	240	26.3	131	30.1	109	22.8
	Tertiary or University	Count	544	59.6	257	59.1	287	60.0
Weight (kg)		Mean (SE)	72.1 (0.4)		81.2 (0.5)		63.6 (0.5)	
Height (cm)		Mean (SE)	169.5 (0.3)		176.2 (0.3)		163.1 (0.3)	
BMI (kg/m^2)		Mean (SE)	25.07 (0.12)		26.22 (0.16)		23.98 (0.18)	
BMI class (kg/m^2)	Underweight	Count	28	2.8	3	0.6	25	4.8
	Normal weight	Count	513	50.9	188	38.6	325	62.5
	Overweight	Count	351	34.9	218	44.8	133	25.6
	Obese	Count	115	11.4	78	16.0	37	7.1

The contribution of foods and beverages in detail to water intake (g/day) and energy intake (kcal/day) are presented in Table 2. Mean water intake was 3387 g/day (SE 46), while for males, was 3531 g/day (SE 71), and for females was 3253 g/day (SE 58). Beverage contribution to water intake was 78%, 80%, and 78% for the total sample, males, and females respectively. Mean energy intake was 1911 kcal/day (SE 26) for the total sample, 1975 kcal/day (SE 45) for males, and 1852 kcal/day (SE 31) for females, while the contribution of beverages to total energy intake was 24%, 26%, and 22% for the total sample, males, and females respectively. Finally, water was the most popular beverage consumed, followed by hot beverages, alcoholic drinks, and milk (Table 2).

Table 3 presents the contribution of foods and beverages in detail to water intake (g/day) and energy intake (kcal/day) by age groups for each gender. Differences were observed between two age groups for both genders for total water intake ($p < 0.001$), for water from beverages ($p < 0.001$) and for total beverages consumption ($p < 0.001$). Differences were also observed for beverage types, in particular for fruit and vegetable juices, for caloric soft drinks, for water, and for other non-alcoholic beverages.

Correlations between water intake, energy intake, and beverage consumption were highlighted in Table 4. Total water intake was strongly correlated with energy intake from beverages and total energy intake ($r = 0.636$, $r = 0.618$), while water intake from beverages was correlated moderately with energy intake from beverages ($r = 0.589$). Positive correlations were observed amongst total water intake and water intake from beverages ($r = 0.914$), and beverage weight ($r = 0.957$). Fruit and vegetable juice, alcoholic drinks, and water had a moderate correlation with total water ($r = 0.389$, 0.461 and 0.687, respectively). Additionally, caloric soft drinks and alcoholic drinks had a moderate correlation with total energy intake ($r = 0.309$, $r = 0.516$). The variety score was positively correlated with total water intake and water intake from beverages ($p < 0.001$ in both cases).

Table 5 presents detailed characteristics for the population of study B.

Table 2. Contribution of food and beverages to total water and energy intake of subjects using the WBQ (n = 1092).

		Total Weight Consumed (g/Day) GRAMS				Contribution to Energy Intake (kcal/Day) KCAL				Contribution to Water Intake (g/Day) WATER			
	Count	Total	Male	Female	p^1	Total	Male	Female	p^2	Total	Male	Female	p^3
		1107	532	575		1107	532	575		1107	532	575	
All food and drink Mean (SE)		3387 (46)	3531 (71)	3253 (58)	<0.01	1911 (26)	1975 (45)	1852 (31)	0.02	3254 (43)	3404 (66)	3116 (55)	0.001
Food only Mean (SE)		831 (14)	817 (22)	843 (18)	0.37	1453 (21)	1471 (35)	1437 (26)	0.43	706 (12)	683 (19)	727 (16)	0.07
Beverages only Mean (SE)		2668 (40)	2826 (62)	2522 (50)	<0.01	460 (12)	508 (20)	416 (12)	<0.001	2551 (39)	2725 (61)	2390 (50)	<0.001
Hot beverages Mean (SE)		283 (9)	261 (12)	304 (12)	0.12	149 (4)	141 (7)	157 (6)	0.08	330 (9)	307 (13)	351 (13)	0.02
Milk Mean (SE)		176 (6)	175 (10)	178 (8)	0.84	115 (5)	113 (6)	116 (6)	0.66	160 (6)	158 (9)	162 (7)	0.69
Fruit and Vegetable Juices Mean (SE)		128 (8)	138 (12)	119 (11)	0.23	65 (4)	69 (6)	61 (5)	0.34	119 (7)	126 (11)	112 (9)	0.34
Caloric soft drink Mean (SE)		71 (5)	89 (8)	54 (5)	<0.001	27 (2)	34 (3)	21 (2)	<0.001	64 (4)	80 (7)	48 (4)	<0.001
Diet soft drink Mean (SE)		58 (4)	57 (6)	58 (6)	0.86	5 (0)	7 (1)	4 (0.4)	<0.001	52 (4)	47 (5)	57 (7)	0.25
Alcohol Mean (SE)		267 (17)	310 (29)	227 (18)	0.14	95 (8)	140 (15)	54 (5)	<0.001	146 (13)	215 (26)	82 (8)	<0.001
Water Mean (SE)		1671 (30)	1779 (43)	1571 (40)	<0.001	-	-	-	<0.01	1671 (30)	1779 (43)	1571 (40)	<0.001
Other non-alcoholic beverages Mean (SE)		15 (2)	20 (3)	10 (1)	<0.01	3 (0)	5 (1)	5 (1)		9 (1)	14 (2)	5 (1)	<0.001

p-values derived through Student's t-test between genders.

Table 3. Total water intake and beverage consumption (g/day) by age group of subjects using the WBQ (n = 1092).

	Male				Female			
	Age Group (Years)				Age Group (Years)			
		18-64	65-75	p¹		18-64	65-75	p²
	(A)	(B)	(C)		(D)	(E)	(F)	
	532	419	103		575	466	104	
Total Water intake from food and beverages mean (SE)	3404 (66)	3568 (75)	3030 (104)	<0.001	3116 (55)	3243 (62)	2658 (110)	<0.001
Water from food mean (SE)	683 (19)	683 (22)	738 (33)	0.24	727 (16)	738 (17)	693 (42)	0.27
Water from beverages mean (SE)	2725 (61)	2886 (69)	2315 (100)	<0.001	2390 (50)	2505 (57)	1997 (83)	<0.001
Total beverages consumption mean (g/day) (SE)	2826 (62)	3012 (70)	2323 (97)	<0.001	2522 (50)	2656 (56)	1997 (84)	<0.001
of which (g/day)								
Hot beverages mean (g/day) (SE)	307 (13)	265 (13)	269 (30)	0.89	351 (13)	317 (14)	260 (26)	0.08
Milk mean (g/day) (SE)	158 (9)	179 (11)	178 (19)	0.98	162 (7)	180 (9)	174 (20)	0.76
Fruit and Vegetable Juices mean (g/day) (SE)	126 (11)	158 (14)	72 (12)	<0.001	112 (9)	131 (13)	74 (15)	0.04
Caloric soft drink mean (g/day) (SE)	80 (7)	101 (10)	49 (8)	<0.001	48 (4)	61 (6)	26 (7)	<0.001
Diet soft drink mean (g/day) (SE)	47 (5)	56 (6)	65 (17)	0.62	57 (4)	61 (6)	43 (16)	0.21
Alcohol mean (g/day) (SE)	215 (26)	329 (34)	264 (58)	0.34	82 (8)	255 (21)	91 (21)	<0.001
Water mean (g/day) (SE)	1779 (43)	1900 (50)	1442 (61)	<0.001	1571 (40)	1640 (47)	1323 (62)	<0.01
Other non-alcoholic beverages mean (g/day) (SE)	14 (2)	25 (4)	1 (1)	<0.001	5 (1)	11 (6)	2 (2)	0.07

p-values derived through Student's t-test age groups.

Table 4. Partial correlations between water intake, energy intake and beverage consumption adjusted for age, gender, body weight, and physical activity using the WBQ (n = 1092).

	Total Water (from Food and Beverages) (g/Day)	Total Water from Beverages (g/Day)	Total Water from Food (g/Day)	Total Food Weight (g/Day)	Total Beverages Weight (g/Day)	Total Energy (kcal)	Total Energy from Food (kcal/Day)	Total Energy (kcal/Day)	Total Energy from Food (kcal/Day)	Total Energy (kcal/Day) from Beverages
Total water (g/day) (from food and beverages)	1	0.914 **	0.371 **	0.461 **	0.957 **	0.618 **	0.354 **	0.618 **	0.354 **	0.636 **
Total water (g/day) from beverages	0.914 **	1	0.117 **	0.167 **	0.958 **	0.493 **	0.089 **	0.493 **	0.089 **	0.589 **
Total water (g/day) from food	0.371 **	0.117 **	1	0.808 **	0.146 **	0.337 **	0.730 **	0.337 **	0.730 **	0.143 **
Total food weight (g/day)	0.461 **	0.167 **	0.808 **	1	0.184 **	0.370 **	0.781 **	0.370 **	0.781 **	0.238 **
Total beverages weight (g/day)	0.957 **	0.958 **	0.146 **	0.184 **	1	0.563 **	0.136 **	0.563 **	0.136 **	0.627 **
Total energy (kcal)	0.618 **	0.493 **	0.337 **	0.370 **	0.563 **	1	0.438 **	1	0.438 **	0.523 **
Total energy (kcal) from food	0.354 **	0.089 **	0.730 **	0.781 **	0.136 **	0.438 **	1	0.438 **	1	0.189 **
Total energy (kcal) from beverages	0.636 **	0.589 **	0.143 **	0.238 **	0.627 **	0.523 **	0.189 **	0.523 **	0.189 **	1
(1) Hot beverages (g/day)	0.297 **	0.222 **	0.165 **	0.235 **	0.252 **	0.144 **	0.153 **	0.144 **	0.153 **	0.395 **
(2) Milk (g/day)	0.147 **	0.111 **	0.165 **	0.172 **	0.107 **	0.104 **	0.156 **	0.104 **	0.156 **	0.229 **
(3) Fruit and vegetable juice (g/day)	0.389 **	0.379 **	0.082 *	0.097 **	0.400 **	0.309 **	0.097 **	0.309 **	0.097 **	0.568 **
(4) Caloric soft drink (g/day)	0.224 **	0.230 **	-0.038	0.028	0.239 **	0.216 **	0.038	0.216 **	0.038	0.355 **
(5) Diet soft drink (g/day)	0.162 *	0.086 *	-0.002	0.069 *	0.157 **	0.152 **	0.011	0.152 **	0.011	0.118 **
(6) Alcoholic drinks (g/day)	0.461 **	0.347 **	0.077 *	0.065	0.490 **	0.516 **	0.117 **	0.516 **	0.117 **	0.658 **
(7) Water (g/day)	0.687 **	0.804 **	0.049	0.05	0.744 **	0.219 **	-0.005	0.219 **	-0.005	0.034
(8) Other non-alcoholic beverages (g/day)	0.191 **	0.083 *	0.017	0.146 **	0.164 **	0.135 **	0.064	0.135 **	0.064	0.110 **
Variety score	0.160 **	0.170 **	0.007	0.112 **	0.190 **	0.136 **	0.096 **	0.136 **	0.096 **	0.194 **

** Correlation is significant at the 0.01 level; * Correlation is significant at the 0.05 level.

Table 5. Descriptive characteristics of subjects that completed seven-day diaries (n = 178).

			Total	%	Male	%	Female	%
		Total	178	100	91	51.1	87	48.9
Age group (years)	18–39	Count	103	57.9	56	61.5	47	54
	40–64	Count	75	42.1	35	38.5	40	46
Unemployed		Count	23	13.1	11	12	12	14.1
Level of physical activity	Inactive	Count	109	61.2	58	63.4	51	59.0
	Active	Count	69	38.8	33	36.6	36	41.0
Level of education	Primary or less	Count	1	1	0	0	1	2.7
	Secondary	Count	2	2	1	1.6	1	2.7
	Tertiary or University	Count	95	96.9	60	98.4	35	94.6
Tobacco	Yes	Count	41	23	20	22	21	24.1
	No	Count	137	77	71	78	66	75.9
Weight (kg)		Mean (SE)	75.53 (3.38)		82.89 (6.62)		68.44 (1.57)	
Height (cm)		Mean (SE)	1.70 (0.01)		1.73 (0.01)		1.67 (0.01)	
BMI Class (kg/m^2)	Normal weight	Count	104	58.4	50	55.4	53	61.3
	Overweight	Count	48	26.8	26	28.4	22	25.3
	Obese	Count	26	14.8	15	16.2	12	13.3

The contribution of foods and beverages to water (g/day) and energy intake (kcal/day) is presented in Table 6 for males, females, and totally. Mean daily water intake was 2349 g (SE 59), while for males it was 2517 g (SE 91), and for females it was 2174 g (SE 71). Beverages were the main contributors to water intake (79% for males, and 76% for females). The contribution of all types of beverages to water intake was similar for males and females (p values are provided in Table 6). Mean energy intake was 1780 kcal/day (SE 36), while the contribution of foods to total energy intake was approximately 78% for the total sample.

Table 6. Contribution of foods and beverages to water and energy intake using seven-day diaries ($n = 178$).

		Contribution to Water Intake (g/Day)			p^1	Contribution to Energy Intake (kcal/Day)			p^2
		Total	Male	Female		Total	Male	Female	
	Count	178	91	87		178	91	87	
All food and drink	Mean	2349	2517	2174	0.003	1780	1890	1667	0.002
	(SE)	(59)	(91)	(71)		(36)	(51)	(46)	
Food only	Mean	504	501	508	0.848	1551	1594	1425	0.005
	(SE)	(17)	(21)	(27)		(31)	(47)	(37)	
Beverages only	Mean	1826	1990	1653	0.003	206	216	194	0.199
	(SE)	(57)	(90)	(63)		(9)	(12)	(12)	
Hot beverages	Mean	286	282	291	0.779	127	125	129	0.779
	(SE)	(17)	(22)	(26)		(8)	(10)	(12)	
Milk	Mean	119	116	122	0.721	117	114	120	0.721
	(SE)	(8)	(12)	(12)		(8)	(12)	(11)	
Fruit and vegetable juice	Mean	63	57	69	0.272	36	32	39	0.272
	(SE)	(6)	(8)	(8)		(3)	(5)	(4)	
Caloric soft drink	Mean	27	30	24	0.486	12	13	11	0.486
	(SE)	(4)	(5)	(6)		(2)	(2)	(3)	
Diet soft drink	Mean	23	33	12	0.075	1	1	0	0.075
	(SE)	(6)	(10)	(5)		(0)	(0)	(0)	
Alcoholic drinks	Mean	81	84	77	0.696	142	147	136	0.696
	(SE)	(9)	(12)	(12)		(15)	(21)	(22)	
Water	Mean	1170	1310	1023	0.007	-	-	-	-
	(SE)	(54)	(86)	(61)		-	-	-	
Other beverages	Mean	18	23	12	0.096	5	6	3	0.096
	(SE)	(3)	(6)	(2)		(1)	(2)	(1)	

p-values derived through Student's *t*-test between genders.

Males had a higher total water intake and water intake from beverages ($p = 0.003$ for both) as presented in Table 6. Moreover, males consumed more beverages than females (1999 g against 1692 g), which reflect a higher consumption of water (tap or bottled) ($p = 0.007$). Water was by far the most popular beverage consumed for both genders, followed by hot beverages, milk, and alcoholic drinks.

In Table 7 are presented the intakes of water, energy and beverage type the first three days of the experiment, as well as during the seven-day period. Total water intake, water intake from beverages, and energy intake decreased in the extended period of the study. The seven-day period revealed a higher variety score for beverages consumed of 5 (SD 1) and a higher intake of alcoholic drinks.

Table 7. Water and energy intake of subjects the first three days and the seven days of the experiment using day diaries (*n* = 178).

Variable	3 Days	7 Days	*p*
Total water intake (mL/day)	2412 (63)	2351 (59)	0.005
Water intake from beverages (mL/day)	1869 (60)	1826 (57)	0.027
Water intake from foods (mL/day)	535 (19)	505 (17)	0.009
Total energy intake (kcal/day)	1818 (38)	1775 (35)	0.017
Energy intake from beverages (kcal/day)	201 (9)	207 (9)	NS
Energy intake from foods (kcal/day)	1573 (36)	1512 (31)	0.011
Hot beverages (mL/day)	302 (19)	290 (17)	NS
Milk (mL/day)	138 (11)	143 (10)	NS
Fruit and vegetable juice (mL/day)	79 (8)	72 (8)	NS
Caloric soft drinks (mL/day)	29 (6)	31 (4)	MS
Diet soft drinks (mL/day)	28 (8)	26 (7)	NS
Alcoholic drinks (mL/day)	85 (10)	100 (11)	0.036
Water (mL/day)	1233 (55)	1176 (54)	0.004
Other beverages (mL/day)	16 (3)	20 (4)	0.159
Variety score	4	5	0.0001

p-values derived through Student's *t*-test between three and seven days of the experiment.

Total water intake was strongly correlated with beverage weight (*r* = 0.953) and water from beverages (*r* = 0.952). The correlation of total water intake with water from foods was very weak (*r* = 0.29, Table 8). Total water intake from all sources was correlated weakly with total energy intake (*r* = 0.265), and water intake from beverages is also correlated weakly with energy intake from beverages (*r* = 0.230). Milk, fruit and vegetable juice, alcoholic drinks, and caloric soft drinks had a moderate correlation with total energy from beverages (*r* = 0.46, 0.43, 0.43, and 0.24, respectively). The variety score of beverages consumed in a day was positively correlated with total water intake (*r* = 0.169), water and energy intake from beverages (*r* = 0.214 and 0.316, respectively).

Finally, in the present study the classification of total water intake is presented in Table 9. Seventy-five percent of males from study A and 40% from study B followed the scientific opinion of EFSA for adequate daily water intake (2.5 L/day; Criterion 1). The adherence of females (2.0 L/day; Criterion 1) was 83% in the sample of study A and 62% in study B. Ninety-six percent of the subjects from study A and 80% of subjects from study B fulfilled Criterion 2 (1 g of water per 1 kcal of energy intake).

Table 8. Partial correlations between water intake, energy intake, and beverage consumption adjusted for age, gender, body weight, and activity from seven-day diaries (*n* = 178).

	Total Water Intake (g/Day)	Total Water from Beverages (g/Day)	Total Water from Food (g/Day)	Total Beverages Weight (g/Day)	Total Energy (kcal/Day)	Total Energy from Beverages (kcal/Day)	Total Energy from Food (kcal/Day)
Total water (from food and beverages) (g/day)	1	0.952 **	0.291 **	0.953 **	0.265 **	0.213 *	0.222 **
Water from beverages (g/day)	0.952 **	1	0.006	0.959 **	0.142	0.230 **	0.094
Water from food (g/day)	0.291 **	0.006	1	0.142	0.407 **	0.013	0.446 **
Beverage weight (g/day)	0.953 **	0.959 **	0.142	1	0.189 *	0.291 **	0.140
Total energy (kcal)	0.265 **	0.142	0.407 **	0.189 *	1	0.394 **	0.885 **
Energy from beverages (kcal)	0.213 *	0.230 **	0.013	0.291 **	0.394 **	1	0.146
Energy from food (kcal)	0.222 **	0.094	0.446 **	0.140	0.885 **	0.146	1
(1) Hot beverages (g/day)	0.092	0.116	−0.048	0.131	−0.078	−0.101	−0.020
(2) Milk (g/day)	0.080	0.010	0.211 *	0.100	0.199 *	0.460 **	0.089
(3) Fruit and vegetable juice (g/day)	0.273 **	0.286 **	−0.030	0.314 **	0.277 **	0.428 **	0.145
(4) Caloric soft drink (g/day)	0.147	0.098	0.219 **	0.206 *	0.239 **	0.376 **	0.167 *
(5) Diet soft drink (g/day)	0.140	0.145	−0.006	0.145	−0.002	−0.005	0.066
(6) Alcoholic drinks (g/day)	0.254 **	0.279 **	−0.005	0.276 **	0.125	0.433 **	0.039
(7) Water (g/day)	0.898 **	0.909 **	0.115	0.919 **	0.110	0.085	0.094
(8) Other beverages (g/day)	0.251 **	0.245 **	0.077	0.265 **	0.161	0.264 **	0.074
Variety score	0.167 *	0.214 *	−0.098	0.250 **	0.121	0.316 **	0.053

** Correlation is significant at the 0.01 level; * Correlation is significant at the 0.05 level.

Table 9. Combined classification for the total water intake (TWI) following established criteria.

Classification of Total Water Intake	Study	Males	Females
CRITERION 1 (%)	A	75	83
	B	40	62
CRITERION 2 (%)	A	97	96
	B	79	81
CRITERION 3 (1 and 2) (%)	A	74	80
	B	40	60

(1) Criterion 1: TWI > 2.5 L males, > 2 L females (aged 14 to 75 years); (2) Criterion 2: Ratio of total water/total energy intakes > 1; (3) Criterion 3: Both criteria.

4. Discussion

The present study reports and comments on data for water intake from all sources (foods and beverages) using the WBQ, a semi-quantified food and fluid frequency questionnaire (study A) and a seven-day diary record (study B) in healthy Greek adults aged 18–75 years living in the metropolitan area of Athens.

The main finding of our study is that total water intake was 3254 (SE 43) g/day in study A and 2349 (SE 59) g/day in study B. This finding draws attention not only because it contributes data for water intake in Greece, but also because it reveals deviation in findings when using different research tools.

Total water intake in other countries ranges from 1488 mL/day in China to 3563 mL/day in the USA [4–7,9,10,21–24]. Deviation in water intake in different countries may reflect between country differences in dietary habits, lifestyle choices, and environmental conditions [25], but also between study differences in the choice of method used to evaluate water intake.

The research tools that are used in most studies are three- or seven-day diary records, or 24 h recall or food frequency questionnaires [24], but commonly these are designed to evaluate food intake and not water intake; studies in large population groups, such as the European Prospective Investigation into Cancer and Nutrition (EPIC) study and the National Health and Nutrition Examination Survey (NHANES) study, have been designed to assess macro and micronutrient intakes and not total water or beverages intake. Therefore, they may not fully capture water intake because the consumption of some beverages is underestimated by the individual or the interviewer [13]. For example, the food intake diaries or 24 h recalls record eating occasions around meals and snacks, but not all drinking occasions, while fluid-specific, records report two more drinking occasions per day not with meals or snacks. These are less likely to be included in a 24 h recall [26]. A growing number of studies having as their primary outcome the estimation of total water intake is now published [3,8,23,24,27]. Research tools that are designed specifically to record water intake exist [18,21,24]. It appears that these report a higher total fluid intake compared to tools that are not specifically designed to record water intake [21,24].

In data presented herein, this observation is confirmed. In study A the WBQ, which registers in detail all sources of fluid consumption, recorded a higher water intake by approximately 900 mL/day than in study B, although subjects completing the seven-day diaries were instructed to record all drinking occasions. The difference between study A and B may be attributed to a variety of factors: WBQ was administered to 1092 subjects while the seven-day diaries were administered to 178 subjects, although of the same distribution in terms of age, sex, season, and location; WBQ records water intake for beverages for the previous month, while seven-day diaries record water intake for one week; WBQ, designed specifically for recording fluid intake, embeds a food frequency questionnaire with 23 questions for beverage intake including all types of hot and cold beverages, alcoholic, and non-alcoholic beverages, that are usually consumed in Greece; questions in the WBQ were expressed as the number of glasses, while continuous data (mL per drinking occasion) were collected in seven-day diary records; the seven-day diary was part of an elaborate protocol including 24 h urine collection for all seven days. This systematic urine collection in study B may be intruding and may alter routine behavior, including drinking.

There is not yet a gold standard method to assess water intake. Contributing to the discussion on the appropriateness of research tools evaluating water intake, the exposure study of Mons, et al. [28] concluded that the best method to collect water intake data is a 3–4 days diary record or, if not feasible, two or more 24 h recalls are preferable to food frequency questionnaires. It must be noted that the WBQ was validated with three-day diary records [18]. Mons, et al. [28] also suggests that an extended period may result to less accurate reporting. In order to confirm this argument we retrospectively analyzed diary records from study B and compared the recordings of three and in seven days. We observed a decreased total water intake and water intake from beverages in seven days. Others [29–31] also supported that food frequency questionnaires report a higher water intake than the diary records.

International organizations define adequate water intake based on data collected in various population groups. In Europe, EFSA [2] defines adequate water intake from all sources at 2 L for females and 2.5 L per day for males. In the USA, based on daily dietary recruitment (DRI), Institute of Medicine (IOM) suggests adequate intake range 2.7–3.7 L per day in adults, with men to require 1 L more [32]. Adequate intake may be adjusted when water requirements are increased according to physical activity levels and environmental conditions [32–34]. It may be expected that new data collected using improved validated methodology specific for evaluating water intake in different population groups and in different countries may lead to resetting values for adequate water intake by different organizations.

The discrepancy of results obtained from different tools is clearly confusing, when it comes to observing compliance with EFSA adequate intakes. For example, 83% of females and 75% of males from study A, and 62% of females and 40% of males from study B, complied with the EFSA adequate water intake. In the study of Ferreira-Pego, et al. [24], averaging data from 13 countries, 40% of men and 60% of women complied with the EFSA adequate intakes for water intake from fluids. In the ANIBES study [23] performed in Spain, 21% of women and 12% of men complied with EFSA adequate intakes. In general, women exhibit a healthier pattern of eating and food choices than men [35]. Women seem to be more reflective about health issues and foods. Adults that adopt a healthier dietary pattern usually have a healthier fluid pattern (higher consumption of water and total fluids) [36].

Another important finding is that, despite differences in volumes when recording total water intake using the WBQ and seven-day diaries in study A and B, respectively, the contribution in water intake of foods and beverages, as well as of types of beverages, was similar in both studies. The importance of all sources, i.e., drinking water or beverages or moisture in solid foods in hydration [36] should be highlighted. This finding signifies that WBQ and seven-day diaries may evaluate the subjects' choices in a similar manner. In particular, the contribution of beverages to total water intake was 78% in WBQ study and seven-day diaries study of foods was 22%, respectively. This finding accords with the scientific opinion of EFSA [2]. Similar findings in the contribution of foods and beverages to water intake were observed in the UK [5] and Indonesian [4] populations.

Beverages that were consumed in larger volumes in both studies A and B were water, by almost 10-fold, followed by hot beverages and milk. This finding is in accordance with the study of Armstrong, et al. [37] in which water consumed in similar volumes, as well as the study of Perrier, et al. [38] with water being the major contributor to fluid intake. These findings were not observed in the UK population, with hot beverages being the most popular beverage. The variety in beverage choice has been considered a factor linked to water intake. An important finding from our study is that the variety score, using both tools, is positively correlated with total water intake ($p < 0.001$, $p = 0.005$ respectively) and water intake from beverages ($p < 0.001$, $p = 0.005$ respectively).

The results of this study may be exploited in view of a number of limitations. The WBQ that was used in study A estimates the usual food intake over a month, but details of intake are not measured, such as the size of the portion consumed. In addition, retrospective methods, such as 24 h recall and food frequency questionnaires, depend on memory and recall ability of the applicant [27]. Both methodologies require updated and extended information for food composition data, which is limited in Greece. It should be noted that subjects of study B that completed the seven-day diaries had to follow a demanding protocol that required the collection of samples from all urination on a 24 h basis for seven consecutive days. It appears that approaches such as three- or seven-day diary records that require a collection of a large amount of data from the subject results in reduced compliance and may underestimate the fluid intake [26]. New research developments that introduce electronic recording of dietary intake [28] attempt to maximize the compliance of the subject; however, these are not yet used extensively in water intake.

5. Conclusions

In conclusion, water intake using the WBQ recorded a higher water intake than the seven-day diaries in a sample of Greek adults, yet both methodologies found that the beverages that were consumed in larger volumes were water, hot beverages, and milk. This work implies caution when interpreting data obtained from different approaches and highlights the need for concerted efforts towards developing a robust, validated methodology for the evaluation of water intake in the general population.

Acknowledgments: The study was financially supported by a Grant from the European Hydration Institute to the Canarian Foundation Science and Technology Park of the University of Las Palmas de Gran Canaria. The funding sponsors had no role in the design of the study, the collection, analysis, or interpretation of the data, writing of the manuscript, or in the decision to publish the results.

Author Contributions: A.A., O.M., A.K. and M.K. analyzed the data, drafted and wrote the paper.

Conflicts of Interest: The authors declare no conflict of interest.

References

1. European Food Safety Authority (EFSA). Scientific Opinion on the substantiation of health claims related to water and maintenance of normal physical and cognitive functions (ID 1102, 1209, 1294, 1331), maintenance of normal thermoregulation (ID 1208) and "basic requirement of all living things" (ID 1207) pursuant to Article 13(1) of Regulation (EC) NO 1924/2006. *EFSA J.* **2011**, *9*, 2075–2091.
2. European Food Safety Authority (EFSA). Scientific opinion on dietary reference values for water. *EFSA J.* **2010**, *8*, 1459–1507.
3. Malisova, O.; Athanasatou, A.; Pepa, A.; Husemann, M.; Domnik, K.; Braun, H.; Mora-Rodriguez, R.; Ortega, J.F.; Fernandez-Elias, V.E.; Kapsokefalou, M. Water intake and hydration indices in healthy european adults: The european hydration research study (EHRS). *Nutrients* **2016**, *8*. [CrossRef] [PubMed]
4. Bardosono, S.; Monrozier, R.; Permadhi, I.; Manikam, N.R.; Pohan, R.; Guelinckx, I. Total fluid intake assessed with a 7-day fluid record versus a 24-h dietary recall: A crossover study in indonesian adolescents and adults. *Eur. J. Nutr.* **2015**, *54*, 17–25. [CrossRef] [PubMed]
5. Gibson, S.; Shirreffs, S.M. Beverage consumption habits "24/7" among british adults: Association with total water intake and energy intake. *Nutr. J.* **2013**, *12*, 1–13. [CrossRef] [PubMed]
6. Manz, F.; Johner, S.A.; Wentz, A.; Boeing, H.; Remer, T. Water balance throughout the adult life span in a german population. *Br. J. Nutr.* **2012**, *107*, 1673–1681. [CrossRef] [PubMed]
7. O'Connor, L.; Walton, J.; Flynn, A. Water intakes and dietary sources of a nationally representative sample of irish adults. *J. Hum. Nutr. Diet.* **2014**, *27*, 550–556. [CrossRef] [PubMed]
8. Malisova, O.; Bountziouka, V.; Panagiotakos, D.; Zampelas, A.; Kapsokefalou, M. Evaluation of seasonality on total water intake, water loss and water balance in the general population in greece. *J. Hum. Nutr. Diet.* **2013**, *26*, 90–96. [CrossRef] [PubMed]
9. Bellisle, F.; Thornton, S.N.; Hebel, P.; Denizeau, M.; Tahiri, M. A study of fluid intake from beverages in a sample of healthy french children, adolescents and adults. *Eur. J. Clin. Nutr.* **2010**, *64*, 350–355. [CrossRef] [PubMed]
10. Drewnowski, A.; Rehm, C.D.; Constant, F. Water and beverage consumption among adults in the united states: Cross-sectional study using data from nhanes 2005–2010. *BMC Public Health* **2013**, *13*, 1068. [CrossRef] [PubMed]
11. Westerterp, K.R.; Plasqui, G.; Goris, A.H. Water loss as a function of energy intake, physical activity and season. *Br. J. Nutr.* **2005**, *93*, 199–203. [CrossRef] [PubMed]
12. Gandy, J. Water intake: Validity of population assessment and recommendations. *Eur. J. Nutr.* **2015**, *54*, 11–16. [CrossRef] [PubMed]
13. Nielsen, S.J.; Popkin, B.M. Changes in beverage intake between 1977 and 2001. *Am. J. Prev. Med.* **2004**, *27*, 205–210. [CrossRef] [PubMed]
14. Duffey, K.J.; Huybrechts, I.; Mouratidou, T.; Libuda, L.; Kersting, M.; De Vriendt, T.; Gottrand, F.; Widhalm, K.; Dallongeville, J.; Hallstrom, L.; et al. Beverage consumption among european adolescents in the helena study. *Eur. J. Clin. Nutr.* **2012**, *66*, 244–252. [CrossRef] [PubMed]

15. Farajian, P.; Panagiotakos, D.B.; Risvas, G.; Micha, R.; Tsioufis, C.; Zampelas, A. Dietary and lifestyle patterns in relation to high blood pressure in children: The greco study. *J. Hypertens.* **2015**, *33*, 1174–1181. [CrossRef] [PubMed]

16. Trichopoulou, A.; Gnardellis, C.; Lagiou, A.; Benetou, V.; Naska, A.; Trichopoulos, D. Physical activity and energy intake selectively predict the waist-to-hip ratio in men but not in women. *Am. J. Clin. Nutr.* **2001**, *74*, 574–578. [PubMed]

17. Pitsavos, C.; Panagiotakos, D.B.; Chrysohoou, C.; Stefanadis, C. Epidemiology of cardiovascular risk factors in greece: Aims, design and baseline characteristics of the attica study. *BMC Public Health* **2003**, *3*, 32. [CrossRef] [PubMed]

18. Malisova, O.; Bountziouka, V.; Panagiotakos, D.B.; Zampelas, A.; Kapsokefalou, M. The water balance questionnaire: Design, reliability and validity of a questionnaire to evaluate water balance in the general population. *Int. J. Food Sci. Nutr.* **2012**, *63*, 138–144. [CrossRef] [PubMed]

19. Craig, C.L.; Marshall, A.L.; Sjostrom, M.; Bauman, A.E.; Booth, M.L.; Ainsworth, B.E.; Pratt, M.; Ekelund, U.; Yngve, A.; Sallis, J.F.; et al. International physical activity questionnaire: 12-country reliability and validity. *Med. Sci. Sports Exerc.* **2003**, *35*, 1381–1395. [CrossRef] [PubMed]

20. Willet, W.C. Issues in analysis and presentation of dietary data. In *Nutritional Epidemiology*, 2nd ed.; Oxford University Press: New York, NY, USA, 1998; pp. 321–346.

21. Ma, G.; Zhang, Q.; Liu, A.; Zuo, J.; Zhang, W.; Zou, S.; Li, X.; Lu, L.; Pan, H.; Hu, X. Fluid intake of adults in four chinese cities. *Nutr. Rev.* **2012**, *70*, S105–S110. [CrossRef] [PubMed]

22. Tani, Y.; Asakura, K.; Sasaki, S.; Hirota, N.; Notsu, A.; Todoriki, H.; Miura, A.; Fukui, M.; Date, C. The influence of season and air temperature on water intake by food groups in a sample of free-living japanese adults. *Eur. J. Clin. Nutr.* **2015**, *69*, 907–913. [CrossRef] [PubMed]

23. Nissensohn, M.; Sanchez-Villegas, A.; Ortega, R.M.; Aranceta-Bartrina, J.; Gil, A.; Gonzalez-Gross, M.; Varela-Moreiras, G.; Serra-Majem, L. Beverage consumption habits and association with total water and energy intakes in the spanish population: Findings of the anibes study. *Nutrients* **2016**, *8*. [CrossRef] [PubMed]

24. Ferreira-Pego, C.; Guelinckx, I.; Moreno, L.A.; Kavouras, S.A.; Gandy, J.; Martinez, H.; Bardosono, S.; Abdollahi, M.; Nasseri, E.; Jarosz, A.; et al. Total fluid intake and its determinants: Cross-sectional surveys among adults in 13 countries worldwide. *Eur. J. Nutr.* **2015**, *54*, 35–43. [CrossRef] [PubMed]

25. Vergne, S. Methodological aspects of fluid intake records and surveys. *Nutr. Today* **2012**, *47*, S7–S10. [CrossRef]

26. Sebastian, R.S.; Wilkinson Enns, C.; Goldman, J.D.; Moshfegh, A.J. Change in methodology for collection of drinking water intake in what we eat in america/national health and nutrition examination survey: Implications for analysis. *Public Health Nutr.* **2012**, *15*, 1190–1195. [CrossRef] [PubMed]

27. Mora-Rodriguez, R.; Ortega, J.F.; Fernandez-Elias, V.E.; Kapsokefalou, M.; Malisova, O.; Athanasatou, A.; Husemann, M.; Domnik, K.; Braun, H. Influence of physical activity and ambient temperature on hydration: The european hydration research study (EHRS). *Nutrients* **2016**, *8*. [CrossRef] [PubMed]

28. Mons, M.N.; van der Wielen, J.M.; Blokker, E.J.; Sinclair, M.I.; Hulshof, K.F.; Dangendorf, F.; Hunter, P.R.; Medema, G.J. Estimation of the consumption of cold tap water for microbiological risk assessment: An overview of studies and statistical analysis of data. *J. Water Health* **2007**, *5*, 151–170. [CrossRef] [PubMed]

29. Robertson, B.; Forbes, A.; Sinclair, M.; Black, J.; Veitch, M.; Pilotto, L.; Kirk, M.; Fairley, C.K. How well does a telephone questionnaire measure drinking water intake? *Aust. N. Zeal. J. Public Health* **2000**, *24*, 619–622. [CrossRef]

30. Kaur, S.; Nieuwenhuijsen, M.J.; Ferrier, H.; Steer, P. Exposure of pregnant women to tap water related activities. *Occup. Environ. Med.* **2004**, *61*, 454–460. [CrossRef] [PubMed]

31. Levallois, P.; Guevin, N.; Gingras, S.; Levesque, B.; Weber, J.P.; Letarte, R. New patterns of drinking-water consumption: Results of a pilot study. *Sci. Total Environ.* **1998**, *209*, 233–241. [CrossRef]

32. Medicine, I.O. *Panel on Dietary Reference Intakes for Electrolytes and Water: Dietary Reference Intakes for Water, Potassium, Sodium, Chloride and Sulfate*; National Academies Press: Washington, DC, USA, 2005.

33. Greenleaf, J.E.; Bernauer, E.M.; Juhos, L.T.; Young, H.L.; Morse, J.T.; Staley, R.W. Effects of exercise on fluid exchange and body composition in man during 14-day bed rest. *J. Appl. Physiol. Respir. Environ. Exerc. Physiol.* **1977**, *43*, 126–132. [PubMed]

34. Gunga, H.C.; Maillet, A.; Kirsch, K.; Rocker, L.; Gharib, C.; Vaernes, R. European isolation and confinement study. Water and salt turnover. *Adv. Space Biol. Med.* **1993**, *3*, 185–200. [PubMed]

35. Beards, A.; Bryman, A.; Keil, T.; Goode, J.; Haslam, C.; Lanchashire, E. Women, men and food: The significance of gender for nutritional attitudes and choices. *Brit. Food J.* **2002**, *104*, 470–491. [CrossRef]

36. Duffey, K.J.; Popkin, B.M. Adults with healthier dietary patterns have healthier beverage patterns. *J. Nutr.* **2006**, *136*, 2901–2907. [PubMed]

37. Armstrong, L.E.; Johnson, E.C.; Munoz, C.X.; Swokla, B.; Le Bellego, L.; Jimenez, L.; Casa, D.J.; Maresh, C.M. Hydration biomarkers and dietary fluid consumption of women. *J. Acad. Nutr. Diet.* **2012**, *112*, 1056–1061. [CrossRef] [PubMed]

38. Perrier, E.; Vergne, S.; Klein, A.; Poupin, M.; Rondeau, P.; Le Bellego, L.; Armstrong, L.E.; Lang, F.; Stookey, J.; Tack, I. Hydration biomarkers in free-living adults with different levels of habitual fluid consumption. *Br. J. Nutr.* **2013**, *109*, 1678–1687. [CrossRef] [PubMed]

nutrients

MDPI

Article

Beverage Consumption Patterns among Norwegian Adults

Mari Mohn Paulsen *, Jannicke Borch Myhre and Lene Frost Andersen

Department of Nutrition, Institute of Basic Medical Sciences, University of Oslo, P.O. Box 1046 Blindern, Oslo 0317, Norway; j.b.myhre@medisin.uio.no (J.B.M.); l.f.andersen@medisin.uio.no (L.F.A.)
* Correspondence: m.m.paulsen@medisin.uio.no; Tel.: +47-957-72-048

Received: 29 June 2016; Accepted: 6 September 2016; Published: 13 September 2016

Abstract: Beverages may be important contributors for energy intake and dietary quality. The purpose of the study was to investigate how beverage consumption varies between different meals (breakfast, lunch, dinner, supper/evening meal, snacks) and between weekdays and weekend-days in Norwegian adults. A cross-sectional dietary survey was conducted among Norwegian adults (n = 1787) in 2010–2011. Two telephone-administered 24 h recalls were used for dietary data collection. Breakfast was the most important meal for milk and juice consumption, dinner for sugar-sweetened beverages and wine, and snacks for water, coffee, artificially sweetened beverages, and beer. Consumption of sugar-sweetened and artificially sweetened beverages did not differ between weekdays and weekend-days among consumers. The average intake of wine and beer (men only) was higher on weekend-days. Higher age was positively associated with wine consumption and negatively associated with consumption of water, sugar-sweetened, and artificially sweetened beverages. Higher education was associated with consumption of water, beer, and wine, whereas lower education was associated with sugar-sweetened beverage consumption. Beverage consumption patterns among Norwegian adults vary between different meal types and in subgroups of the population. Alcohol consumption was higher on weekend-days. Knowledge regarding beverage consumption patterns in the population should be considered when revising dietary guidelines in the future.

Keywords: beverage consumption pattern; meal types; food based dietary guide lines; alcohol consumption; sugar-sweetened beverages

1. Introduction

Beverages may be important contributors for energy intake and overall dietary quality, in the same way as food [1–3]. We know, for instance, that milk is one of the most important contributors of calcium intake [4–7], while sugar-sweetened beverages contribute, in large part, to the intake of added sugar, especially among youths [6,8]. Sugar-sweetened beverage consumption has been associated with the worldwide obesity epidemic [9–11], although systematic reviews have highlighted the need for better randomized controlled trials, to investigate a causal effect [12,13]. High alcohol consumption has been associated with several acute and chronic conditions in a dose-response relationship [14]. Earlier studies have indicated a J-shaped association for alcohol consumption and all-cause mortality [15]. Recent studies have, in contrast, demonstrated that only women older than 65 years had lower mortality with low alcohol consumption [16]. A newly-published meta-analysis did not find any protective effects of a low-to-moderate alcohol consumption on all-cause mortality, compared to non-drinkers [17].

In the Norwegian food-based dietary guidelines (FBDGs), two of the twelve guidelines concern beverage intake; one regards avoidance of beverages and foods rich in added sugar on an everyday basis and one recommends drinking water when thirsty [18]. The same is found in international guidelines [19]. In Norway the consumption of sugar-sweetened beverages has been reduced from 63 to 55 liters per inhabitant from 2010 to 2014 [8]. The same trend is seen in Britain and the USA [20,21]. There are also specific advices concerning alcohol intake and the health authorities recommend reducing the consumption of alcohol-containing beverages [22]. Despite this, the consumption of alcoholic beverages in Norway has increased since the year 2000. The intake of wine per capita was at the highest level registered ever in 2013, while beer has had a slight reduction since the top levels in 2009 [8].

Despite dietary recommendations and knowledge regarding health effects of the consumption of different beverages, there is scarce knowledge concerning which meals and weekdays different beverages are consumed. There are few systematic analyses of overall beverage patterns and trends at the national and international level. It has been suggested that public health advice and strategies to change dietary intake need to focus on meal types to be understandable and usable by the population [23]. Kearney and coworkers describe that a consideration of eating patterns in the general population, including beverage consumption, is necessary when developing FBDGs [24]. Information regarding the distribution of food and beverage intake from different meals may provide important information for development and revision of FBDGs, understand habits, and for tailoring dietary interventions to the population [25].

Dietary behavior varies among different subgroups of the population and several studies have described an association between socio-economic position and dietary habits [26–28]. Less literature is published regarding beverage consumption habits and background variables in general, although the association with higher intakes of sugar-sweetened beverages in groups with lower socioeconomic status is well described [29–32]. Knowledge concerning how beverage consumption varies in relation to the background variables age, gender, education, smoking habits, and body mass index (BMI) may contribute to more specific and tailored beverage recommendations to the population. It may also be useful in understanding habits and designing dietary interventions.

The aim of the present paper was to investigate the consumption of beverage types across meals, beverage intake during weekdays and weekend-days, and how beverage intake is associated with gender, age, education, smoking, and BMI.

2. Materials and Methods

2.1. Design and Participants

The present study was based on data from a Norwegian national dietary survey, Norkost 3, conducted in 2010–2011. The design and methodologies have earlier been described in detail [33]. A representative sample of the adult (18–70 years) Norwegian population (*n* = 5000) was randomly selected from the National register and asked to complete two 24 h recalls administered by telephone approximately four weeks apart. Data were collected about all days of the week in the study, but not for each individual. The distribution of interviews across the days of the weeks was the following: Mondays (21%), Tuesdays (18%), Wednesdays (18%), Thursdays (10%), Fridays (7%), Saturdays (7%), and Sundays (19%).

Of the 5000 persons invited, 153 were unavailable for contact. In total, 1787 participants completed two recalls (37% participation rate). Only participants completing both 24 h recalls were included in the analyses.

Every 25th participant was randomly selected to receive 3000.00 NOK. Feedback regarding the individual participant's dietary composition was offered to those who wanted such feedback.

Verbal informed consent was collected from all participants. The study (2009/1318b) was approved by the Regional Committee for Medical and Health Research Ethics, 13 October 2009, and conducted according to the guidelines laid down in the Declaration of Helsinki.

2.2. Assessment of Beverage Intake

The 24 h recalls assessing food and beverage intake were performed by trained interviewers using a dietary assessment system (KBS version 7.0, University of Oslo/clave, Oslo, Norway) which is linked directly to a food composition database based on the Norwegian food composition table from 2006 [34]. Before starting the interview, the participants were asked if the previous day was considered a normal day with regard to food and beverage intake. Seventy-three percent of the recall days were considered as normal days by the participants. The respondents were encouraged to give detailed information regarding portion sizes of foods and beverages consumed. Amounts were quantified by household measures and aids in the form of a booklet including pictures of foods in different portion sizes and glasses/cups in different sizes. The booklet was sent by mail to all invited participants together with the invitation letter. The interviewers used a checklist of commonly forgotten food and drink items at the end of the interview to reduce the risk of underreporting.

2.3. Meal Types and Categorization of Beverage Types

Meal types were categorized as breakfast, lunch, dinner, supper, or snacks. Snacks also included only a beverage and intake of supplements. The most important meal for each beverage type was defined as the meal type with the highest average consumption in grams of the beverage type in question.

The beverage types included in the analyses were water, coffee, tea, milk, fruit juice, sugar-sweetened beverages, artificially sweetened beverages, beer, and wine. Water included both tap and bottled water. Sugar-sweetened beverages included soft drinks and squash with added sugar. Artificially sweetened beverages included soft drinks and squash with artificial sweeteners or without added sugar. The beer and wine included were all alcohol-containing.

2.4. Background Variables

Body mass index (BMI) was calculated based on self-reported weight (in kilograms) and height (in meters), as weight divided by the square of height (kg/m^2). The continuous BMI variable was divided into two categories; "low and normal weight" (BMI < 25 kg/m^2) and "overweight" (BMI ≥ 25 kg/m^2). Level of education was reported into eight categories, but was merged to two categories: "high school, technical school, trade school or lower" and "university or college". The continuous age variable was categorized into three age groups: 18–34 years, 35–54 years, and 55–70 years. Smoking habits were categorized into: "smokers" (daily/occasional smokers) and "non-smokers" (never-smokers and previous smokers). Interest in a healthy diet was reported into five categories ranging from "no interest" to "very high interest", and this variable was categorized into: "no, low, or moderate interest" or "high or very high interest".

2.5. Days of the Week

For the analyses regarding differences between weekdays and weekend days the days of the week were categorized as either weekday or weekend day. All meals during Monday to Thursday were categorized as weekday meals, whereas all meals during Saturdays and Sundays were categorized as weekend meals. It was assumed that dinner, supper, and snacks on Fridays were more like weekend meals and, therefore, categorized as weekend meals. While breakfast and lunch meals on Fridays were assumed to be more like weekday meals and, therefore, categorized as weekday meals.

2.6. Statistical Analyses

Statistical analyses were performed using Stata version 14.0 (StataCorp LP, College Station, TX, USA) and IBM SPSS Statistics 20.0 (IBM Corporation, Armonk, NY, USA). The analyses were performed separately for each type of beverage and all tests were two-sided. The data contained repeated measurements for each participant as the same participant could contribute with more than one meal to the analyses. To adjust for the dependency in the data due to repeated measurements for each participant, mixed models with total daily intake in grams of each beverage type as outcome variables were used with a variance component (random intercept) for participants. These adjustments were performed for the analyses of beverage consumption for different meals and differences in intake of selected beverage types between weekdays and weekend days.

To identify the most important meal for each beverage type in each gender, meal type (breakfast, lunch, dinner, supper, and snacks) was added as an independent variable to the mixed model. Differences between genders in the most important meal were tested. In cases with significant differences between genders, men and women were analyzed separately.

As the data contained a high number of zeros (meaning that the person had not consumed the beverage type in question for the respective meal or for the day in question), causing a violation of the assumption of normally distributed residuals, case bootstrapping with 1000 repetitions was performed for analyzes of average beverage consumption to different meals. The results are presented as adjusted means, bootstrap 95% confidence intervals, and bootstrap *p*-values. For some of the meal types the number of consumers of certain beverage types (e.g., beer for breakfast, tea for dinner) was zero or very small. In these specific cases, estimation of a 95% confidence interval was not possible.

In the analyses of differences between weekdays and weekend-days only consumers of the different beverage types were included. Adjustments were made for the categorical variables gender, BMI, normal day, smoking, interest in a healthy diet, education, and age.

To analyze the associations between background characteristics of the study participants and beverage consumption logistic regression was used (The participants were categorized as "users" or "non-users" of the different beverage types and these dichotomous variables were the dependent variables in the analyses. The models were adjusted for BMI, education, age, interest in a healthy diet, and smoking.

3. Results

3.1. Characteristics of the Study Population

Table 1 shows the background characteristics of the participants in the Norkost 3 survey. Fifty-two percent of the study participants were women and the mean age was 45 years for women and 47 years for men (age range 18–70 for both genders). In the Norkost 3 study, a higher percentage belonged to the highest age interval and a lower percentage to the youngest age interval, compared to the general population. The proportion with higher education was larger and the proportion of smokers was lower in Norkost 3 than in the general population [25].

Table 1. Background characteristics of the study population in Norkost 3 (*n* = 1787).

	Men (*n* = 862)		Women (*n* = 925)	
	n	%	*n*	%
Age group (*n* = 1787)				
18–34 years	199	23	208	22
35–54 years	355	41	461	50
55–70 years	308	36	256	28
BMI (*n* = 1756)				
<25 kg/m^2	344	40	544	61
≥25 kg/m^2	517	60	351	39
Education level (*n* = 1784)				
High school, technical school, trade school or lower	432	50	414	45
University or college	429	50	509	55
Interest in a healthy diet (*n* = 1786)				
No, low or moderate	447	52	335	36
High or very high	414	48	590	64
Smoking habits (*n* = 1787)				
Non-smokers	686	80	724	78
Smokers	176	20	201	22

3.2. Patterns of Beverage Consumption Related to Meals

Table 2 shows mean daily intake of beverages from each meal. The average intake to the most important meal was not different between genders for any of the beverage types, except for tea. Men had the highest intake of tea from breakfast, while women had the highest tea intake from snacks.

Milk and fruit juices were mainly consumed for breakfast. Dinner was the most important meal for sugar-sweetened beverages and wine, whereas snacks contributed to the highest intake of water, coffee, artificially sweetened beverages, and beer.

Table 2. Shows mean daily intake of beverages from each meal.

	Breakfast		Lunch		Dinner		Supper		Snack	
	Mean (g)	95% CI	Mean (g)	95% CI	Mean (g)	95% CI	Mean (g)	95% CI	Mean (g)	95% CI
Water	120 *	112, 129	128 *	120, 136	266 *	255, 278	73 *	66, 80	476	454, 499
Coffee	121 *	113, 128	76 *	70, 81	24 *	20, 27	18 *	14, 21	282	267, 298
Tea men	36	29, 42	27 *	22, 32	1 *	NA	11 *	8, 15	33	25, 41
Tea women	57 *	49, 64	53 *	46, 60	7 *	4, 10	36 *	31, 41	85	73, 96
Milk	125	118, 132	47 *	43, 52	32 *	29, 35	45 *	41, 50	37 *	33, 42
Fruit juice	55	50, 59	21 *	18, 24	7 *	6, 9	8 *	6, 10	15 *	13, 17
Sugar sweetened beverages	3 *	1, 4	12 *	10, 15	50	45, 56	11 *	9, 14	41 *	36, 46
Artificially sweetened beverages	5 *	4, 7	12 *	10, 15	38 *	34, 43	12 *	10, 15	44	37, 50
Beer	0 *	NA	1 *	NA	26 *	19, 33	9 *	5, 12	47	36, 58
Wine	0 *	NA	1 *	NA	22	19, 25	6 *	4, 7	17 *	14, 20

* $p \leq 0.001$ for difference in average intake between most important meal (bold numbers) and the other meals, tested with mixed models. NA: Not applicable because of zero or small values for average consumption. Mean (grams) and 95% confidence interval (95% CI).

The average intake to the most important meal was not different between genders for any of the beverage types, except for tea. Men had the highest intake of tea from breakfast, while women had the highest tea intake from snacks.

Milk and fruit juices were mainly consumed for breakfast. Dinner was the most important meal for sugar-sweetened beverages and wine, whereas snacks contributed to the highest intake of water, coffee, artificially sweetened beverages, and beer.

3.3. Patterns of Beverage Consumption on Weekdays vs. Weekend Days

The proportion of participants consuming sugar-sweetened beverages, artificially sweetened beverages, beer, and wine on one or both recall days are presented in Table 3. On average, 34% of the participants were consumers of sugar-sweetened beverages, with the proportion being higher for men.

Table 3. Proportion of participants consuming sugar-sweetened beverages, artificially sweetened beverages, beer, and wine on one and/or both recall days.

	Sugar-Sweetened Beverages		Artificially Sweetened Beverages		Beer		Wine	
	%	n	%	n	%	n	%	n
Women	28.8	260	26.2	242	9.2	85	22.1	204
Men	41.0	353	22.2	191	21.1	182	18.1	156

Figure 1 illustrates mean intakes of sugar-sweetened beverages, artificially sweetened beverages, beer and wine on weekdays and weekend-days for men and women (consumers only).

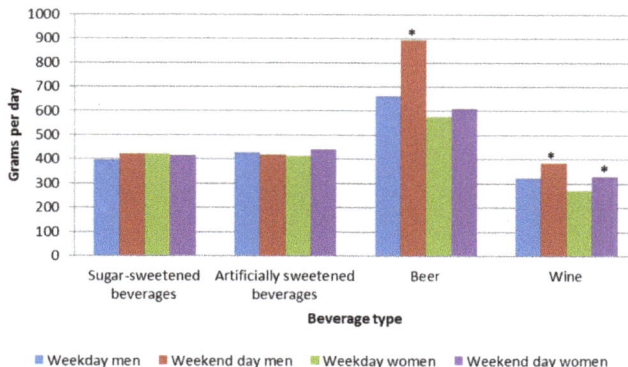

Figure 1. Average consumption in grams of sugar-sweetened beverages (n = 353 men and 260 women), artificially sweetened beverages (n = 191 men and 242 women), beer (n = 182 men and 85 women), and wine (n = 156 men and 204 women) among consumers of the selected beverage types on weekdays and weekend days. * p < 0.05 for difference between weekdays and weekend days. Tested with mixed models.

The average consumption of both types of beverages among consumers was about 4 dL per day. The intakes of sugar-sweetened beverages and artificially sweetened beverages did not differ between weekdays and weekend days.

The average beer intake among consumers was 26% higher for men on weekend days than on weekdays, 891 g/day vs. 661 g/day, respectively (p = 0.028). For female beer consumers, no differences in beer intake were observed between weekdays and weekend days. Wine intake was higher on weekend days, compared to weekdays for both men (p = 0.044) and women (p = 0.016), the differences were rather modest; 16% (63 g) in men and 17% (57 g) in women.

3.4. Background Variables Associated with Intake of Different Types of Beverages

Table 4 shows how background characteristics were associated with users and non-users of different beverage types.

In general, water was consumed by a high proportion of participants (more than 90%) in all of the analyzed groups. Women were more frequent water drinkers with 92% higher odds of having consumed water on one or both recall days, compared to men. The oldest age group (55–70 years) had lower odds for consuming water than the younger participants (18–34 years) and there was a significant trend for less water consumption with increasing age. Additionally, those having a higher education and those reporting to have an interest for a healthy diet were more likely to be water consumers.

Milk consumption was not associated with any of the background variables analyzed, whereas juice intake was associated with being young, having a normal or low BMI, having a university or college education, and being a non-smoker.

Coffee intake showed a strong association with age. The oldest age group in the study population had almost five times higher odds of drinking coffee, compared to the youngest age group. Participants interested in a healthy diet also had higher odds of being a coffee consumer, compared to participants with no, low or moderate interest. Smokers had 70% higher odds of consuming coffee, compared to non-smokers.

Tea consumption was associated with all background variables analyzed. The factors associated with tea drinking were being a woman, being in the oldest age group, having a normal or low BMI, having a higher education, being interested in a healthy diet, and being a non-smoker.

Table 4. Background characteristics associated with users and non-users of different beverage types.

Background Variables	Water n (%)	Water OR (95% CI)	Milk n (%)	Milk OR (95% CI)	Juice n (%)	Juice OR (95% CI)	Coffee n (%)	Coffee OR (95% CI)	Tea n (%)	Tea OR (95% CI)
Gender										
Men	809 (94)	1.00	737 (86)	1.00	393 (46)	1.00	720 (84)	1.00	242 (28)	1.00
Women	900 (97)	**1.92 (1.16–3.19)**	764 (83)	0.78 (0.54–1.13)	465 (50)	1.03 (0.84–1.23)	731 (79)	0.69 (0.53–0.90)	493 (53)	**2.76 (2.24–3.41)**
Age (years)										
18–34	397 (98)	1.00	352 (87)	1.00	218 (54)	1.00	263 (65)	1.00	141 (35)	1.00
35–54	780 (96)	0.48 (0.23–1.00)	680 (83)	0.81 (0.57–1.15)	409 (50)	0.87 (0.68–1.12)	681 (84)	**2.70 (2.0–3.6)**	356 (44)	**1.41 (1.07–1.84)**
55–70	532 (94)	**0.42 (0.20–0.88)**	469 (83)	0.78 (0.54–1.13)	231 (41)	**0.67 (0.51–0.88)**	507 (90)	**4.9 (3.4–7.1)**	238 (42)	**1.62 (1.2–2.2)**
p trend		0.028		0.207		0.003		<0.001		0.002
BMI										
<25 kg/m²	874 (97)	1.00	760 (84)	1.00	496 (55)	1.00	722 (80)	1.00	424 (47)	1.00
≥25 kg/m²	804 (94)	0.71 (0.43–1.17)	718 (84)	0.98 (0.75–1.29)	350 (41)	**0.63 (0.51–0.77)**	707 (83)	0.89 (0.68–1.16)	297 (35)	**0.70 (0.57–0.87)**
Education										
No or lower degree	790 (93)	1.00	709 (84)	1.00	323 (38)	1.00	670 (79)	1.00	282 (33)	1.00
University or college	916 (98)	**2.46 (1.47–4.14)**	789 (84)	1.00 (0.77–1.30)	535 (57)	**2.03 (1.67–2.48)**	778 (83)	1.26 (0.98–1.63)	451 (48)	**1.58 (1.28–1.95)**
Interest in healthy diet										
No, low or moderate	732 (94)	1.00	649 (83)	1.00	345 (44)	1.00	601 (77)	1.00	254 (33)	1.00
High or very high	976 (97)	**1.81 (1.11–2.96)**	851 (85)	1.21 (0.93–1.58)	513 (51)	1.17 (0.96–1.43)	849 (85)	**1.57 (1.2–2.0)**	481 (48)	**1.46 (1.18–1.80)**
Smoking habits										
Non-smokers	1362 (97)	1.00	1186 (84)	1.00	702 (50)	1.00	1129 (80)	1.00	632 (45)	1.00
Smokers	1709 (92)	**0.48 (0.29–0.78)**	315 (84)	0.97 (0.60–1.02)	156 (41)	**0.78 (0.61–0.99)**	322 (85)	**1.7 (1.2–2.4)**	103 (27)	**0.46 (0.36–0.61)**

Table 4. *Cont.*

Background Variables	n (%)	OR (95% CI) Sugar-sweetened beverages [1]	n (%)	OR (95% CI) Artificially sweetened beverages [2]	n (%)	OR (95% CI) Beer	n (%)	OR (95% CI) Wine
Gender								
Men	353 (41)	1.00	191 (22)	1.00	182 (21)	1.00	156 (18)	1.00
Women	260 (28)	**0.57 (0.46–0.71)**	242 (26)	**1.38 (1.10–1.75)**	85 (9)	**0.34 (0.25–0.46)**	204 (22)	1.13 (0.88–1.15)
Age (years)								
18–34	221 (54)	1.00	113 (28)	1.00	69 (17)	1.00	41 (10)	1.00
35–54	260 (32)	**0.43 (0.33–0.56)**	225 (28)	0.95 (0.72–1.25)	120 (15)	0.91 (0.65–1.28)	165 (20)	**2.28 (1.56–3.33)**
55–70	132 (23)	**0.24 (0.18–0.33)**	95 (17)	**0.47 (0.34–0.65)**	78 (14)	0.81 (0.56–1.17)	154 (27)	**3.78 (2.57–5.57)**
p trend		**<0.001**		**<0.001**		0.255		**<0.001**
BMI								
<25 kg/m^2	318 (35)	1.00	185 (21)	1.00	140 (16)	1.00	206 (23)	1.00
≥25 kg/m^2	287 (34)	0.95 (0.76–1.18)	239 (28)	**1.70 (1.35–2.15)**	123 (14)	0.76 (0.58–1.01)	148 (17)	**0.66 (0.51–0.85)**
Education								
No or lower degree	343 (41)	1.00	223 (26)	1.00	115 (14)	1.00	130 (15)	1.00
University or college	270 (29)	**0.65 (0.53–0.81)**	209 (22)	0.83 (0.66–1.04)	151 (16)	**1.43 (1.08–1.89)**	230 (25)	**1.67 (1.29–2.15)**
Interest in healthy diet								
No, low or moderate	345 (44)	1.00	211 (27)	1.00	131 (17)	1.00	120 (15)	1.00
High or very high	267 (27)	**0.56 (0.45–0.69)**	222 (22)	**0.79 (0.63–0.98)**	136 (14)	0.89 (0.67–1.17)	240 (24)	**1.48 (1.14–1.91)**
Smoking habits								
Non-smokers	472 (34)	1.00	328 (23)	1.00	189 (13)	1.00	282 (20)	1.00
Smokers	141 (37)	1.05 (0.81–1.35)	105 (28)	1.17 (0.90–1.54)	78 (21)	**1.79 (1.31–2.43)**	78 (21)	1.17 (0.87–1.58)

All analyses are adjusted for all background variables. Bold numbers represents statistical significant values. [1] Includes sugar-sweetened soft drinks and squash drinks; [2] Includes soft drinks and squash drinks without sugar and/or artificial sweeteners.

For sugar-sweetened beverages, women were less likely to consume such beverages than men. The oldest age group had 76% lower odds of sugar-sweetened beverage consumption compared to the youngest participants. Participants with higher education and participants with high or very high interest in a healthy diet also had lower odds of being consumers of sugar-sweetened beverages.

In contrast to the gender differences observed for sugar-sweetened beverages, women had 38% higher odds of consuming artificially sweetened beverages compared to men. Participants in the oldest age group had 53% lower odds of drinking artificially sweetened beverages, while participants being overweight had higher odds of consuming artificially sweetened beverages, compared to participants with a normal or low BMI. People interested in a healthy diet had 21% lower odds of consuming artificially sweetened beverages, compared to people with no, low or moderate interest.

Women were less likely to have consumed beer than men. Having a university or college education was associated with 43% higher odds of drinking beer. Smokers were more likely to be beer consumers than non-smokers.

With regard to wine, participants in the oldest age group were almost four times more likely to be wine consumers compared to the youngest participants. Wine consumption was less prevalent among participants with a BMI ≥ 25 kg/m^2 compared to those with a BMI < 25 kg/m^2. Wine consumption was also positively associated with an interest of having a healthy diet, compared to having no, low, or moderate interest.

4. Discussion

The results showed that, in a Norwegian setting, breakfast was the most important meal for the intake of milk and juice. For tea, the main contributing meal differed between men and women, with breakfast being the most important meal for men and snacks being the most important meal for women. Dinner was the most important meal for sugar-sweetened beverages and wine, whereas snacks were the most important meal for water, coffee, artificially sweetened beverages, and beer. The intake of wine was higher on weekend days than on weekdays among consumers. The same accounts for beer intake among men. Higher age was found to have a strong association with consumption of coffee, tea, and wine, whereas younger age was associated with consuming water and sugar-sweetened beverages. Higher education was associated with consumption of water, juice, tea, and alcohol-containing beverages (beer and wine), whereas no education or education of lower degree was associated with consumption of sugar-sweetened beverages.

4.1. Patterns of Beverage Consumption Related to Meals

Milk and fruit juices, together with coffee and tea, have also been previously found to be the most commonly consumed beverages for breakfast in Norway and the Scandinavian countries. This is described in the survey "Eating patterns, a day in the life of Nordic people", where computer assisted telephone interviews (CATI) were performed among 4800 Scandinavian individuals above 15 years of age [35].

Dinner was the most important meal for intake of sugar-sweetened beverages and wine. The average intake of sugar-sweetened beverages among all participants was 1/2 dL each day for dinner. One third (34%) of the participants were consumers of sugar-sweetened beverages. Among consumers the average daily intake was about 4 dL. The Norwegian health authorities recommend drinking water at meals and between meals because sugar-sweetened beverages increase the risk of obesity, tooth decay, and acid damage to teeth [22].

Snacks were the most important meal for water consumption in our study. A reason for this may be that water is regularly drunk between meals when thirsty and in association with physical activities. Snacks were also the most important meal for coffee, beer and artificially sweetened beverages. Coffee is a beverage that may be frequently consumed in social settings and at work. Beer may also be associated with social hang-outs in some groups of the population. Sieri et al. [36] found that alcohol was drunk outside main meals in most of the ten countries participating in the

European Prospective Investigation into Cancer and Nutrition (EPIC) study. Italy was an exception to this, where most of the alcohol intake was consumed during meals [36]. Snacks were also found to be the most important meal for alcoholic drinks among 6000 participants in The Netherlands, Ireland, and the UK [24]. In a study of fluid intake in the French population most beverages were ingested during the main meals breakfast, lunch, and dinner, and only small amounts were consumed between meals [37]. This deviates somewhat from our results, where the highest average intake of several beverage types, particularly water and coffee, were consumed as part of snacks.

4.2. Patterns of Beverage Consumption on Weekdays Compared to Weekend Days

We observed that the average intakes of wine among wine-consumers (both men and women) and beer (men only) were higher during weekend days, compared to weekdays. This complies with results from a British study by Gibson and coworkers, where higher consumption of alcoholic drinks was observed during weekends, especially Saturdays [38]. Among almost 12,000 U.S. adults it was also found that energy intake from alcohol was higher on Saturdays, compared to weekdays [39]. For women, beer intake was not significantly higher on weekend days compared to weekdays in our study. Sieri et al. [36] found that alcohol consumption, particularly among women, increased markedly during the weekend in nearly all centers participating in the EPIC study. Exceptions from this were some centers in Germany and Spain for men and Italy for women. Among U.S. adults it was found, in contrast, that the weekend-weekday difference in energy intake from alcohol was larger among male adults than among women [39]. It seems like consumption habits with regard to wine and beer on weekdays compared to weekend days varies between different countries. Therefore, it may be reasonable to evaluate the situation in each country when giving public health advice.

Surprisingly, we did not find any differences in the intake of sugar-sweetened and artificially sweetened beverages between weekdays and weekend days among consumers. There is scarce literature published regarding consumption of such beverages among adults. Among almost 800 Danish children and adolescents the intake of sugar-sweetened beverages was found to be higher during the weekend, compared to weekdays [40]. A national representative survey among Norwegian children found that the intake of sugar-sweetened soft drinks was significantly higher during weekend days, compared to weekdays among four-year old children and school children in 4th and 8th grade [41]. Among 1500 Norwegian adolescents and their parents, the intake of sugar-sweetened beverages was found to be low during weekdays, but doubled during weekend days [42]. In a study among almost 12,000 U.S. adults from 2003–2012 the authors found that energy intake from sugar-sweetened beverages was higher on weekend days compared to weekdays. This difference was larger among men than women [39]. Since the weekend constitutes almost one third of the week, improvement of the composition of foods and beverages consumed during weekends will contribute to improve the total dietary quality.

4.3. Background Variables Associated with the Intake of Different Types of Beverages

Our results implied that water consumption was more prevalent among younger participants and participants having a higher education. This corresponds partly to data from the National Health and Nutrition Examination Surveys (NHANES) from 1999–2006 among more than 4000 U.S. adult participants, where the researchers found that water intake declined with increasing age and higher education was associated with higher water consumption [43]. We also found that women and participants being interested in a healthy diet had higher odds of consuming water.

We observed no associations between milk intake and background variables. Canadian data from 35,000 participants in 2004 described that the proportion of adults who reported drinking milk tended to rise with increasing age. The same study also found that juice consumption was associated with younger age groups [44]. This corresponds to the results from the present study as the odds of juice consumption were significantly lower in the oldest, compared to the youngest, age group.

Coffee intake was associated with higher age, being interested in a healthy diet and smoking in our study. Sousa and Macedo da Costa also found a positive association between coffee intake and higher age among Brazilian adults, but this association was only found for men [45]. A Canadian study of beverage consumption found that coffee consumption peaked at ages 31–50 years and, thereby, decreased with increasing age [44]. Smoking has also been found to be associated with coffee consumption in several other studies [46–48].

Tea consumption was associated with all factors analyzed in our study; being a woman, being in the oldest age group, having a normal or low BMI, having higher education, being interested in a healthy diet, and being a non-smoker. Higher tea consumption with increasing age was also reported in the aforementioned Canadian study [44]. A study among almost 6000 university students in Taiwan found that having a higher BMI was a significant predictor of tea drinking [49], which contrasts with our results. De Castro and Taylor describe an association between cigarette smoking and frequent consumption of coffee and tea among 650 U.S. adults [46]. This complies with our results for coffee, but is opposite of our results for tea consumers, where smokers had 54% lower odds of consuming tea, compared to non-smokers.

Consumption of sugar-sweetened beverages dropped sharply at older ages in both the present and other studies [30,44]. Mullie et al. [30] found that high age, high BMI, non-smoking, and income were negatively related to consumption of sugar-sweetened beverages. Our results indicated that participants with university or college education had lower odds of consuming sugar-sweetened beverages. The association between consumption of sugar-sweetened beverages and lower or no education has also been found in other studies [29,31,32]. Liu and coworkers [50] described that, compared to college educated individuals, the odds of consuming sugar-sweetened beverages was more than three times greater for those with high school education or less. Why a lower socioeconomic position is associated with higher consumption of sugar-sweetened beverages is not clear, but it has been argued that the low cost and aggressive marketing in low-income areas could be an explanation [30]. It is well documented that low socioeconomic position is associated with a clustering of unhealthy lifestyles, such as smoking, unhealthy dietary patterns, and obesity [51]. Drinking sugar-sweetened beverages regularly can be seen as an unhealthy habit due to the high energy-content and the low nutritional value [30].

In a study among almost 2000 military men in Belgium, high BMI and trying to lose weight were found to be positively related to consumption of artificially sweetened beverages [30]. This corresponds to our results where participants with a BMI of 25 kg/m^2 or higher had 70% higher odds of consuming artificially sweetened beverages, compared to participants with a normal or low BMI. This may indicate that people being overweight or obese are drinking more artificially sweetened beverages in an attempt to lose weight [30].

Men in the present study had higher odds of drinking beer compared to women, and the percentage of wine consumers increased with increasing age. The same associations have also been described in the Canadian population [44]. In a study in the older population in Spain from 2008–2010 alcohol consumption was significantly more frequent among men, compared to women [52]. De Castro and Taylor [46] found that cigarette smoking was associated with alcohol consumption among 600 adults in Texas, USA. We found the same tendency for beer consumers, but not for wine consumers.

4.4. Strengths and Limitations

The detailed information about types and amounts of beverage intakes and meal types are the major strengths of the Norkost 3 survey, in addition to the relatively large sample size. A limitation of the study is the fairly low participation rate of 37%, which limits the generalizability of the results [53]. The proportion of participants in the Norkost 3 study with a college/university education was higher than in the general population [33]. We may assume that a study population with higher education has healthier beverage consumption habits, compared to the general population with lower education. An association between higher education and healthier diets has been found in several studies [27,28,33]. The consumption of sugar-sweetened beverages may have been underestimated in the present study due to the high percentage of participants with a college/university education. A higher percentage of the participants in Norkost 3 belonged to the highest age interval and a lower percentage to the youngest interval, compared to the general population. The background characteristics of the participants in the Norkost 3 survey, compared to the characteristics of the general population have earlier been described in detail [33].

Self-reported surveys collecting the intake of fluids are open to potential bias due to over- or under-reporting of certain fluid types [54]. The use of 24 h recall or food frequency questionnaire (FFQ) has been reported to underestimate fluid intakes by as much as 500 mL/day. The reason for this is that fluids are often consumed outside mealtimes and not perceived as a food [29,55]. The 24 h recall method relies on the participants' ability and willingness to correctly inform the interviewer about all eating and drinking events that occurred on the preceding day [53]. In the present study pure drinking meals were defined as snacks (pure drinking meals representing about 40% of meals defined as snacks). There is some evidence that snacks are more likely to be underreported than main meals [56], if this is the case in the present study total beverage intake may have been underestimated. Alcohol consumption [57] and soft drink consumption [58] have been described, in particular, as being subject to underreporting. The interviewers in the Norkost 3 survey were thoroughly trained on interview techniques and to remind the participants about forgotten food or drink items, which may have reduced the underreporting of snack events [53].

Body weight was self-reported, which may be a limitation for the validity of the estimated BMI because self-reported weight tends to be underestimated [59,60]. This may have contributed to misclassification of participants as normal weight participants and a reduction in the difference between the two groups [53].

4.5. Practical Implications

The findings from the present study provide insight into the beverage consumption pattern to different meals among a group of Norwegian adults and in different subgroups of the study population. This insight may be useful when developing and revising dietary recommendations. Holmback et al. has suggested that the inclusion of meal-based recommendations may be an advantage in FBDG [23].

Still, the data in Norkost 3 were collected in 2010–2011, and beverage consumption habits in the population may have changed somewhat during the last 5–6 years.

Age and education seemed to be highly associated with consumption of certain beverage types. Being a young adult (18–34 years) was associated with consumption of sugar-sweetened beverages, artificially sweetened beverages, and water, whereas being older was associated with wine consumption. Having a higher education seemed to be associated with a healthier beverage consumption pattern, including water and less sugar-sweetened beverages. On the other hand, higher education was associated with beer and wine consumption. Knowledge about how beverage consumption is associated with age and education helps us understand habits in subgroups of the population. More knowledge from research on these associations may be used when tailoring interventions regarding consumption of sugar-sweetened and alcoholic beverages in the future.

5. Conclusions

Beverage consumption patterns in the Norwegian adult population varied between different meal types. Breakfast was the most important meal type for intake of milk and juice, and dinner for sugar-sweetened beverages and wine, whereas snacks contributed most to intakes of water, coffee, artificially sweetened beverages, and beer. Alcohol consumption was higher on weekend days, compared to weekdays among consumers. Higher education was associated with a healthier beverage consumption pattern, but also more frequent alcohol consumption. Higher age was strongly associated with consumption of coffee, tea and wine, whereas younger age was associated with consumption of water and sugar-sweetened beverages. Knowledge regarding beverage consumption patterns in the population and in subgroups of the population may be considered when revising FBDGs in the future.

Acknowledgments: The authors would like to thank the participants of the Norkost 3 survey.

Author Contributions: M.M.P., J.B.M. and L.F.A. formulated the research questions. M.M.P. carried out the data analyses, assisted by J.B.M., and drafted the first manuscript. J.B.M. and L.F.A. assisted and provided advice at all stages of the work. All authors read and approved the final manuscript.

Conflicts of Interest: The authors declare no conflict of interest. The founding sponsors had no role in the design of the study; in the collection, analyses, or interpretation of data; in the writing of the manuscript, and in the decision to publish the results.

References

1. Kerver, J.M.; Yang, E.J.; Obayashi, S.; Bianchi, L.; Song, W.O. Meal and snack patterns are associated with dietary intake of energy and nutrients in US adults. *J. Am. Diet. Assoc.* **2006**, *106*, 46–53. [CrossRef] [PubMed]
2. Pobocik, R.S.; Trager, A.; Monson, L.M. Dietary patterns and food choices of a population sample of adults on Guam. *Asia Pac. J. Clin. Nutr.* **2008**, *17*, 94–100. [PubMed]
3. Venci, B.; Hodac, N.; Lee, S.Y.; Shidler, M.; Krikorian, R. Beverage consumption patterns and micronutrient and caloric intake from beverages in older adults with mild cognitive impairment. *J. Nutr. Gerontol. Geriatr.* **2015**, *34*, 399–409. [CrossRef] [PubMed]
4. Coudray, B. The contribution of dairy products to micronutrient intakes in France. *J. Am. Coll. Nutr.* **2011**, *30*, 410S–414S. [CrossRef] [PubMed]
5. Drewnowski, A. The contribution of milk and milk products to micronutrient density and affordability of the US Diet. *J. Am. Coll. Nutr.* **2011**, *30*, 422S–428S. [CrossRef] [PubMed]
6. Huth, P.J.; Fulgoni, V.L.; Keast, D.R.; Park, K.; Auestad, N. Major food sources of calories, added sugars, and saturated fat and their contribution to essential nutrient intakes in the US Diet: Data from the national health and nutrition examination survey (2003–2006). *Nutr. J.* **2013**, *12*, 116. [CrossRef] [PubMed]
7. Vissers, P.A.; Streppel, M.T.; Feskens, E.J.; de Groot, L.C. The contribution of dairy products to micronutrient intake in The Netherlands. *J. Am. Coll. Nutr.* **2011**, *30*, 415S–421S. [CrossRef] [PubMed]
8. The Norwegian Directorate of Health. Utviklingen I Norsk Kosthold 2015. Available online: https://helsedirektoratet.no/Lists/Publikasjoner/Attachments/1021/Utviklingen-i-norsk-kosthold-2015-IS-2382.pdf (accessed on 10 December 2015).
9. Hu, F.B.; Malik, V.S. Sugar-sweetened beverages and risk of obesity and type 2 diabetes: Epidemiologic evidence. *Physiol. Behav.* **2010**, *100*, 47–54. [CrossRef] [PubMed]
10. Malik, V.S.; Schulze, M.B.; Hu, F.B. Intake of sugar-sweetened beverages and weight gain: A systematic review. *Am. J. Clin. Nutr.* **2006**, *84*, 274–288. [PubMed]
11. Woodward-Lopez, G.; Kao, J.; Ritchie, L. To what extent have sweetened beverages contributed to the obesity epidemic? *Public Health Nutr.* **2011**, *14*, 499–509. [CrossRef] [PubMed]
12. Gibson, S. Sugar-sweetened soft drinks and obesity: A systematic review of the evidence from observational studies and interventions. *Nutr. Res. Rev.* **2008**, *21*, 134–147. [CrossRef] [PubMed]
13. Mattes, R.D.; Shikany, J.M.; Kaiser, K.A.; Allison, D.B. Nutritively sweetened beverage consumption and body weight: A systematic review and meta-analysis of randomized experiments. *Obes. Rev.* **2011**, *12*, 346–365. [CrossRef] [PubMed]
14. Rehm, J.; Baliunas, D.; Borges, G.L.; Graham, K.; Irving, H.; Kehoe, T.; Parry, C.D.; Patra, J.; Popova, S.; Poznyak, V. The relation between different dimensions of alcohol consumption and burden of disease: An overview. *Addiction* **2010**, *105*, 817–843. [CrossRef] [PubMed]
15. Holman, C.; English, D.R.; Milne, E.; Winter, M.G. Meta-analysis of alcohol and all-cause mortality: A validation of nhmrc recommendations. *Med. J. Aust.* **1996**, *164*, 141–145. [PubMed]
16. Knott, C.S.; Coombs, N.; Stamatakis, E.; Biddulph, J.P. All cause mortality and the case for age specific alcohol consumption guidelines: Pooled analyses of up to 10 population based cohorts. *BMJ* **2015**, *350*, h384. [CrossRef] [PubMed]

17. Stockwell, T.; Zhao, J.; Panwar, S.; Roemer, A.; Naimi, T.; Chikritzhs, T. Do "moderate" drinkers have reduced mortality risk? A systematic review and meta-analysis of alcohol consumption and all-cause mortality. *J. Stud. Alcohol Drugs* **2016**, *77*, 185–198. [CrossRef] [PubMed]

18. The Norwegian Directorate of Health. Kostråd for å Fremme Folkehelsen og Forebygge Kroniske Sykdommer: Metodologi og Vitenskapelig Kunnskapsgrunnlag. Available online: https://fido.nrk.no/5070725ea6c90cbb7d02b12dd53955b754904a13a5ba80e83464533b457f8e0f/Kosthold.pdf (accessed on 10 December 2015).

19. Food and Agriculture Organization of the United Nations. Food-Based Dietary Guidelines. Available online: http://www.fao.org/nutrition/nutrition-education/food-dietary-guidelines/en/ (accessed on 8 January 2016).

20. Kit, B.K.; Fakhouri, T.H.; Park, S.; Nielsen, S.J.; Ogden, C.L. Trends in sugar-sweetened beverage consumption among youth and adults in the United States: 1999–2010. *Am. J. Clin. Nutr.* **2013**, *98*, 180–188. [CrossRef] [PubMed]

21. Ng, S.W.; Ni Mhurchu, C.; Jebb, S.A.; Popkin, B.M. Patterns and trends of beverage consumption among children and adults in great britain, 1986–2009. *Br. J. Nutr.* **2012**, *108*, 536–551. [CrossRef] [PubMed]

22. The Norwegian Directorate of Health. Anbefalinger om Kosthold, Ernæring og Fysisk Aktivitet. Available online: https://helsedirektoratet.no/publikasjoner/anbefalinger-om-kosthold-ernering-og-fysisk-aktivitet (accessed on 8 January 2016).

23. Holmback, I.; Ericson, U.; Gullberg, B.; Wirfalt, E. Five meal patterns are differently associated with nutrient intakes, lifestyle factors and energy misreporting in a sub-sample of the Malmo Diet and Cancer Cohort. *Food Nutr. Res.* **2009**. [CrossRef] [PubMed]

24. Kearney, J.M.; Hulshof, K.F.; Gibney, M.J. Eating patterns—Temporal distribution, converging and diverging foods, meals eaten inside and outside of the home—Implications for developing FBDG. *Public Health Nutr.* **2001**, *4*, 693–698. [CrossRef] [PubMed]

25. Myhre, J.B.; Loken, E.B.; Wandel, M.; Andersen, L.F. Meal types as sources for intakes of fruits, vegetables, fish and whole grains among Norwegian adults. *Public Health Nutr.* **2015**, *18*, 2011–2021. [CrossRef] [PubMed]

26. Darmon, N.; Drewnowski, A. Does social class predict diet quality? *Am. J. Clin. Nutr.* **2008**, *87*, 1107–1117. [PubMed]

27. Hjartaker, A.; Lund, E. Relationship between dietary habits, age, lifestyle, and socio-economic status among adult Norwegian women. The Norwegian Women and Cancer Study. *Eur. J. Clin. Nutr.* **1998**, *52*, 565–572. [CrossRef] [PubMed]

28. Johansson, L.; Thelle, D.S.; Solvoll, K.; Bjorneboe, G.E.; Drevon, C.A. Healthy dietary habits in relation to social determinants and lifestyle factors. *Br. J. Nutr.* **1999**, *81*, 211–220. [CrossRef] [PubMed]

29. Han, E.; Powell, L.M. Consumption patterns of sugar-sweetened beverages in the United States. *J. Acad. Nutr. Diet.* **2013**, *113*, 43–53. [CrossRef] [PubMed]

30. Mullie, P.; Aerenhouts, D.; Clarys, P. Demographic, socioeconomic and nutritional determinants of daily versus non-daily sugar-sweetened and artificially sweetened beverage consumption. *Eur. J. Clin. Nutr.* **2012**, *66*, 150–155. [CrossRef] [PubMed]

31. Park, S.; Blanck, H.M.; Sherry, B.; Brener, N.; O'Toole, T. Factors associated with sugar-sweetened beverage intake among United States high school students. *J. Nutr.* **2012**, *142*, 306–312. [CrossRef] [PubMed]

32. Rehm, C.D.; Matte, T.D.; Van Wye, G.; Young, C.; Frieden, T.R. Demographic and behavioral factors associated with daily sugar-sweetened soda consumption in New York City adults. *J. Urban Health* **2008**, *85*, 375–385. [CrossRef] [PubMed]

33. Myhre, J.B.; Loken, E.B.; Wandel, M.; Andersen, L.F. Eating location is associated with the nutritional quality of the diet in Norwegian adults. *Public Health Nutr.* **2014**, *17*, 915–923. [CrossRef] [PubMed]

34. Norwegian Food Safety Authority; Norwegian Directorate of Health; University of Oslo. The Norwegian Food Composition Table. Available online: http://www.matportalen.no/verktoy/the_norwegian_food_composition_table/old_tables (accessed on 23 October 2015).

35. Kjærnes, U. *Eating Patterns: A Day in the Lives of Nordic Peoples*; National Instititute for Consumer Research: Lysaker, Norway, 2001.

36. Sieri, S.; Agudo, A.; Kesse, E.; Klipstein-Grobusch, K.; San-Jose, B.; Welch, A.A.; Krogh, V.; Luben, R.; Allen, N.; Overvad, K.; et al. Patterns of alcohol consumption in 10 European countries participating in the European Prospective Investigation Into Cancer and Nutrition (EPIC) project. *Public Health Nutr.* **2002**, *5*, 1287–1296. [CrossRef] [PubMed]

37. Bellisle, F.; Thornton, S.N.; Hebel, P.; Denizeau, M.; Tahiri, M. A study of fluid intake from beverages in a sample of healthy French children, adolescents and adults. *Eur. J. Clin. Nutr.* **2010**, *64*, 350–355. [CrossRef] [PubMed]

38. Gibson, S.; Shirreffs, S.M. Beverage consumption habits "24/7" among British adults: Association with total water intake and energy intake. *Nutr. J.* **2013**, *12*, 9. [CrossRef] [PubMed]

39. An, R. Weekend-weekday differences in diet among US Adults, 2003–2012. *Ann. Epidemiol.* **2016**, *26*, 57–65. [CrossRef] [PubMed]

40. Rothausen, B.W.; Matthiessen, J.; Hoppe, C.; Brockhoff, P.B.; Andersen, L.F.; Tetens, I. Differences in Danish children's diet quality on weekdays v. Weekend days. *Public Health Nutr.* **2012**, *15*, 1653–1660. [CrossRef] [PubMed]

41. Lillegaard, I.T.L.; Øverby, N.; Andersen, L.F. Er det forskjell på hva barn spiser på hverdager og i helgen. *Barn* **2003**, *2*, 89–98.

42. Bjelland, M.; Lien, N.; Grydeland, M.; Bergh, I.H.; Anderssen, S.A.; Ommundsen, Y.; Klepp, K.I.; Andersen, L.F. Intakes and perceived home availability of sugar-sweetened beverages, fruit and vegetables as reported by mothers, fathers and adolescents in the HEIA (HEalth in Adolescents) study. *Public Health Nutr.* **2011**, *14*, 2156–2165. [CrossRef] [PubMed]

43. Kant, A.K.; Graubard, B.I.; Atchison, E.A. Intakes of plain water, moisture in foods and beverages, and total water in the adult US population—Nutritional, meal pattern, and body weight correlates: National Health and Nutrition Examination Surveys 1999–2006. *Am. J. Clin. Nutr.* **2009**, *90*, 655–663. [CrossRef] [PubMed]

44. Garriguet, D. Beverage consumption of Canadian adults. *Health Rep.* **2008**, *19*, 23–29. [PubMed]

45. Sousa, A.G.; da Costa, T.H. Usual coffee intake in Brazil: Results from the national dietary survey 2008–9. *Br. J. Nutr.* **2015**, *113*, 1615–1620. [CrossRef] [PubMed]

46. De Castro, J.M.; Taylor, T. Smoking status relationships with the food and fluid intakes of free-living humans. *Nutrition* **2008**, *24*, 109–119. [CrossRef] [PubMed]

47. McPhillips, J.B.; Eaton, C.B.; Gans, K.M.; Derby, C.A.; Lasater, T.M.; McKenney, J.L.; Carleton, R.A. Dietary differences in smokers and nonsmokers from two southeastern New England communities. *J. Am. Diet. Assoc.* **1994**, *94*, 287–292. [CrossRef]

48. Whichelow, M.J.; Erzinclioglu, S.W.; Cox, B.D. A comparison of the diets of non-smokers and smokers. *Br. J. Addict.* **1991**, *86*, 71–81. [CrossRef] [PubMed]

49. Tseng, H.C.; Wang, C.J.; Cheng, S.H.; Sun, Z.J.; Chen, P.S.; Lee, C.T.; Lin, S.H.; Yang, Y.K.; Yang, Y.C. Tea-drinking habit among new university students: Associated factors. *Kaohsiung J. Med. Sci.* **2014**, *30*, 98–103. [CrossRef] [PubMed]

50. Liu, J.L.; Han, B.; Cohen, D.A. Associations between eating occasions and places of consumption among adults. *Appetite* **2015**, *87*, 199–204. [CrossRef] [PubMed]

51. Mullie, P.; Clarys, P.; Hulens, M.; Vansant, G. Dietary patterns and socioeconomic position. *Eur. J. Clin. Nutr.* **2010**, *64*, 231–238. [CrossRef] [PubMed]

52. Leon-Munoz, L.M.; Galan, I.; Donado-Campos, J.; Sanchez-Alonso, F.; Lopez-Garcia, E.; Valencia-Martin, J.L.; Guallar-Castillon, P.; Rodriguez-Artalejo, F. Patterns of alcohol consumption in the older population of Spain, 2008–2010. *J. Acad. Nutr. Diet.* **2015**, *115*, 213–224. [CrossRef] [PubMed]

53. Myhre, J.B.; Loken, E.B.; Wandel, M.; Andersen, L.F. The contribution of snacks to dietary intake and their association with eating location among Norwegian adults—Results from a cross-sectional dietary survey. *BMC Public Health* **2015**, *15*, 369. [CrossRef] [PubMed]

54. Guelinckx, I.; Ferreira-Pego, C.; Moreno, L.A.; Kavouras, S.A.; Gandy, J.; Martinez, H.; Bardosono, S.; Abdollahi, M.; Nasseri, E.; Jarosz, A.; et al. Intake of water and different beverages in adults across 13 countries. *Eur. J. Nutr.* **2015**, *54*, 45–55. [CrossRef] [PubMed]

55. Nissensohn, M.; Ruano, C.; Serra-Majem, L. Validation of beverage intake methods vs. Hydration biomarkers; a short review. *Nutr. Hosp.* **2013**, *28*, 1815–1819. [PubMed]

56. Poppitt, S.D.; Swann, D.; Black, A.E.; Prentice, A.M. Assessment of selective under-reporting of food intake by both obese and non-obese women in a metabolic facility. *Int. J. Obes. Relat. Metab. Disord.* **1998**, *22*, 303–311. [CrossRef] [PubMed]

57. Stockwell, T.; Donath, S.; Cooper-Stanbury, M.; Chikritzhs, T.; Catalano, P.; Mateo, C. Under-reporting of alcohol consumption in household surveys: A comparison of quantity-frequency, graduated-frequency and recent recall. *Addiction* **2004**, *99*, 1024–1033. [CrossRef] [PubMed]

58. Krebs-Smith, S.M.; Graubard, B.I.; Kahle, L.L.; Subar, A.F.; Cleveland, L.E.; Ballard-Barbash, R. Low energy reporters vs others: A comparison of reported food intakes. *Eur. J. Clin. Nutr.* **2000**, *54*, 281–287. [CrossRef] [PubMed]

59. Nyholm, M.; Gullberg, B.; Merlo, J.; Lundqvist-Persson, C.; Rastam, L.; Lindblad, U. The validity of obesity based on self-reported weight and height: Implications for population studies. *Obesity* **2007**, *15*, 197–208. [CrossRef] [PubMed]

60. Scribani, M.; Shelton, J.; Chapel, D.; Krupa, N.; Wyckoff, L.; Jenkins, P. Comparison of bias resulting from two methods of self-reporting height and weight: A validation study. *JRSM Open* **2014**. [CrossRef] [PubMed]

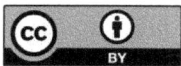

nutrients

MDPI

Article

Fructose Beverage Consumption Induces a Metabolic Syndrome Phenotype in the Rat: A Systematic Review and Meta-Analysis

Carla R. Toop and Sheridan Gentili *

School of Pharmacy and Medical Sciences, Sansom Institute for Health Research, University of South Australia, Adelaide 5000, SA, Australia; carla.toop@mymail.unisa.edu.au
* Correspondence: Sheridan.Gentili@unisa.edu.au; Tel.: +61-8-8302-2452

Received: 27 July 2016; Accepted: 13 September 2016; Published: 20 September 2016

Abstract: A high intake of refined carbohydrates, particularly the monosaccharide fructose, has been attributed to the growing epidemics of obesity and type-2 diabetes. Animal studies have helped elucidate the metabolic effects of dietary fructose, however, variations in study design make it difficult to draw conclusions. The aim of this study was to review the effects of fructose beverage consumption on body weight, systolic blood pressure and blood glucose, insulin and triglyceride concentrations in validated rat models. We searched Ovid Embase Classic + EmbaseMedline and Ovid Medline databases and included studies that used adolescent/adult male rats, with fructose beverage consumption for >3 weeks. Data from 26 studies were pooled by an inverse variance weighting method using random effects models, expressed as standardized mean differences (SMD) with 95% confidence intervals (CI). Overall, 10%–21% w/v fructose beverage consumption was associated with increased rodent body weight (SMD, 0.62 (95% CI: 0.18, 1.06)), systolic blood pressure (SMD, 2.94 (95% CI: 2.10, 3.77)) and blood glucose (SMD, 0.77 (95% CI: 0.36, 1.19)), insulin (SMD, 2.32 (95% CI: 1.57, 3.07)) and triglyceride (SMD, 1.87 (95% CI: 1.39, 2.34)) concentrations. Therefore, the consumption of a low concentration fructose beverage is sufficient to cause early signs of the metabolic syndrome in adult rats.

Keywords: fructose; beverage; rat; metabolic syndrome; meta-analysis; diabetes; obesity

1. Introduction

A high intake of refined carbohydrates and sweeteners, including sucrose and high fructose corn syrup (HFCS), have been attributed to the growing epidemics of obesity and type-2 diabetes (T2D) in Western society [1]. Current evidence suggests that the consumption of added dietary sugars (including sucrose and HFCS) is currently stable or decreasing [2], however, it still remains high. It is estimated that Australians consume approximately 46.83 kg of sugar per year, while Americans consume on average 68.57 kg per year [3]. This translates to between 26.8% and 39.3% of daily energy consumed from added sugar (based on 2000 Cal/day). Furthermore, sugar consumption is high in both children and adolescents [4], which has been identified as contributing to the alarming rates of T2D and obesity observed in this population [5]. Specifically, the monosaccharide fructose has been identified as a key component of added sugars contributing to these epidemics. Despite the evidence, there is still confusion surrounding whether the consumption of fructose at physiologically relevant concentrations contributes to the development of metabolic disease. This is not surprising due to the varying outcomes found by studies investigating the effects of fructose consumption on human metabolic health [6–8].

While the western diet is typically low in free fructose, the main dietary sources of fructose are sucrose, HFCS, fruits and honey. Despite having the same chemical formula as glucose, hepatic fructose metabolism is different [9]. In the rodent, chronic consumption of fructose at high concentrations is known to give rise to ectopic fat deposition, insulin resistance, T2D and elevated blood pressure [9]. The evidence associated with lower concentration fructose beverage consumption, however, is less clear [6].

Fructose feeding is an established experimental model for inducing the metabolic syndrome in rats [10,11]; however, studies vary significantly in fructose delivery and the administered concentration. The concentration of fructose administered as a component of chow itself is generally supraphysiological and ranges between 60%–70% w/w or 0.6–0.7 g/g chow [10,12–21], whereas the concentration of fructose beverages can often vary anywhere between 10%–30% w/v or 0.1–0.3 g fructose/mL water [22–45]. Despite the reported effects on metabolic health, studies investigating the effect of high concentrations of fructose in chow or as a beverage report no effect of fructose consumption on rodent body weight [10,12,46,47], while others report an increase in body weight [22,23,27,29,30,38–41,43,48,49]. Furthermore, while these studies give an understanding of the effects associated with excess fructose intake, the physiological outcomes associated with supraphysiological concentrations of fructose cannot be used to extrapolate the effects to human health. Thus, the effect of lower concentration fructose beverage consumption at concentrations similar to those found in sugar-sweetened beverages (~10% w/v) must be clarified in a rodent model.

To provide consistent evidence of the metabolic effects of fructose, we undertook a systematic review and meta-analysis of experimental animal studies to assess the effect of low concentration fructose beverage administration on rodent body weight, systolic blood pressure and blood glucose, insulin and triglyceride concentrations. To our knowledge, this is the first meta-analysis to explore the effects of administration of a fructose beverage in a rodent model.

2. Materials and Methods

2.1. Literature Search

We searched Ovid Embase Classic + EmbaseMedline and Ovid Medline for articles published within the last 10 years with medical subject headings (MeSH) terms fructose, rat or rats, and weight. Only articles published in English were included in the study. From this, 1317 eligible articles were identified, of which 371 were identified as duplicates. The remaining 946 articles were reviewed for inclusion in the analysis. The exclusion search criteria included: conference abstracts, review articles, studies utilizing pregnant rodents, studies completed on rodents during the lactation or weaning periods, studies conducted during rodent development (i.e., fetuses or offspring less than 8 weeks of age), HFCS feeding, and citations which did not list fructose or body weight in the title or abstract (Figure 1).

2.2. Study Selection

Of the remaining 139 citations, only studies which used male adolescent/adult rodents (>8 weeks of age) were included in the analysis, in which fructose alone (not in combination with glucose or as sucrose or HFCS) was administered in a beverage where the concentration was provided. Of these, studies that included numerical data (mean ± standard deviation) on at least two of; final body weight, systolic blood pressure and blood glucose, insulin and triglyceride concentrations were included (26 studies in total as summarized in Figure 1 and Table 1).

2.3. Data Collected

We collected the mean and standard deviation data for body weight (g), systolic blood pressure (mmHg), blood glucose (mmol/L), blood insulin (pmol/L) and blood triglyceride (mmol/L) concentrations in animals exposed to control and fructose as reported in the publications. Where required, the glucose, insulin and triglyceride concentrations were converted to the above listed units. Where reported, the major findings of fructose on each biological measure is summarized in Table 1.

Table 1. Characteristics and major outcome measures of studies included in the meta-analysis, including the effects of fructose beverage consumption on male body weight, systolic blood pressure and blood glucose, insulin and triglyceride concentrations.

Citation	Fructose Concentration (% *w/v*)	Duration of Intervention (Weeks)	*n* (% of Control)	Body Weight	Systolic Blood Pressure	Blood Glucose	Blood Insulin	Blood Triglycerides
						Summary of Findings: Effect of Fructose Relative to Control		
Ge et al. 2016 [23]	10	5	16 (50)	Significant increase	Data not reported	No effect	Significant increase	Significant increase
Prince et al. 2016 [24]	10	8	16 (50)	No effect	Data not reported	No effect	Data not reported	Significant increase
Ibrahim et al. 2015 [22]	10	20	14 (57.1) *	Significant increase (raw data not provided)	Data not reported	Significant increase	Significant increase	Significant increase
Litterio et al. 2015 [25]	10	8	18 (55.6)	No effect	Significant increase	Data not reported	Data not reported	Data not reported
Peredo et al. 2015 [26]	10	9	12 (50)	No effect	Significant increase	No effect	Significant increase	Significant increase
Al-Rasheed et al. 2014 [27]	10	8	20 (50)	Significant increase	Data not reported	Significant increase	Data not reported	Significant increase (raw data not provided)
Castro et al. 2014 [28]	10	3	40 (50)	No effect	Data not reported	No effect	Significant increase	Significant increase
Mahmoud and Elshazly, 2014 [29]	10	12	10 (50) *	Significant increase (raw data not provided)	Significant increase	Significant increase	Significant increase	Significant increase
Cardinali et al. 2013 [30]	10	8	16 (50)	Significant increase	Significant increase	Data not reported	Data not reported	Significant increase
Farina et al. 2013 [31]	10	3	20 (50) *	No effect	Data not reported	No effect	No effect	Significant increase
Larsen et al. 2013 [32]	10	26	12 (50)	No effect	Data not reported	No effect	No effect	No effect
Zarfeshani et al. 2012 [33]	21	10	12 (50)	No effect	Data not reported	No effect	Data not reported	No effect
Maïztegui et al. 2011 [34]	10	3	40 (50)	No effect	Data not reported	No effect	Significant increase	Significant increase
Shahraki et al. 2011 [35]	10	8	19 (47.4)	No effect (raw data not provided)	Data not reported	No effect	No effect	Significant increase

Table 1. *Cont.*

Citation	Fructose Concentration (% w/v)	Duration of Intervention (Weeks)	n (% of Control)	Body Weight	Systolic Blood Pressure	Blood Glucose	Blood Insulin	Blood Triglycerides
					Summary of Findings: Effect of Fructose Relative to Control			
Francini et al. 2010 [50]	10	3	30 (50)	No effect	Data not reported	Significant increase	Significant increase	Significant increase
Giani et al. 2010 [36]	10	6	16 (50)	No effect	Significant increase	No effect	Significant increase	Data not reported
Atanasovska et al. 2009 [37]	10	12	28 (42.9)	No effect	Significant increase	Data not reported	Significant increase	Significant increase
Bi et al. 2009 [38]	10	32	30 (40)	Significant increase (raw data not provided)	Data not reported	No effect	Significant increase	Significant increase
Bi et al. 2008 [49]	10	38	21 (57.1)	Significant increase	Significant increase	No effect	Significant increase	Significant increase
Tan et al. 2008 [39]	10	32	21 (57.1)	Significant increase	Significant increase	No effect	Significant increase	Significant increase
Xing et al. 2008 [40]	10	34.7	21 (57.1)	Significant increase (raw data not provided)	Significant increase	No effect	Significant increase	Significant increase
Jalal et al. 2007 [41]	10	8	34 (29.4)	Significant increase	Data not reported	Significant increase	Data not reported	Significant increase
Sanchez-Lozada et al. 2007 [42]	10	8	14 (50)	No effect	Significant increase	No effect	Data not reported	No effect
Yadav et al. 2007 [43]	21	8	12 (50)	Significant increase	Data not reported	Significant increase	Significant increase	Significant increase
Xi et al. 2007 [44]	10	8	20 (50)	No effect	Significant increase	No effect	Significant increase	Significant increase
Shalam et al. 2006 [45]	10	2.86	12 (50)	Data not reported	Data not reported	Significant increase	Significant increase	Significant increase (raw data not provided)

* Where animal numbers per group were given as a range, the smallest number has been reported and used in the analysis.

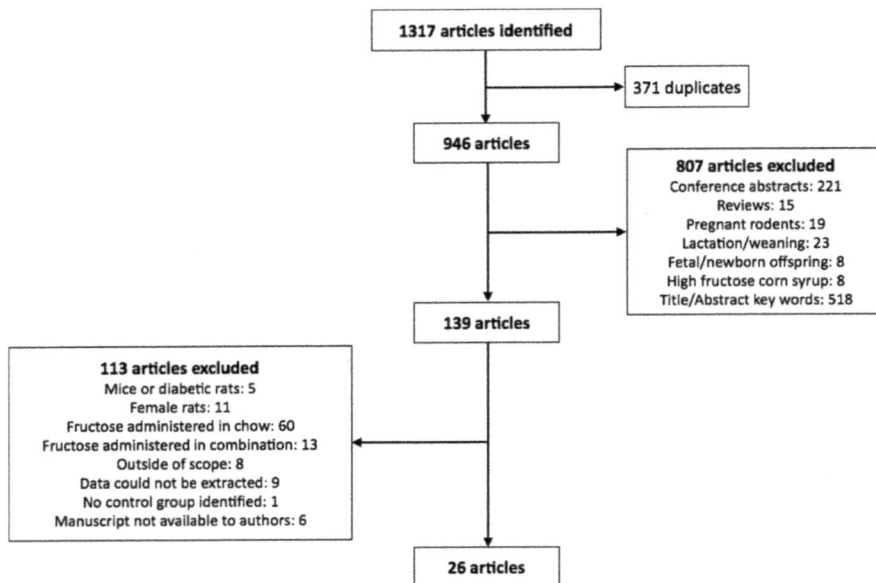

Figure 1. Flowchart of studies selected for the meta-analysis.

2.4. Statistical Analysis

Data were expressed as standardized mean differences (SMD) with 95% confidence intervals (CI). Heterogeneity was assessed with the Q and I^2 statistics. Q values $p < 0.10$ and $I^2 \geq 85\%$ were taken to indicate heterogeneity [51]. For all analyses, a random-effects model was used due to the significant heterogeneity associated with study design, rodent strain (not assessed as part of this analysis) and the duration of intervention. Where possible, the effects of study duration (fructose consumption for $\leq$12 weeks versus >12 weeks) on fructose-induced changes in body weight, systolic blood pressure and blood glucose, insulin and triglyceride concentrations were determined. All analyses were completed in R-Studio using the meta package (R-Studio version 0.99.491: Integrated Development for R. RStudio, Inc., Boston, MA, USA; meta package version 4.3-2) [52].

3. Results

3.1. Study Characteristics

This analysis only included studies in which fructose was administered as a beverage to adolescent or adult male rodents. Fructose was supplied at a concentration of either 10% w/v (24 studies) or 20%–21% w/v (two studies), and was administered for a period ranging from 2.9 to 38 weeks (Table 1). A seminal study by Hwang et al. showed that the metabolic syndrome can be induced after only 2 weeks of fructose consumption at a concentration of 60% of daily calories [10]. However, consumption of fructose at such supraphysiological concentrations is rare in humans. When planning this study our intention was to group all studies, independent of study duration. However, whilst collating the data we noted divergent study durations of either less than or greater than 12 weeks (refer to summary statistics in Table 2). We found no difference in the concentration of fructose administered or the sample size between the two groups, therefore data were split for all subsequent analyses. Of the 26 studies identified, 20 reported raw data on final body weight following fructose consumption. Of these, 35.0% reported that fructose consumption significantly increased rodent body weight at the end of the study period (Table 1). Similarly, of the 23 studies that reported blood glucose concentration, only 30.4% reported a significant effect of fructose consumption. Significant increases in blood insulin, blood triglycerides and systolic blood pressure were reported in 84.2%, 87.5% and 100%, respectively, for studies in which this data were reported (Table 1).

Table 2. Summary statistics (mean (95% CI)) of fructose beverage concentration (% w/v), study duration and sample size (as a percentage of control) split for study duration ($\leq$12 weeks or >12 weeks).

	Less Than or Equal to 12 Weeks (n = 20)	Greater Than 12 Weeks (n = 6)
Fructose beverage concentration (% w/v)	11.1 (9.5, 12.8)	10 *
Study duration (weeks)	7.0 (5.7, 8.4)	30.5 (23.7, 37.2)
Sample size (% of control)	48.8 (46.4, 51.1)	53.1 (45.7, 60.4)

* Fructose concentration was the same in all studies (10% w/v).

3.2. Effect of Fructose on Rodent Body Weight and Systolic Blood Pressure

When all studies that reported mean body weight and standard deviation were combined, there was an overall effect of fructose consumption on rodent body weight (Figure 2; SMD, 0.62 (95% CI: 0.18, 1.06); z = 2.79; p = 0.005). It is important to note, however, the high degree of heterogeneity across these studies (I^2 = 75.9% (95% CI: 62.9, 84.3)). There was no effect of study duration (between group difference p = 0.944) on rodent body weight.

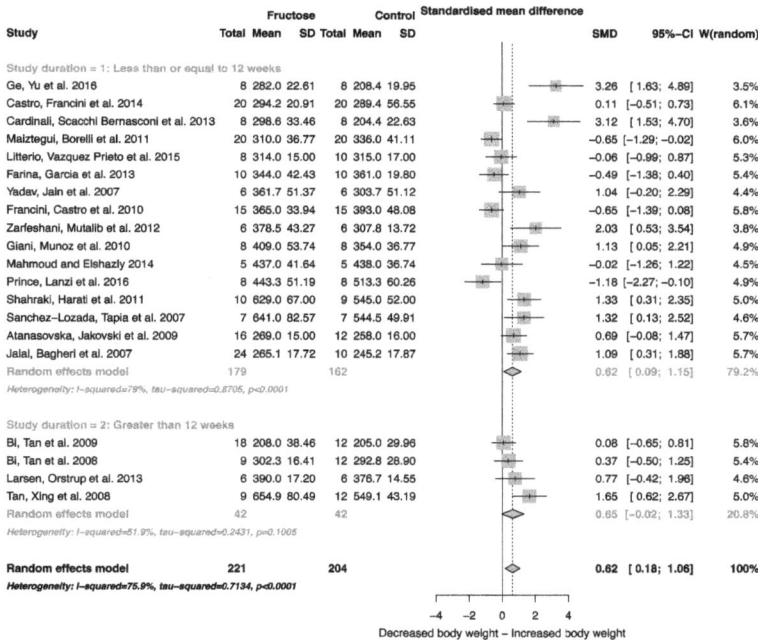

Figure 2. Forest plots of the effect of fructose consumption on adult male rodent body weight (mean and standard deviation (SD), split by study duration. The pooled effects estimates are represented by three diamonds; one for studies of 12 weeks or less, one for studies of greater than 12 weeks, and one representing the combined effect. Data are presented as standardized mean differences (SMD) with 95% confidence interval (CI). p-Values are for the inverse variance random effects models with DerSimonian-Laird estimator for Tau^2. Inter-study heterogeneity was tested by Cochran's Q at a significance of p < 0.10 and quantified by I^2.

Fructose consumption was associated with a strong effect on systolic blood pressure (SMD, 2.94 (95% CI: 2.10, 3.77); $z = 6.91$, $p < 0.0001$; Figure 3). Furthermore, there was a significant effect of study duration on systolic blood pressure (between group difference $p = 0.0002$), with fructose consumption for greater than 12 weeks resulting in a significant increase in systolic blood pressure when compared to less than or equal to 12 weeks (Figure 3).

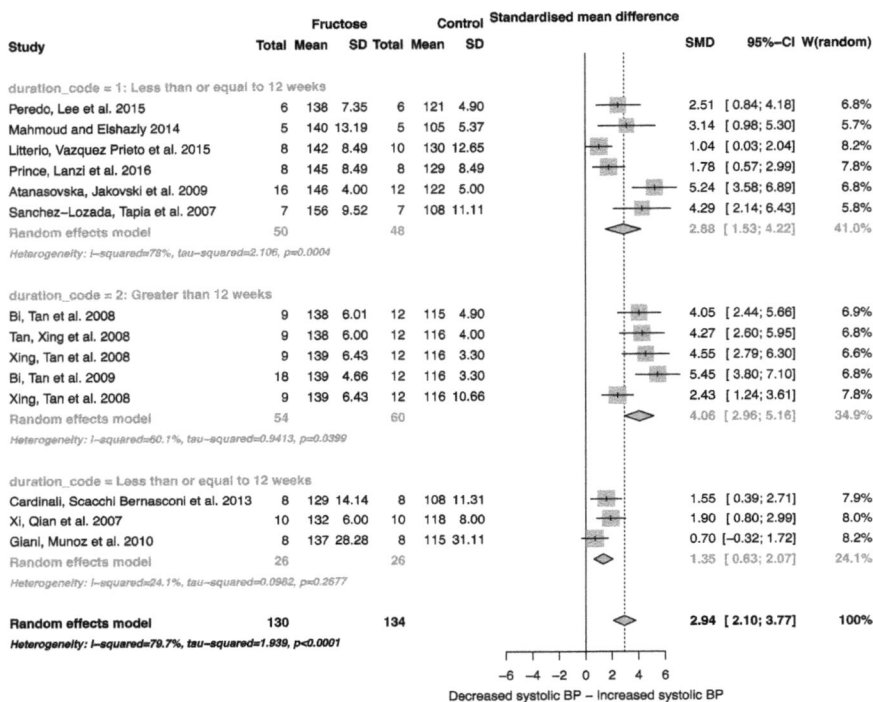

Figure 3. Forest plots of the effect of fructose consumption on adult male systolic blood pressure (mean and standard deviation (SD)), split by study duration. The pooled effects estimates are represented by three diamonds; one for studies of 12 weeks or less, one for studies of greater than 12 weeks, and one representing the combined effect. Data are presented as standardized mean differences (SMD) with 95% confidence interval (CI). *p*-Values are for the inverse variance random effects models with DerSimonian-Laird estimator for Tau^2. Inter-study heterogeneity was tested by Cochran's Q at a significance of $p < 0.10$ and quantified by I^2.

3.3. Effect of Fructose on Rodent Blood Glucose, Insulin and Triglyceride Concentrations

The effect of fructose consumption on blood glucose, insulin and triglyceride concentrations is summarized in Figures 4–6, respectively. Overall, there was an effect of fructose consumption on blood glucose (Figure 4; SMD, 0.77 (95% CI: 0.36, 1.19); $z = 3.64$, $p = 0.003$), insulin (Figure 5; SMD, 2.32 (95% CI: 1.57, 3.07); $z = 6.09$, $p < 0.0001$) and triglyceride (Figure 6; SMD, 1.87 (95% CI: 1.39, 2.34); $z = 7.70$, $p < 0.0001$) concentrations. Subgroup analysis showed no effect of study duration on blood glucose (between group difference $p = 0.9332$) or insulin (between group difference $p = 0.2042$). Interestingly, the subgroup analysis suggested an effect of study duration on blood triglyceride concentration (between group difference $p = 0.037$), with fructose beverage consumption for greater than 12 weeks resulting in a significant decrease in blood triglyceride concentration when compared to less than or equal to 12 weeks (Figure 6).

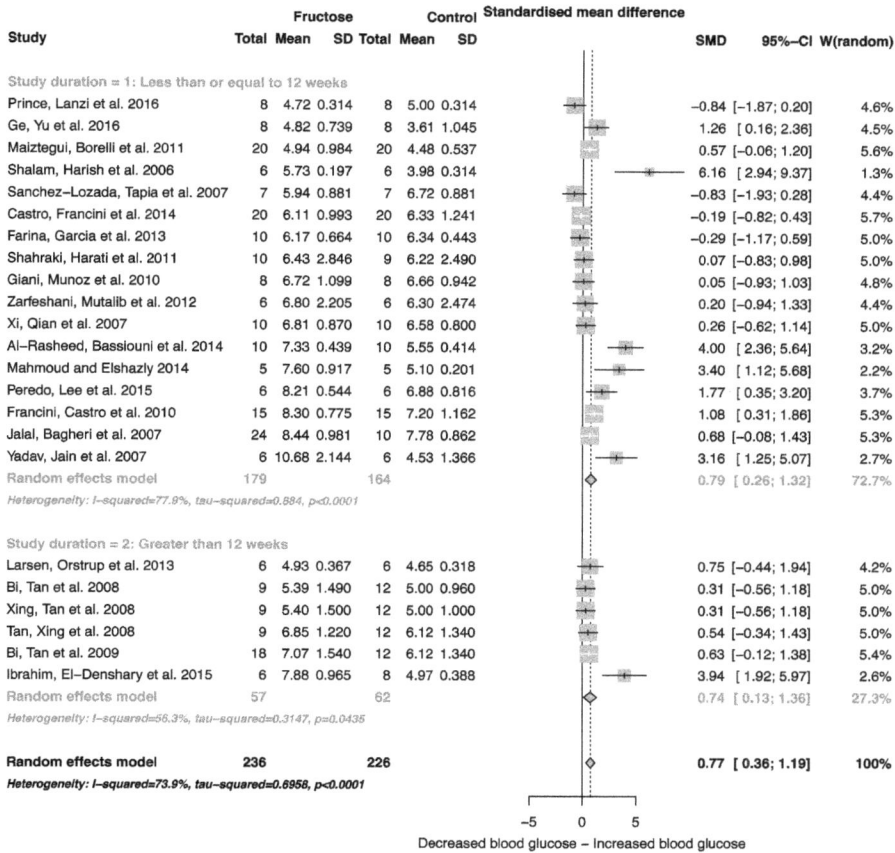

Figure 4. Forest plots of the effect of fructose consumption on adult male rodent blood glucose concentration (mean and standard deviation (SD)), split by study duration. The pooled effects estimates are represented by three diamonds; one for studies of 12 weeks or less, one for studies of greater than 12 weeks, and one representing the combined effect. Data are presented as standardized mean differences (SMD) with 95% confidence interval (CI). *p*-Values are for the inverse variance random effects models with DerSimonian-Laird estimator for Tau^2. Inter-study heterogeneity was tested by Cochran's *Q* at a significance of $p < 0.10$ and quantified by I^2.

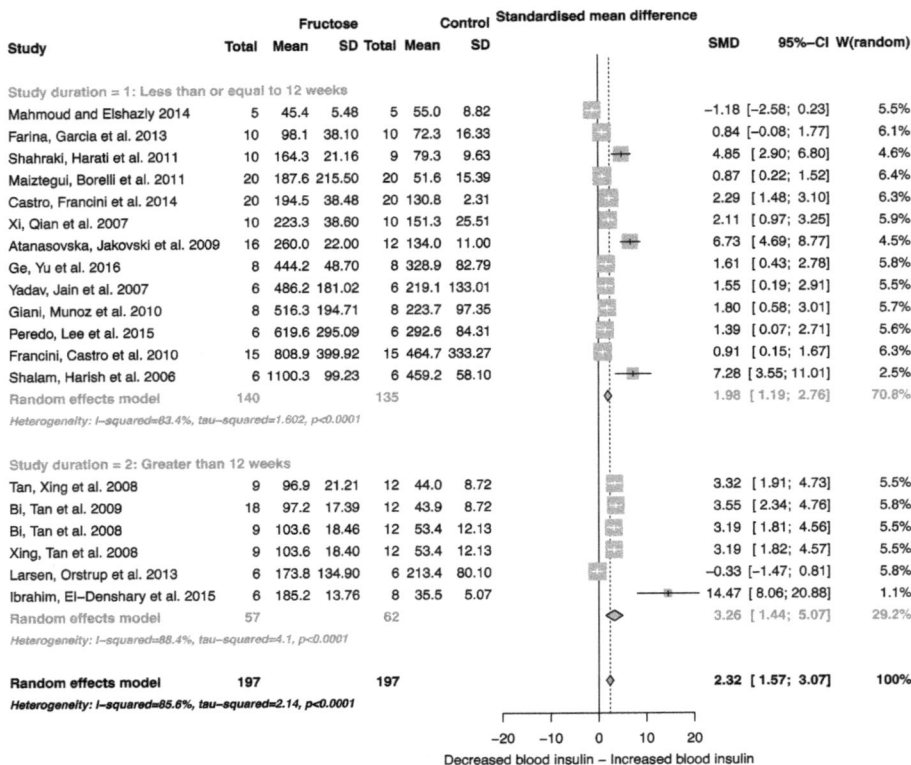

Study	Total	Fructose Mean	SD	Control Total	Mean	SD		SMD	95%–CI	W(random)
Study duration = 1: Less than or equal to 12 weeks										
Mahmoud and Elshazly 2014	5	45.4	5.48	5	55.0	8.82		−1.18	[−2.58; 0.23]	5.5%
Farina, Garcia et al. 2013	10	98.1	38.10	10	72.3	16.33		0.84	[−0.08; 1.77]	6.1%
Shahraki, Harati et al. 2011	10	164.3	21.16	9	79.3	9.63		4.85	[2.90; 6.80]	4.6%
Maiztegui, Borelli et al. 2011	20	187.6	215.50	20	51.6	15.39		0.87	[0.22; 1.52]	6.4%
Castro, Francini et al. 2014	20	194.5	38.48	20	130.8	2.31		2.29	[1.48; 3.10]	6.3%
Xi, Qian et al. 2007	10	223.3	38.60	10	151.3	25.51		2.11	[0.97; 3.25]	5.9%
Atanasovska, Jakovski et al. 2009	16	260.0	22.00	12	134.0	11.00		6.73	[4.69; 8.77]	4.5%
Ge, Yu et al. 2016	8	444.2	48.70	8	328.9	82.79		1.61	[0.43; 2.78]	5.8%
Yadav, Jain et al. 2007	6	486.2	181.02	6	219.1	133.01		1.55	[0.19; 2.91]	5.5%
Giani, Munoz et al. 2010	8	516.3	194.71	8	223.7	97.35		1.80	[0.58; 3.01]	5.7%
Peredo, Lee et al. 2015	6	619.6	295.09	6	292.6	84.31		1.39	[0.07; 2.71]	5.6%
Francini, Castro et al. 2010	15	808.9	399.92	15	464.7	333.27		0.91	[0.15; 1.67]	6.3%
Shalam, Harish et al. 2006	6	1100.3	99.23	6	459.2	58.10		7.28	[3.55; 11.01]	2.5%
Random effects model	140			135				1.98	[1.19; 2.76]	70.8%
Heterogeneity: I–squared=83.4%, tau–squared=1.602, p<0.0001										
Study duration = 2: Greater than 12 weeks										
Tan, Xing et al. 2008	9	96.9	21.21	12	44.0	8.72		3.32	[1.91; 4.73]	5.5%
Bi, Tan et al. 2009	18	97.2	17.39	12	43.9	8.72		3.55	[2.34; 4.76]	5.8%
Bi, Tan et al. 2008	9	103.6	18.46	12	53.4	12.13		3.19	[1.81; 4.56]	5.5%
Xing, Tan et al. 2008	9	103.6	18.40	12	53.4	12.13		3.19	[1.82; 4.57]	5.5%
Larsen, Orstrup et al. 2013	6	173.8	134.90	6	213.4	80.10		−0.33	[−1.47; 0.81]	5.8%
Ibrahim, El–Denshary et al. 2015	6	185.2	13.76	8	35.5	5.07		14.47	[8.06; 20.88]	1.1%
Random effects model	57			62				3.26	[1.44; 5.07]	29.2%
Heterogeneity: I–squared=88.4%, tau–squared=4.1, p<0.0001										
Random effects model	**197**			**197**				**2.32**	**[1.57; 3.07]**	**100%**
Heterogeneity: I–squared=85.6%, tau–squared=2.14, p<0.0001										

Standardised mean difference

−20 −10 0 10 20

Decreased blood insulin – Increased blood insulin

Figure 5. Forest plots of the effect of fructose consumption on adult male rodent blood insulin concentration (mean and standard deviation (SD)), split by study duration. The pooled effects estimates are represented by three diamonds; one for studies of 12 weeks or less, one for studies of greater than 12 weeks, and one representing the combined effect. Data are presented as standardized mean differences (SMD) with 95% confidence interval (CI). *p*-Values are for the inverse variance random effects models with DerSimonian-Laird estimator for Tau^2. Inter-study heterogeneity was tested by Cochran's Q at a significance of $p < 0.10$ and quantified by I^2.

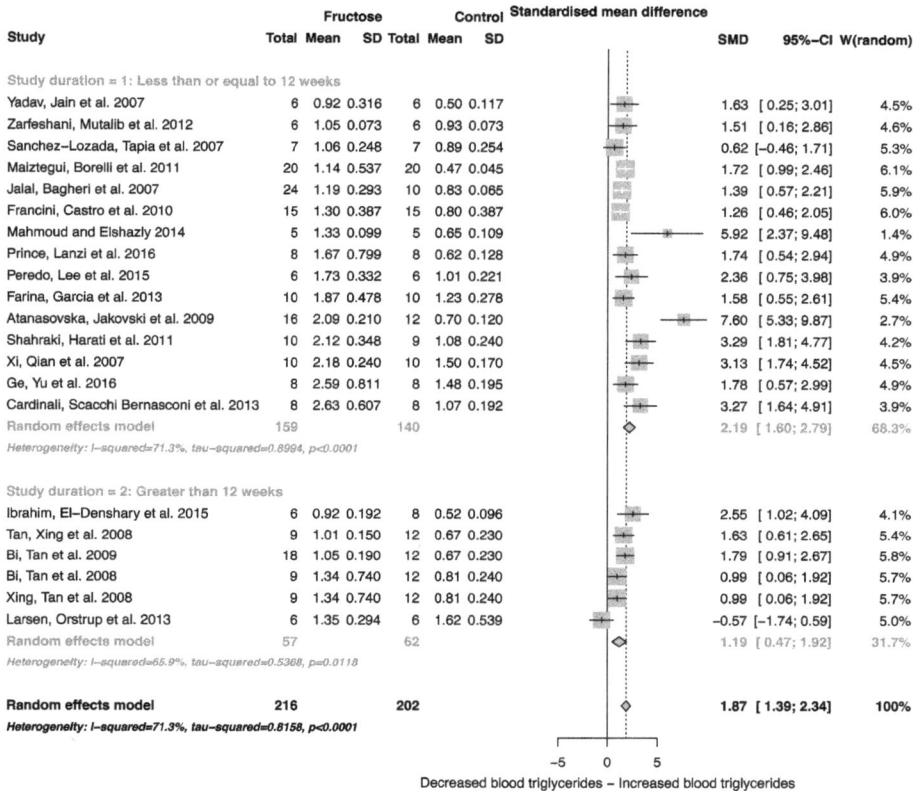

Study	Fructose			Control			Standardised mean difference	SMD	95%–CI	W(random)
	Total	Mean	SD	Total	Mean	SD				
Study duration = 1: Less than or equal to 12 weeks										
Yadav, Jain et al. 2007	6	0.92	0.316	6	0.50	0.117		1.63	[0.25; 3.01]	4.5%
Zarfeshani, Mutalib et al. 2012	6	1.05	0.073	6	0.93	0.073		1.51	[0.16; 2.86]	4.6%
Sanchez–Lozada, Tapia et al. 2007	7	1.06	0.248	7	0.89	0.254		0.62	[−0.46; 1.71]	5.3%
Maiztegui, Borelli et al. 2011	20	1.14	0.537	20	0.47	0.045		1.72	[0.99; 2.46]	6.1%
Jalal, Bagheri et al. 2007	24	1.19	0.293	10	0.83	0.065		1.39	[0.57; 2.21]	5.9%
Francini, Castro et al. 2010	15	1.30	0.387	15	0.80	0.387		1.26	[0.46; 2.05]	6.0%
Mahmoud and Elshazly 2014	5	1.33	0.099	5	0.65	0.109		5.92	[2.37; 9.48]	1.4%
Prince, Lanzi et al. 2016	8	1.67	0.799	8	0.62	0.128		1.74	[0.54; 2.94]	4.9%
Peredo, Lee et al. 2015	6	1.73	0.332	6	1.01	0.221		2.36	[0.75; 3.98]	3.9%
Farina, Garcia et al. 2013	10	1.87	0.478	10	1.23	0.278		1.58	[0.55; 2.61]	5.4%
Atanasovska, Jakovski et al. 2009	16	2.09	0.210	12	0.70	0.120		7.60	[5.33; 9.87]	2.7%
Shahraki, Harati et al. 2011	10	2.12	0.348	9	1.08	0.240		3.29	[1.81; 4.77]	4.2%
Xi, Qian et al. 2007	10	2.18	0.240	10	1.50	0.170		3.13	[1.74; 4.52]	4.5%
Ge, Yu et al. 2016	8	2.59	0.811	8	1.48	0.195		1.78	[0.57; 2.99]	4.9%
Cardinali, Scacchi Bernasconi et al. 2013	8	2.63	0.607	8	1.07	0.192		3.27	[1.64; 4.91]	3.9%
Random effects model	159			140				2.19	[1.60; 2.79]	68.3%
Heterogeneity: I-squared=71.3%, tau-squared=0.8994, p<0.0001										
Study duration = 2: Greater than 12 weeks										
Ibrahim, El–Denshary et al. 2015	6	0.92	0.192	8	0.52	0.096		2.55	[1.02; 4.09]	4.1%
Tan, Xing et al. 2008	9	1.01	0.150	12	0.67	0.230		1.63	[0.61; 2.65]	5.4%
Bi, Tan et al. 2009	18	1.05	0.190	12	0.67	0.230		1.79	[0.91; 2.67]	5.8%
Bi, Tan et al. 2008	9	1.34	0.740	12	0.81	0.240		0.99	[0.06; 1.92]	5.7%
Xing, Tan et al. 2008	9	1.34	0.740	12	0.81	0.240		0.99	[0.06; 1.92]	5.7%
Larsen, Orstrup et al. 2013	6	1.35	0.294	6	1.62	0.539		−0.57	[−1.74; 0.59]	5.0%
Random effects model	57			62				1.19	[0.47; 1.92]	31.7%
Heterogeneity: I-squared=65.9%, tau-squared=0.5368, p=0.0118										
Random effects model	**216**			**202**				**1.87**	**[1.39; 2.34]**	**100%**
Heterogeneity: I-squared=71.3%, tau-squared=0.8158, p<0.0001										

−5 0 5
Decreased blood triglycerides − Increased blood triglycerides

Figure 6. Forest plots of the effect of fructose consumption on adult male rodent blood triglyceride concentration (mean and standard deviation (SD)), split for study duration. The pooled effects estimates are represented by three diamonds; one for studies of 12 weeks or less, one for studies of greater than 12 weeks, and one representing the combined effect. Data are presented as standardized mean differences (SMD) with 95% confidence interval (CI). *p*-Values are for the inverse variance random effects models with DerSimonian-Laird estimator for Tau^2. Inter-study heterogeneity was tested by Cochran's Q at a significance of $p < 0.10$ and quantified by I^2.

4. Discussion

Fructose is commonly used in experimental animal models to induce features of the metabolic syndrome [10,11,53], however, the physiological impact of fructose varies depending on the concentration administered and the route of administration. This variation in study design has led to inconsistencies in the published effects of fructose consumption, which has made it difficult to extrapolate and understand the impact that fructose may have on human health. This study has shown that low concentration fructose beverage consumption, independent of variations in study design and duration, results in an increase in rodent body weight, systolic blood pressure and blood glucose, insulin and triglyceride concentrations.

The meta-analysis presented confirms that, within the limits of the studies undertaken, fructose beverage consumption at concentrations consistent with sugar-sweetened beverages (~10% w/v), results in an increase in rodent body weight, independent of study duration. Furthermore, we have shown that fructose beverage consumption is associated with increased blood triglyceride concentration and, together, this may suggest that the increase in body weight reported may be due to increased adipose tissue mass. Fructose feeding in rodents is commonly associated with increased hepatic de novo lipogenesis, leading to increased plasma triglycerides [12,14], non-esterified fatty acids (NEFA) [54] and very low-density lipoprotein (VLDL) cholesterol [16,19]. Furthermore, it is associated with increased hepatic lipogenic gene expression [16,55]. Fructose-induced increases in hepatic fatty acid synthesis are associated with increased ectopic fat deposition in a number of peripheral tissues including the liver. This may contribute to the increase in liver weight reported in several studies [17,48], and acts to promote hepatic inflammation and oxidative stress [17,55]. Interestingly, only a few rodent studies have reported an overall increase in body adipose tissue mass following fructose consumption [48,56,57], despite its known lipogenic effects.

Elevated plasma uric acid concentration is associated with fructose metabolism, and in addition to increased fat mass, is known to mediate cardiorenal disease risk [58,59]. Consistent with this, we report an increase in systolic blood pressure associated with fructose administration. Unlike body weight, blood pressure was reported to increase in all studies included in the analysis, and the magnitude of the change was dependent on the duration of the study. The standardized mean difference for systolic blood pressure was two-fold higher in studies that lasted for longer than 12 weeks. Interestingly, in studies greater than 12 weeks, the subgroup analysis suggested an almost two-fold decrease in blood triglyceride concentration. Although there was no overall effect of study duration on body weight, this decrease could be linked to a change in body composition, specifically increased body fat mass or ectopic fat deposition.

Consumption of fructose is also associated with increased plasma glucose and insulin concentrations. Unlike glucose, the uptake and metabolism of fructose in the liver is virtually unregulated (see Regnault et al. [60] for review). As a result, excess fructose is rapidly converted into fatty acids and triglycerides through the induction of lipogenesis-promoting transcription factors sterol regulatory binding protein 1c (SREBP-1c) and carbohydrate response element binding protein (ChREBP) [61]. While insulin resistance is one of the main outcomes associated with long-term fructose feeding [62], short-term feeding has been shown to induce a transient insulin resistant state [9] that can significantly impact on insulin-mediated glucose metabolism, contributing to the development of insulin resistance and T2D. This transient insulin resistant state is believed to contribute to the loss of inhibition of gluconeogenic pathways [9], driving an increase in hepatic glucose output independent of pre- and postprandial blood glucose concentrations. The analysis presented herein suggests that the consumption of fructose, independent of duration, results in elevated blood glucose and insulin concentrations. This may contribute to the development of insulin resistance, and may eventually manifest as T2D.

As indicated in Figures 2–6, there was a high degree of heterogeneity in all analyses conducted. We did not control for rodent strain in this analysis, which may account for the variability observed (Wistar-albino, 19 studies; Wistar-Kyoto, 1 study; Sprague-Dawley, 6 studies). To our knowledge, there have been no studies focused on rat strain-specific differences in fructose metabolism. Furthermore, two of the 26 studies used in this analysis reported fasting blood glucose, insulin and triglyceride concentrations collected after an overnight fast, which potentially contributed to the variability observed. This study was unable to control for the volume of beverage consumed per day, and it has been reported that rodents demonstrate increased intake when sugar is supplied in the form of a beverage when compared to chow [63]. Although a low concentration fructose beverage was provided to rodents in all studies included in this analysis, the volume consumed per day may have resulted in the daily caloric intake from fructose being higher than the beverage itself. However, this is consistent with human consumption of added sugars, as previously highlighted.

In conclusion, we observed that, independent of subtle study variations, consumption of a 10%–21% fructose beverage results in increased body weight in adult male rodents. This increase is accompanied by elevated systolic blood pressure and higher blood glucose, insulin and triglyceride concentrations. Furthermore, systolic blood pressure and blood triglyceride concentrations are sensitive to the duration of the fructose intervention, such that systolic blood pressure is elevated in long-term studies (over 12 weeks), while blood triglyceride concentrations are reduced. The physiological effects associated with low concentration fructose beverage consumption are consistent with development of the metabolic syndrome. Whilst we acknowledge that humans rarely consume fructose in isolation, we are consuming more fructose as either sucrose or HFCS than ever before. Understanding the metabolic effects of fructose, in isolation and when consumed with glucose, is critical to our understanding of metabolic disease. Rodent studies utilizing physiologically relevant fructose doses (~10% w/w), compared to those utilizing supraphysiological doses (~60% w/w), are important in allowing us to better elucidate the cellular mechanisms contributing to the development of type 2 diabetes, obesity and cardiovascular disease. This analysis confirms that administration of supraphysiological concentrations of fructose in rodent studies is not required to induce characteristics of the metabolic syndrome phenotype.

Acknowledgments: No funding was received for the conduct of this research. S.G. receives salary support from the University of South Australia.

Author Contributions: C.T. and S.G. conceived and designed the experiments; C.T. and S.G. performed the experiments; C.T. and S.G. analyzed the data; C.T. and S.G. wrote the paper.

Conflicts of Interest: The authors declare no conflict of interest.

References

1. Johnson, R.K.; Appel, L.J.; Brands, M.; Howard, B.V.; Lefevre, M.; Lustig, R.H.; Sacks, F.; Steffen, L.M.; Wylie-Rosett, J.; American Heart Association Nutrition Committee of the Council on Nutrition, Physical Activity, and Metabolism and the Council on Epidemiology and Prevention. Dietary sugars intake and cardiovascular health: A scientific statement from the American heart association. *Circulation* **2009**, *120*, 1011–1020. [CrossRef] [PubMed]
2. Wittekind, A.; Walton, J. Worldwide trends in dietary sugars intake. *Nutr. Res. Rev.* **2014**, *27*, 330–345. [CrossRef] [PubMed]
3. Goran, M.I.; Ulijaszek, S.J.; Ventura, E.E. High fructose corn syrup and diabetes prevalence: A global perspective. *Glob. Public Health* **2013**, *8*, 55–64. [CrossRef] [PubMed]
4. Newens, K.J.; Walton, J. A review of sugar consumption from nationally representative dietary surveys across the world. *J. Hum. Nutr. Diet.* **2015**, *29*, 224–240. [CrossRef] [PubMed]
5. Ruff, R.R. Sugar-sweetened beverage consumption is linked to global adult morbidity and mortality through diabetes mellitus, cardiovascular disease and adiposity-related cancers. *Evid.-Based Med.* **2015**, *20*, 223–224. [CrossRef] [PubMed]
6. Wang, D.; Sievenpiper, J.L.; de Souza, R.J.; Cozma, A.I.; Chiavaroli, L.; Ha, V.; Mirrahimi, A.; Carleton, A.J.; Di Buono, M.; Jenkins, A.L.; et al. Effect of fructose on postprandial triglycerides: A systematic review and meta-analysis of controlled feeding trials. *Atherosclerosis* **2014**, *232*, 125–133. [CrossRef] [PubMed]
7. Livesey, G.; Taylor, R. Fructose consumption and consequences for glycation, plasma triacylglycerol, and body weight: Meta-analyses and meta-regression models of intervention studies. *Am. J. Clin. Nutr.* **2008**, *88*, 1419–1437. [PubMed]
8. Kelishadi, R.; Mansourian, M.; Heidari-Beni, M. Association of fructose consumption and components of metabolic syndrome in human studies: A systematic review and meta-analysis. *Nutrition* **2014**, *50*, 503–510. [CrossRef] [PubMed]
9. Lustig, R.H. Fructose: It's "alcohol without the buzz". *Adv. Nutr. (Bethesda, MD)* **2013**, *4*, 226–235. [CrossRef] [PubMed]
10. Hwang, I.S.; Ho, H.; Hoffman, B.B.; Reaven, G.M. Fructose-induced insulin resistance and hypertension in rats. *Hypertension* **1987**, *10*, 512–516. [CrossRef] [PubMed]
11. Leibowitz, A.; Rehman, A.; Paradis, P.; Schiffrin, E.L. Role of t regulatory lymphocytes in the pathogenesis of high-fructose diet–induced metabolic syndrome. *Hypertension* **2013**, *61*, 1316–1321. [CrossRef] [PubMed]
12. Ackerman, Z.; Oron-Herman, M.; Grozovski, M.; Rosenthal, T.; Pappo, O.; Link, G.; Sela, B.A. Fructose-induced fatty liver disease: Hepatic effects of blood pressure and plasma triglyceride reduction. *Hypertension* **2005**, *45*, 1012–1018. [CrossRef] [PubMed]

13. Bezerra, R.; Ueno, M.; Silva, M.; Tavares, D.; Carvalho, C.; Saad, M. A high fructose diet affects the early steps of insulin action in muscle and liver of rats. *J. Nutr.* **2000**, *130*, 1531–1535. [PubMed]

14. Huang, B.W.; Chiang, M.T.; Yao, H.T.; Chiang, W. The effect of high-fat and high-fructose diets on glucose tolerance and plasma lipid and leptin levels in rats. *Diabetes Obes. Metab.* **2004**, *6*, 120–126. [CrossRef] [PubMed]

15. Huang, D.; Dhawan, T.; Young, S.; Yong, W.H.; Boros, L.G.; Heaney, A.P. Fructose impairs glucose-induced hepatic triglyceride synthesis. *Lipids Health Dis.* **2011**, *10*, 20. [CrossRef] [PubMed]

16. Koo, H.Y.; Wallig, M.A.; Chung, B.H.; Nara, T.Y.; Cho, B.H.; Nakamura, M.T. Dietary fructose induces a wide range of genes with distinct shift in carbohydrate and lipid metabolism in fed and fasted rat liver. *Biochim. Biophys. Acta* **2008**, *1782*, 341–348. [CrossRef] [PubMed]

17. Kawasaki, T.; Igarashi, K.; Koeda, T.; Sugimoto, K.; Nakagawa, K.; Hayashi, S.; Yamaji, R.; Inui, H.; Fukusato, T.; Yamanouchi, T. Rats fed fructose-enriched diets have characteristics of nonalcoholic hepatic steatosis. *J. Nutr.* **2009**, *139*, 2067–2071. [CrossRef] [PubMed]

18. Catena, C.; Giacchetti, G.; Novello, M.; Colussi, G.; Cavarape, A.; Sechi, L.A. Cellular mechanisms of insulin resistance in rats with fructose-induced hypertension. *Am. J. Hypertens.* **2003**, *16*, 973–978. [CrossRef]

19. Taghibiglou, C.; Carpentier, A.; van Iderstine, S.C.; Chen, B.; Rudy, D.; Aiton, A.; Lewis, G.F.; Adeli, K. Mechanisms of hepatic very low density lipoprotein overproduction in insulin resistance. Evidence for enhanced lipoprotein assembly, reduced intracellular ApoB degradation, and increased microsomal triglyceride transfer protein in a fructose-fed hamster model. *J. Biol. Chem.* **2000**, *275*, 8416–8425. [PubMed]

20. Kannappan, S.; Jayaraman, T.; Rajasekar, P.; Ravichandran, M.K.; Anuradha, C.V. Cinnamon bark extract improves glucose metabolism and lipid profile in the fructose-fed rat. *Singap. Med. J.* **2006**, *47*, 858–863.

21. Hirano, T.; Mamo, J.C.; Poapst, M.E.; Kuksis, A.; Steiner, G. Impaired very low-density lipoprotein-triglyceride catabolism in acute and chronic fructose-fed rats. *Am. J. Physiol.* **1989**, *256*, E559–E565. [PubMed]

22. Ibrahim, S.M.; El-Denshary, E.S.; Abdallah, D.M. Geraniol, alone and in combination with pioglitazone, ameliorates fructose-induced metabolic syndrome in rats via the modulation of both inflammatory and oxidative stress status. *PLoS ONE* **2015**, *10*, e0117516. [CrossRef] [PubMed]

23. Ge, C.X.; Yu, R.; Xu, M.X.; Li, P.Q.; Fan, C.Y.; Li, J.M.; Kong, L.D. Betaine prevented fructose-induced NAFLD by regulating LXRα/PPARα pathway and alleviating ER stress in rats. *Eur. J. Pharmacol.* **2016**, *770*, 154–164. [CrossRef] [PubMed]

24. Prince, P.D.; Lanzi, C.R.; Toblli, J.E.; Elesgaray, R.; Oteiza, P.I.; Fraga, C.G.; Galleano, M. Dietary (−)-epicatechin mitigates oxidative stress, no metabolism alterations, and inflammation in renal cortex from fructose-fed rats. *Free Radic. Biol. Med.* **2016**, *90*, 35–46. [CrossRef] [PubMed]

25. Litterio, M.C.; Vazquez Prieto, M.A.; Adamo, A.M.; Elesgaray, R.; Oteiza, P.I.; Galleano, M.; Fraga, C.G. (−)-epicatechin reduces blood pressure increase in high-fructose-fed rats: Effects on the determinants of nitric oxide bioavailability. *J. Nutr. Biochem.* **2015**, *26*, 745–751. [CrossRef] [PubMed]

26. Peredo, H.A.; Lee, H.; Donoso, A.S.; Andrade, V.; Sanchez Eluchans, N.; Puyo, A.M. A high-fat plus fructose diet produces a vascular prostanoid alterations in the rat. *Auton. Autacoid Pharmacol.* **2015**, *34*, 35–40. [CrossRef] [PubMed]

27. Al-Rasheed, N.; Bassiouni, Y.; Faddah, L.; Mohamad, A.M. Potential protective effects of Nigella sativa and Allium sativum against fructose-induced metabolic syndrome in rats. *J. Oleo Sci.* **2014**, *63*, 839–848. [CrossRef] [PubMed]

28. Castro, M.C.; Francini, F.; Gagliardino, J.J.; Massa, M.L. Lipoic acid prevents fructose-induced changes in liver carbohydrate metabolism: Role of oxidative stress. *Biochim. Biophys. Acta Gen. Subj.* **2014**, *1840*, 1145–1151. [CrossRef] [PubMed]

29. Mahmoud, A.A.; Elshazly, S.M. Ursodeoxycholic acid ameliorates fructose-induced metabolic syndrome in rats. *PLoS ONE* **2014**, *9*, e106993. [CrossRef] [PubMed]

30. Cardinali, D.P.; Scacchi Bernasconi, P.A.; Reynoso, R.; Reyes Toso, C.F.; Scacchi, P. Melatonin may curtail the metabolic syndrome: Studies on initial and fully established fructose-induced metabolic syndrome in rats. *Int. J. Mol. Sci.* **2013**, *14*, 2502–2514. [CrossRef] [PubMed]

31. Farina, J.P.; Garcia, M.E.; Alzamendi, A.; Giovambattista, A.; Marra, C.A.; Spinedi, E.; Gagliardino, J.J. Antioxidant treatment prevents the development of fructose-induced abdominal adipose tissue dysfunction. *Clin. Sci.* **2013**, *125*, 87–97. [CrossRef] [PubMed]

32. Larsen, L.H.; Orstrup, L.K.H.; Hansen, S.H.; Grunnet, N.; Quistorff, B.; Mortensen, O.H. The effect of long-term taurine supplementation and fructose feeding on glucose and lipid homeostasis in Wistar rats. *Adv. Exp. Med. Biol.* **2013**, *776*, 39–50. [PubMed]

33. Zarfeshani, A.; Mutalib, M.S.A.; Khaza'ai, H. Evaluating of high fructose diet to induce hyperglycemia and its inflammatory complications in rats. *Pak. J. Nutr.* **2012**, *11*, 21–26.

34. Maiztegui, B.; Borelli, M.I.; Madrid, V.G.; Del Zotto, H.; Raschia, M.A.; Francini, F.; Massa, M.L.; Flores, L.E.; Rebolledo, O.R.; Gagliardino, J.J. Sitagliptin prevents the development of metabolic and hormonal disturbances, increased β-cell apoptosis and liver steatosis induced by a fructose-rich diet in normal rats. *Clin. Sci.* **2011**, *120*, 73–80. [CrossRef] [PubMed]

35. Shahraki, M.R.; Harati, M.; Shahraki, A.R. Prevention of high fructose-induced metabolic syndrome in male wistar rats by aqueous extract of Tamarindus indica seed. *Acta Med. Iran.* **2011**, *49*, 277–283. [PubMed]

36. Giani, J.F.; Munoz, M.C.; Mayer, M.A.; Veiras, L.C.; Arranz, C.; Taira, C.A.; Turyn, D.; Toblli, J.E.; Dominici, F.P. Angiotensin-(1-7) improves cardiac remodeling and inhibits growthpromoting pathways in the heart of fructose-fed rats. *Am. J. Physiol. Heart Circ. Physiol.* **2010**, *298*, H1003–H1013. [CrossRef] [PubMed]

37. Atanasovska, E.; Jakovski, K.; Kostova, E.; Petlichkovski, A.; Dimitrovski, C.; Bitovska, I.; Kikerkov, I.; Petrovski, O.; Labachevski, N. Effects of rosiglitazone on metabolic parameters and adiponectin levels in fructose-fed rats. *Maced. J. Med. Sci.* **2009**, *2*, 22–29. [CrossRef]

38. Bi, X.P.; Tan, H.W.; Xing, S.S.; Zhong, M.; Zhang, Y.; Zhang, W. Felodipine downregulates serum interleukin-18 levels in rats with fructose-induced metabolic syndrome. *J. Endocrinol. Investig.* **2009**, *32*, 303–307. [CrossRef] [PubMed]

39. Tan, H.W.; Xing, S.S.; Bi, X.P.; Li, L.; Gong, H.P.; Zhong, M.; Zhang, Y.; Zhang, W. Felodipine attenuates vascular inflammation in a fructose-induced rat model of metabolic syndrome via the inhibition of NF-κB activation. *Acta Pharmacol. Sin.* **2008**, *29*, 1051–1059. [CrossRef] [PubMed]

40. Xing, S.S.; Tan, H.W.; Bi, X.P.; Zhong, M.; Zhang, Y.; Zhang, W. Felodipine reduces cardiac expression of IL-18 and perivascular fibrosis in fructose-fed rats. *Mol. Med.* **2008**, *14*, 395–402. [CrossRef] [PubMed]

41. Jalal, R.; Bagheri, S.M.; Moghimi, A.; Rasuli, M.B. Hypoglycemic effect of aqueous shallot and garlic extracts in rats with fructose-induced insulin resistance. *J. Clin. Biochem. Nutr.* **2007**, *41*, 218–223. [CrossRef] [PubMed]

42. Sanchez-Lozada, L.G.; Tapia, E.; Jimenez, A.; Bautista, P.; Cristobal, M.; Nepomuceno, T.; Soto, V.; Avila-Casado, C.; Nakagawa, T.; Johnson, R.J.; et al. Fructose-induced metabolic syndrome is associated with glomerular hypertension and renal microvascular damage in rats. *Am. J. Physiol. Ren. Physiol.* **2007**, *292*, F423–F429. [CrossRef] [PubMed]

43. Yadav, H.; Jain, S.; Sinha, P.R. Antidiabetic effect of probiotic dahi containing lactobacillus acidophilus and lactobacillus casei in high fructose fed rats. *Nutrition* **2007**, *23*, 62–68. [CrossRef] [PubMed]

44. Xi, L.; Qian, Z.; Xu, G.; Zheng, S.; Sun, S.; Wen, N.; Sheng, L.; Shi, Y.; Zhang, Y. Beneficial impact of crocetin, a carotenoid from saffron, on insulin sensitivity in fructose-fed rats. *J. Nutr. Biochem.* **2007**, *18*, 64–72. [CrossRef] [PubMed]

45. Shalam, M.; Harish, M.S.; Farhana, S.A. Prevention of dexamethasone- and fructose-induced insulin resistance in rats by SH-01D, a herbal preparation. *Indian J. Pharmacol.* **2006**, *38*, 419–422. [CrossRef]

46. Light, H.R.; Tsanzi, E.; Gigliotti, J.; Morgan, K.; Tou, J.C. The type of caloric sweetener added to water influences weight gain, fat mass, and reproduction in growing Sprague-Dawley female rats. *Exp. Biol. Med. (Maywood)* **2009**, *234*, 651–661. [CrossRef] [PubMed]

47. Bergheim, I.; Weber, S.; Vos, M.; Kramer, S.; Volynets, V.; Kaserouni, S.; McClain, C.J.; Bischoff, S.C. Antibiotics protect against fructose-induced hepatic lipid accumulation in mice: Role of endotoxin. *J. Hepatol.* **2008**, *48*, 983–992. [CrossRef] [PubMed]

48. Jurgens, H.; Haass, W.; Castaneda, T. Consuming fructose-sweetened beverages increases body adiposity in mice. *Obes. Res.* **2005**, *13*, 1146–1156. [CrossRef] [PubMed]

49. Bi, X.P.; Tan, H.W.; Xing, S.S.; Wang, Z.H.; Tang, M.X.; Zhang, Y.; Zhang, W. Overexpression of TRB3 gene in adipose tissue of rats with high fructose-induced metabolic syndrome. *Endocr. J.* **2008**, *55*, 747–752. [CrossRef] [PubMed]

50. Francini, F.; Castro, M.C.; Schinella, G.; Garcia, M.E.; Maiztegui, B.; Raschia, M.A.; Gagliardino, J.J.; Massa, M.L. Changes induced by a fructose-rich diet on hepatic metabolism and the antioxidant system. *Life Sci.* **2010**, *86*, 965–971. [CrossRef] [PubMed]

51. Higgins, J.P.T.; Thompson, S.G.; Deeks, J.J.; Altman, D.G. Measuring inconsistency in meta-analyses. *BMJ* **2003**, *327*, 557–560. [CrossRef] [PubMed]

52. Schwarzer, G. Meta: General Package for Meta-Analysis. Available online: https://CRAN.R-project.org/package=meta (accessed on 10 February 2016).

53. Liu, J.; Wang, R.; Desai, K.; Wu, L. Upregulation of aldolase B and overproduction of methylglyoxal in vascular tissues from rats with metabolic syndrome. *Cardiovasc. Res.* **2011**, *92*, 494–503. [CrossRef] [PubMed]

54. Bursac, B.N.; Djordjevic, A.D.; Vasiljevic, A.D.; Milutinovic, D.D.; Velickovic, N.A.; Nestorovic, N.M.; Matic, G.M. Fructose consumption enhances glucocorticoid action in rat visceral adipose tissue. *J. Nutr. Biochem.* **2013**, *24*, 1166–1172. [CrossRef] [PubMed]

55. Roglans, N.; Vila, L.; Farre, M.; Alegret, M.; Sanchez, R.M.; Vazquez-Carrera, M.; Laguna, J.C. Impairment of hepatic STAT-3 activation and reduction of PPARα activity in fructose-fed rats. *Hepatology* **2007**, *45*, 778–788. [CrossRef] [PubMed]

56. Shih, C.C.; Lin, C.H.; Lin, W.L.; Wu, J.B. Momordica charantia extract on insulin resistance and the skeletal muscle GLUT4 protein in fructose-fed rats. *J. Ethnopharmacol.* **2009**, *123*, 82–90. [CrossRef] [PubMed]

57. Sandeva Rositsa, V.; Mihaylova Stanislava, M.; Sandeva Gergana, N.; Trifonova Katya, Y.; Popova-Katsarova Ruska, D. Effect of high-fructose solution on body weight, body fat, blood glucose and triglyceride levels in rats. *J. Biomed. Clin. Res.* **2015**, *8*, 5–8. [CrossRef]

58. Nguyen, S.; Choi, H.K.; Lustig, R.H.; Hsu, C.-Y. Sugar sweetened beverages, serum uric acid, and blood pressure in adolescents. *J. Pediatr.* **2009**, *154*, 807–813. [CrossRef] [PubMed]

59. Gao, X.; Qi, L.; Qiao, N.; Choi, H.K.; Curhan, G.; Tucker, K.L.; Ascherio, A. Intake of added sugar and sugar-sweetened drink and serum uric acid concentration in US men and women. *Hypertension* **2007**, *50*, 306–312. [CrossRef] [PubMed]

60. Regnault, T.R.; Gentili, S.; Sarr, O.; Toop, C.R.; Sloboda, D.M. Fructose, pregnancy and later life impacts. *Clin. Exp. Pharmacol. Physiol.* **2013**, *40*, 824–837. [CrossRef] [PubMed]

61. Samuel, V.T. Fructose induced lipogenesis: From sugar to fat to insulin resistance. *Trends Endocrinol. Metab.* **2011**, *22*, 60–65. [CrossRef] [PubMed]

62. Tran, L.T.; Yuen, V.G.; McNeill, J.H. The fructose-fed rat: A review on the mechanisms of fructose-induced insulin resistance and hypertension. *Mol. Cell. Biochem.* **2009**, *332*, 145–159. [CrossRef] [PubMed]

63. Ritze, Y.; Bárdos, G.; D'Haese, J.G.; Ernst, B.; Thurnheer, M.; Schultes, B.; Bischoff, S.C. Effect of high sugar intake on glucose transporter and weight regulating hormones in mice and humans. *PLoS ONE* **2014**, *9*, e101702. [CrossRef] [PubMed]

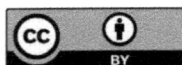

nutrients

MDPI

Article

Total Water Intake from Beverages and Foods Is Associated with Energy Intake and Eating Behaviors in Korean Adults

Kyung Won Lee [1], Dayeon Shin [2] and Won O. Song [1],*

[1] Department of Food Science and Human Nutrition, Michigan State University, 469 Wilson Road, Trout FSHN Building, East Lansing, MI 48824, USA; kyungwon@msu.edu
[2] Department of Nutrition & Dietetics, University of North Dakota, 221 Centennial Dr, Stop 8237, Grand Forks, ND 58202-8237, USA; dayeon.shin@und.edu
* Correspondence: song@msu.edu; Tel.: +1-517-353-3332; Fax: +1-517-353-8963

Received: 12 August 2016; Accepted: 27 September 2016; Published: 4 October 2016

Abstract: Water is essential for the proper functioning of the body. Even though a recommendation exists for adequate water intake for Koreans, studies identifying actual water intake from all beverages and foods consumed daily in the Korean population are limited. Thus, we estimated total water intake from both beverages and foods and its association with energy intake and eating behaviors in Korean adults. We used a nationally representative sample of 25,122 Korean adults aged ≥19 years, from the Korean National Health and Nutrition Examination Survey 2008–2012. We performed multiple regression analyses, adjusting for sociodemographic and health-related variables to investigate the contribution of overall energy and dietary intakes and eating behaviors to total water intake. The mean total water intake excluding plain water was 1071 g (398 g from beverages and 673 g from foods) and the estimated plain water intake was 1.3 L. Among Korean adults, 82% consumed beverages (excluding plain water) and these beverages contributed to 10% of daily energy intake and 32% of total water intake from beverages and foods. For every 100 kcal/day in energy intake, water intake consumed through beverages and foods increased by 18 g and 31 g, respectively. Water intake from beverages and foods was positively associated with energy from fat and dietary calcium, but inversely associated with energy density and energy from carbohydrates. When there was a 5% increase in energy intake from snacks and eating outside the home, there was an increase in water intake from beverages of 13 g and 2 g, respectively. Increased daily energy intake, the number of eating episodes, and energy intake from snacks and eating outside the home predicted higher water intake from beverages and foods. Our results provide evidence suggesting that various factors, including sociodemographic status, dietary intakes, and eating behaviors, could be important contributors to the water intake of Korean adults. Findings from this cross-sectional analysis may provide insight into strategies for promoting adequate water intake among Koreans.

Keywords: water intake; beverage consumption; energy intake; eating behavior; Korean adults

1. Introduction

Water is a crucial nutrient comprising 60% of human body weight [1,2]. It is well documented that water plays an essential role in the heathy functioning of the body, including regulation of body temperature, transport, digestion and absorption of nutrients, and excretion of wastes [3,4]. Water imbalance in the body is associated with adverse health consequences from mild thirst to severe dehydration, delirium, and even death [5]. Plain water intake is the major contributor to total water intake, though the ratios may vary among countries. Water may also be consumed from daily consumption of foods and beverages [2,6].

Many longitudinal and cross-sectional studies have been conducted on water intake in relation to dietary intakes, weight status, and disease. It has been found that increasing one's intake of non-caloric beverages such as plain water and coffee, including the replacement of sugar-sweetened beverages (SSBs) with plain water, is inversely associated with weight gain [7–9] and the risk of type 2 diabetes [10]. A few investigations have suggested inverse associations of the amount of water intake with the risk of chronic kidney disease [11] and negative mood [12]. Additionally, some studies have indicated that water intake from foods and beverages is significantly associated with micronutrient (e.g., vitamins and carotenoids) as well as macronutrient (e.g., carbohydrate, protein, and fat) intakes [2,13,14]. However, most of these prior studies have been conducted in Western countries.

Acknowledging the importance of water intake in maintaining health and preventing disease, many countries suggest recommendations for water intake to encourage the public to drink adequate amounts of water. In the United States (US), the Adequate Intake (AI) of total water was established by adding estimated water intake from foods and beverages obtained from nationally representative data [15]. The European Food Safety Authority recommends an adequate intake of water based on the consideration of the observed national estimates of water intake and the desired urine osmolality [16]. In Korea, recently published the 2015 Dietary Reference Intakes (DRI) for Koreans offer an AI of water for the Korean population. The AI for Korean adults over 19 years of age ranges from 2.1 to 2.6 L/day and 1.8–2.1 L/day for men and women, respectively, with some variations among age groups. The AI of total water for Koreans was estimated by combining water intake from commonly consumed foods and fluid intake, which includes the median value of plain water and beverage intakes (excluding milk and other dairy products) and 200 mL of milk and other dairy products. However, actual water intake from milk and other dairy products as well as water intake from soup, which has a high water content, was not reflected in the calculation of the AI for total water [6].

The beverage industry in Korea has grown and is now a global trend. According to recent statistics on the most frequently consumed foods in Korea, carbonated beverages are ranked third, blended beverages fourth, and fruit/vegetable beverages eighth [17]. Moreover, there is an increasing tendency towards sales of bottled water, coffees, carbonated beverages, and tea-based beverages in Korea [18,19]. Although the importance of beverages including plain water has increased in the Korean diet, there is a limited body of knowledge regarding total water intake and water intake from beverages and foods in Korea. There have been some investigations on water intake and beverage consumption for Koreans, but these were limited to certain regions, small sample sizes [20,21], and specific beverages such as SSBs and coffee [22,23]. Thus, there is no representative picture of total water intake among the Korean population. Moreover, no studies have investigated water intake from the daily consumption of all foods and beverages among Koreans. Basic epidemiological research on estimated water intake from commonly consumed foods and beverages is needed to provide better guidelines for water intake in upcoming DRIs for Koreans.

Given the limited number of studies attempting to quantify total water intake among Korean adults, investigations on the associations of water intake from foods and beverages with dietary intake and meal consumption attributes might help to lay the foundation for future work establishing better recommendations for water intake in Koreans. Therefore, the purpose of this study is (1) to describe water intake from beverages and foods in respect to beverage consumption; (2) to identify certain sociodemographic and health-related characteristics that can predict water intake; and (3) to investigate water intake in relation to energy intake and eating behaviors using a nationally representative sample of Korean adults from the Korea National Health and Nutrition Examination Survey (KNHANES) 2008–2012 data.

2. Methods

2.1. Data Source and Study Sample

The KNHANES conducted by the Korea Centers for Disease Control and Prevention (KCDC) and the Korean Ministry of Health and Welfare provide ongoing surveillance. The KNHANES data were collected to monitor the health and nutritional status among Koreans and to provide meaningful baseline data for health and nutrition policy design in Korea [24,25]. To establish nationally representative samples of the civilian noninstitutionalized population of Korea, the sampling plan of the KNHANES is based on a multi-stage clustered probability design [26].

Data from the KNHANES 2008–2012 were used in this cross-sectional study to identify important contributors of water intake in Korea. All participants who were older than 19 years of age with a nutrition survey including a single 24-h dietary recall and health interview were eligible for inclusion in this study (*n* = 30,642). We excluded those with <500 or >5000 kcal/day of total energy intake (*n* = 469) and pregnant and lactating women (*n* = 612). We also excluded those who had incomplete information on socio-demographic characteristics (*n* = 2816), health-related behaviors (*n* = 1370), and reported implausible total water intake besides plain water intake (>3466 mL) (*n* = 253), for a final analytic sample of 25,122 (10,184 men and 14,938 women).

The KNHANES used in this study was approved by the KCDC Institutional Review Board. All subjects gave their informed consent and participated voluntarily.

2.2. Water Intake Assessment

Four variables reflecting water intake were used in the present study: (1) water intake from beverages excluding plain water; (2) water intake from foods; (3) total water intake from beverages and foods other than plain water; and (4) usual plain water intake. As part of the 24-h dietary recall data, the water content of all beverages and foods consumed by participants in the KNHANES were publicly released [27]. Estimated water intake from beverages were calculated based on the total content of water in all types of fluids such as milk, unsweetened coffee and tea, 100% fruit/vegetable juice, SSBs, alcoholic beverages, and diet beverages. Information on usual plain water intake was collected by asking participants using the food-frequency questionnaire (FFQ)-type question, "How much plain water do you usually drink a day?" after 24-h dietary recalls.

Based on the KNHANES coding scheme [24] and previous classifications of beverages [28–31], we grouped all beverages into six categories (milk, unsweetened coffees/teas, 100% fruit juices, SSBs, alcoholic beverages, and diet beverages). The SSBs category was further divided into five subgroups (sodas, fruit drinks, sweetened coffees/teas, sports/energy drinks, other SSBs). To understand beverage consumption in the Korean adult population, we calculated four estimates (per capita and per consumer): average intake of beverages (mL), average water intake from beverages (g), and the contribution of beverages to daily total energy (%), and total water intake excluding plain water (%).

2.3. Dietary Intake and Eating Behaviors

To describe how each water variable varied according to dietary intakes and eating behaviors, we used several variables that may reflect energy intakes, dietary constituents, and meal consumption behaviors. We estimated total energy intake (kcal/day), % energy from macronutrients (carbohydrate, protein, and fat), dietary fiber, calcium, and sodium consumed [32]. We also used energy density (kcal/g) for all beverages (not including plain water) and foods [2], and estimated the amounts of beverages and all non-beverage foods consumed.

We used several eating behavioral variables based on previous literature [33,34] to assess meal consumption attributes of study subjects in relation to water intake. They were described by the frequency of eating episodes and % energy from main meals and snacks. The KNHANES data provided information on eating episodes reported by survey participants. We identified each eating episode named by respondents with breakfast, lunch, and dinner considered as the main meals. All other non-main meal eating episodes were considered as snacks. Eating episodes reported at different clock times were classified as a single eating episode regardless of the number or quantity of foods or beverages consumed. Based on this information, we estimated the number of total eating episodes, snack and beverage-only episodes, and % energy from main meals and snacks. Length of ingestion period was calculated from the first eating event to the last eating episode reported. Additionally, eating-out behaviors were measured using the information on locations where food and beverages were consumed as collected in the KNHANES. We classified all beverages and foods consumed into two categories based on the eating location and calculated 24-h energy intake at home and outside the home, respectively.

2.4. Potential Covariates

To determine an independent association between all water variables and dietary intakes and eating behavioral factors, potential confounders were included in our statistical model. Socio-demographic variables included: age (19–29, 30–49, 50–64, $\geq$65 years of age); income (income was calculated according to total household income of residents and then divided into quartiles from poorest to wealthiest; low, mid-low, mid-high, or high) [24]; education level (elementary school graduates, middle school graduates, high school graduates, or more than college graduate). Diet and health-related behavioral variables included: smoking status (never smoked, former smoker, or current smoker), the day of recalled intake (Monday-Thursday or Friday-Sunday), regular physical activity (yes or no; having physical activity was defined as walking $\geq$5 times a week for $\geq$30 min each time), and body mass index (BMI; kg/m^2) (calculated as weight in kilograms divided by square of height in meters; $\leq$normal weight, <23; overweight, 23 to <25; or obese, $\geq$25) [35].

2.5. Statistical Analyses

We used SAS (version 9.4, SAS Institute Inc., Cary, NC, USA) for statistical analyses in this study. All statistical tests were two-tailed and $p < 0.05$ were considered statistically significant. We used SURVEY procedure with sample weight, stratum, and primary sampling unit recommended by the KNHANES analytical guidelines to account for unequal selection probabilities resulting from complex survey design and non-response [24,26].

We computed the adjusted means using multiple linear regressions to compare all types of water intake according to sociodemographic and health-related characteristics (Table 1). Frequency (weighted percentage) and means (standard errors) were calculated to depict beverage consumption in Korean adults with regard to the prevalence of consuming different types of beverages and water intake, % total water intake excluding plain water, and % total daily energy from each beverage category (Table 2). Multiple logistic regressions were conducted to determine the associations of sociodemographic and health-related variables with odds of various sorts of beverages. We calculated multivariable-adjusted odds ratios with 95% confidence intervals after controlling for covariates such as sex, age, income, education level, smoking status, the day of recalled intake, regular physical activity (categorical), and total energy intake (continuous) (Table S1). We also conducted multiple linear regression analyses to explore the independent association of energy and dietary intake and eating behaviors with all components of water intake (Tables 3 and 4). For these analyses, important contributors to water intake mentioned above were included in our regression models as covariates.

3. Results

The daily amount of total water intake from beverages and foods was 1071 g (1.1 L) and the mean usual plain water intake was 1.3 L among Korean adults (Table 1). Usual plain water intake reported did not vary depending on sociodemographic characteristics and health-related behaviors, except for smoking status. Current smokers usually consumed more plain water than non-smokers and former smokers ($p < 0.05$). Compared to women, men consumed a higher amount of water from beverages and foods. Age was negatively correlated to water from beverage and total water intake, but positively correlated to water consumed through foods ($p < 0.01$). Income and education levels were positively associated with all water variables ($p < 0.01$). Like usual plain water intake, current smokers consumed higher amounts of water from beverages and total water, but lower amounts of water from foods than non-smokers ($p < 0.01$). Water intake from beverage and total water intake excluding plain water were higher on weekends than weekdays ($p < 0.01$). Those undertaking regular physical activity consumed more water from foods and total water compared with their counterparts ($p < 0.01$), but there was no association with water intake from beverages and usual plain water intake.

Table 1. Water intake by sociodemographic and health-related behaviors in Korean adults, KNHANES 2008–2012 [1].

Independent Variable	n	Water Intake from Beverages [2]	Water Intake from Foods	Total Water Intake Excluding Plain Water	Usual Plain Water Intake
		g	g	g	mL
All, unadjusted	25,122	396 ± 4 [3]	697 ± 4	1093 ± 6	1321 ± 65
All, adjusted for all covariates	25,122	398 ± 5	673 ± 5	1071 ± 7	1281 ± 67
Sex					
Men	10,184	426 ± 6	736 ± 6	1162 ± 10	1303 ± 61
Women	14,938	370 ± 8	610 ± 7	980 ± 11	1259 ± 108
p Value [4]		<0.0001 **	<0.0001 **	<0.0001 **	0.6972
Age (years)					
19–29	2811	456 ± 12	592 ± 9	1048 ± 16	1564 ± 177
30–49	9248	445 ± 7	717 ± 8	1162 ± 11	1245 ± 91
50–64	7086	395 ± 7	762 ± 7	1157 ± 11	1218 ± 86
65+	5977	296 ± 6	621 ± 8	917 ± 11	1098 ± 144
p Value		<0.0001 **	<0.0001 **	<0.0001 **	0.1587
Income					
Q1 (lowest)	6092	379 ± 8	623 ± 7	1002 ± 11	1305 ± 146
Q2	6333	399 ± 7	665 ± 7	1064 ± 10	1408 ± 152
Q3	6354	400 ± 8	686 ± 7	1086 ± 11	1182 ± 85
Q4 (highest)	6343	414 ± 8	718 ± 9	1132 ± 12	1229 ± 100
p Value		0.0053 **	<0.0001 **	<0.0001 **	0.5995
Education level					
≤Elementary school	7014	337 ± 8	595 ± 9	932 ± 12	1415 ± 169
Middle school	2912	384 ± 10	668 ± 10	1052 ± 14	1220 ± 104
High school	8471	414 ± 7	702 ± 7	1116 ± 10	1398 ± 118
≥College	6725	456 ± 8	727 ± 7	1184 ± 11	1091 ± 76
p Value		<0.0001 **	<0.0001 **	<0.0001 **	0.0649
Smoking					
Never	15,302	323 ± 6	691 ± 6	1014 ± 9	1176 ± 77
Former	2863	438 ± 11	699 ± 11	1137 ± 16	1175 ± 133
Current	6957	433 ± 8	628 ± 7	1062 ± 11	1492 ± 109
p Value		<0.0001 **	<0.0001 **	<0.0001 **	0.0260 *
Day of recalled intake					
Monday-Thursday	15,503	398 ± 6	667 ± 6	1053 ± 9	1338 ± 81
Friday-Saturday	9619	398 ± 6	678 ± 6	1089 ± 10	1224 ± 99
p Value		0.0011 **	0.1498	0.0010 **	0.3454
Regular physical activity [5]					
Yes	12,923	385 ± 6	685 ± 6	1083 ± 9	1342 ± 95
No	12,199	411 ± 7	660 ± 6	1059 ± 9	1220 ± 92
p Value		0.9370	<0.0001 **	0.0096 **	0.3487
Body mass index (kg/m²)					
<23	11,227	388 ± 6	656 ± 6	1044 ± 8	1324 ± 118
23 to <25	5957	401 ± 8	682 ± 8	1084 ± 11	1131 ± 88
≥25	7938	405 ± 7	680 ± 7	1085 ± 10	1388 ± 96
p Value		0.0426 *	0.0006 **	0.0001 **	0.0514

[1] Data were from the Korea National Health and Nutrition Examination Surveys (KNHANES). All data except for sample size were weighted accounting for the complex study design according to the directions of the KNHANES analytical guidelines. All covariates shown in the table were added to regression models for all water variables; [2] Water intake from beverages (excluding plain water) and foods were estimated based on a 24-h dietary recall in the KNHANES 2008–2012. Total water intake excluding plain water was a combination of water intake from beverages and foods. Usual plain water intake were estimated from FFQ-type question after collection of the 24-h dietary recalls; [3] All values represented adjusted means ± standard errors (SEs); [4] p Value obtained from the multiple linear regression analyses indicated the significance of the association of each independent variable with all water variables (* $p < 0.05$, ** $p < 0.01$); [5] Having regular physical activity was defined as walking ≥5 time a week for ≥30 min each time.

Korean adults consumed 451.0 ± 4.5 mL of beverages and 395.8 ± 4.0 g of water from beverages per capita each day (Table 2). Beverages other than plain water contributed to about 10% of total energy intakes and 32% of total daily water intake besides plain water. The prevalence of consuming beverages was about 82%. Approximately, 49% of people reported consuming SSBs, more than 32% reported consuming unsweetened coffee/tea, and 26% people reported consumption of milk. The largest per capita beverage consumption were SSBs (139.7 ± 2.2 mL), alcoholic beverages (116.4 ± 2.9 mL), and unsweetened coffee/tea (108.0 ± 2.2 mL). In addition, SSBs (122.5 ± 1.9 g) accounted for the greatest per capita water intake from beverages, followed by unsweetened coffee/tea (100.2 ± 2.1 g), and alcohol beverages (99.2 ± 2.5 g). However, per consumer, both the amount of water from beverages and the percentage of energy consumed as alcoholic beverages were the greatest contributor to water and energy intake from beverages. There was a significant contribution of water intake by unsweetened coffee/tea, although its contribution to total daily energy intakes stayed <1% for both per capita and per consumer. Since diet beverages were rarely consumed by all individuals, meaningful numbers related to this beverage category could not be determined.

The prevalence of consuming different types of beverages according to sociodemographic and health-related characteristics was presented elsewhere (see Table S1). Women were more likely to consume milk, unsweetened coffee/tea, and SSBs ($p < 0.01$), but less likely to have alcohol compared to men ($p < 0.01$). Compared to younger adults (19–29 years of age), the consumption of unsweetened coffee/tea and alcohol was higher in other age groups, however, there was lower milk and 100% fruit juice consumption in adults aged over 30 years compared with younger adults ($p < 0.01$). The prevalence of consuming milk and unsweetened coffee/tea increased with level of income and education. Those with a higher education were more likely to consume milk, unsweetened coffee/tea, and even SSBs ($p < 0.05$). Current smokers and individuals reporting no physical activity were less likely to consume milk but more likely to consume SSBs.

Total daily energy intake was positively correlated to water intake from beverages and foods and total water intake excluding plain water ($p < 0.01$) (Table 3). The 17.8 ± 0.5 g and 30.7 ± 0.5 g increases in water intake from beverages and foods were observed for each 100 kcal increment in energy intake. Energy density (kcal/g) of all beverages and foods were negatively correlated to total water content of beverages and foods ($p < 0.01$). Percent energy as protein was positively related to water intake from foods ($p < 0.01$), but negatively related to water from beverage and total water intake ($p < 0.01$). While percent energy as fat was positively correlated with all water variables ($p < 0.01$), percent energy as carbohydrates was negatively correlated ($p < 0.01$). Dietary fiber and sodium were significantly associated with higher water intake from foods and total water intake ($p < 0.01$), but they showed negative associations with water intake from beverages. Intake of usual plain water had no significant association with water intake from beverages and foods. However, water from foods and beverages were significantly related to each other and to total water intake excluding plain water after adjusting for covariates. All water intake from different types of beverages were positively associated with intake of water from beverages ($p < 0.01$), but such associations were observed in water from foods. The greatest contributors to water intake from beverages were water consumed as alcoholic beverages and 100% fruit juices. When there was a 100 g/day increase in the consumption of alcohols and 100% fruit juices, there was an increase in water consumed through beverages of 90.9 ± 0.8 g and 87.5 ± 4.4 g, respectively.

Table 2. Water and energy intakes from beverages among Korean adults, KNHANES 2008–2012 [1].

Beverage Category	Consumers	Amount of Beverages Consumed		Water Intake from Beverages			% total Daily Energy Intake		% of Total Water Intake Excluding Plain Water	
		per Capita	per Consumer	per Capita	per Consumer		per Capita	per Consumer	per Capita	per Consumer
	n (Weighted %) [2]	mL	mL	g	g		%	%	%	%
Milk	6170 (25.7) [2]	73.5 ± 1.7	276.7 ± 3.8	62.1 ± 1.4	236.1 ± 3.3	2.3 ± 0.1	8.8 ± 0.1	5.6 ± 0.1	21.4 ± 0.2
Unsweetened coffee/tea	7745 (31.9)	108.0 ± 2.2	292.3 ± 4.8	100.2 ± 2.1	272.0 ± 4.5	0.3 ± 0.0	0.9 ± 0.0	8.3 ± 0.2	22.3 ± 0.3
100% fruit juice	1213 (5.2)	13.1 ± 0.6	247.4 ± 7.2	11.7 ± 0.6	222.5 ± 6.6	0.3 ± 0.0	5.4 ± 0.2	1.0 ± 0.0	18.3 ± 0.4
SSBs	11,644 (48.5)	139.7 ± 2.2	287.3 ± 3.2	122.5 ± 1.9	251.9 ± 2.8	3.0 ± 0.0	6.3 ± 0.1	11.2 ± 0.1	23.1 ± 0.2
Soft drink	9354 (37.2)	88.8 ± 1.5	238.1 ± 2.6	78.0 ± 1.3	209.2 ± 2.3	2.0 ± 0.0	5.4 ± 0.1	7.6 ± 0.1	20.5 ± 0.2
Fruit drink	1694 (7.7)	19.9 ± 0.8	251.6 ± 5.7	16.6 ± 0.7	211.6 ± 4.6	0.4 ± 0.0	5.5 ± 0.1	1.4 ± 0.1	18.4 ± 0.4
Sweetened coffee/tea	1771 (9.3)	26.6 ± 1.0	284.9 ± 6.0	23.8 ± 0.9	254.9 ± 5.5	0.5 ± 0.0	5.8 ± 0.1	1.9 ± 0.1	20.1 ± 0.4
Sports/energy drink	165 (0.9)	3.1 ± 0.4	333.7 ± 16.0	2.9 ± 0.3	312.1 ± 15.0	0.0 ± 0.0	4.0 ± 0.2	0.2 ± 0.0	21.9 ± 1.0
Other SSBs	223 (1.0)	1.3 ± 0.1	138.6 ± 6.8	1.2 ± 0.1	121.5 ± 6.0	0.0 ± 0.0	3.3 ± 0.2	0.1 ± 0.0	10.5 ± 0.5
Alcoholic beverages	4630 (20.9)	116.4 ± 2.9	557.2 ± 9.1	99.2 ± 2.5	474.6 ± 8.0	3.6 ± 0.1	17.1 ± 0.2	6.2 ± 0.1	29.7 ± 0.4
Diet beverages	16 (0.1)	0.2 ± 0.1	246.4 ± 30.6	0.2 ± 0.1	241.9 ± 27.9	-	0.2 ± 0.1	-	23.5 ± 3.0
Total beverages	19,900 (82.0)	451.0 ± 4.5	541.5 ± 4.7	395.8 ± 4.0	475.5 ± 4.1	9.6 ± 0.1	11.6 ± 0.1	32.4 ± 0.2	38.7 ± 0.2

[1] Data were from the Korea National Health and Nutrition Examination Surveys (KNHANES). All data except for sample size were weighted accounting for the complex study design according to the directions of the KNHANES analytical guidelines. All values represented adjusted means ± standard errors (SEs), unless otherwise indicated. SSBs, sugar-sweetened beverages; [2] Values represented frequency (weighted percentage).

Table 3. Water intakes from beverages and foods associated with energy and nutrients intakes in Korean adults, KNHANES 2008–2012 [1].

Independent Variable	Water Intake from Beverages [2]	Water Intake from Foods	Total Water Intake Excluding Plain Water
	g	g	g
Energy intake (100 kcal/day)	17.8 ± 0.5 [3,4],**	30.7 ± 0.5 **	48.5 ± 0.6 **
Energy from fat (5%)	21.9 ± 2.2 **	15.6 ± 2.2 **	37.5 ± 3.2 **
Energy from protein (5%)	−11.8 ± 4.2 **	120.2 ± 4.5 **	108.4 ± 6.4 **
Energy from carbohydrate (5%)	−54.1 ± 1.5 **	−4.6 ± 1.6	−59.0 ± 2.1 **
Energy density of all beverages (kcal/g)	−43.9 ± 2.9 **	−1.0 ± 2.8 **	−44.9 ± 3.9 **
Energy density of all non-beverage foods (kcal/g) [5]	−0.8 ± 7.4 **	−530.3 ± 7.2 **	−531.1 ± 9.9 **
Fiber (5 g/day) [5]	−57.4 ± 4.7 **	173.9 ± 5.3 **	116.5 ± 4.4 **
Sodium (100 mg/day) [5]	−1.7 ± 0.1 **	3.4 ± 0.1 **	1.7 ± 0.2 **
Calcium (100 mg/day) [5]	7.1 ± 1.4 **	25.8 ± 1.9 **	32.9 ± 2.5 **
Amount of beverages consumed (100 g/day)	85.0 ± 0.3 **	2.9 ± 0.7 **	87.9 ± 0.8 **
Amount of foods consumed (100 g/day)	2.5 ± 0.6 **	64.1 ± 0.8 **	66.6 ± 1.1 **
Usual plain water intake (100 g/day)	0.0 ± 0.0	0.1 ± 0.1	0.0 ± 0.1
Water in foods (100 g/day)	3.0 ± 0.8 **	-	103.0 ± 0.8 **
Water in beverages (100 g/day)	-	3.1 ± 0.8 **	103.1 ± 0.8 **
Water in milk (100 g/day)	82.4 ± 2.2 **	0.1 ± 2.8	82.5 ± 3.5 **
Water in unsweetened coffee/tea (100 g/day)	83.5 ± 1.3 **	−0.8 ± 1.5	82.7 ± 1.9 **
Water in 100% fruit juice (100 g/day)	87.5 ± 4.4 **	14.1 ± 4.5 **	101.6 ± 6.5 **
Water in SSBs (100 g/day)	78.5 ± 1.5 **	2.5 ± 1.8	81.0 ± 2.4 **
Water in alcoholic beverages (100 g/day)	90.9 ± 0.8 **	4.7 ± 1.1 **	95.5 ± 1.4 **
Water in diet beverages (100 g/day)	32.5 ± 21.5 **	−50.3 ± 27.0	−17.9 ± 31.0

[1] Data were from the Korea National Health and Nutrition Examination Surveys (KNHANES). All data except for sample size were weighted accounting for the complex study design according to the directions of the KNHANES analytical guidelines. Water intake from beverages (excluding plain water) and foods were estimated based on a 24-h dietary recall in the KNHANES 2008–2012. The multiple regression models included covariates including sex, age (continuous), income (low, mid-low, mid-high, or high) and education levels (elementary school graduates, middle school graduates, high school graduates, or more than college graduate), regular physical activity (yes or no), smoking status (non-smoker, former smoker, or current smoker), the day of recalled intake (Monday–Thursday or Friday–Sunday), and body mass index (continuous). SSBs, sugar-sweetened beverages; [2] Water intake from beverages (excluding plain water) and foods were estimated based on a 24-h dietary recall in the KNHANES 2008–2012. Total water intake excluding plain water was a combination of water intake from beverages and foods; [3] All values represented βs ± standard errors (SEs) which were associated with units of measurement given in parentheses for each independent variable (for example, when there was a 100 kcal/day increase in energy intake, water intake from beverage increased by 18 g, water intake from food increased by 31 g, and total water intake excluding plain water increased by 49 g).[4] *p* Values obtained from the multiple linear regression analyses indicate the significance of the association of each independent variable with all water variables (* *p* < 0.05, ** *p* < 0.01); [5] The models also included total daily energy (continuous) intake as an independent variable.

Table 4. Water intakes from beverages and foods associated with eating behaviors in Korean adults, KNHANES 2008–2012 [1].

Independent Variable	Water Intake from Beverages [2]	Water Intake from Foods	Total Water Intake Excluding Plain Water
	g	g	g
Number of different beverage items consumed [3]	211.2 ± 2.7 [4,5],**	−38.5 ± 3.0 **	172.6 ± 3.8 **
Number of different non-beverage food items consumed [3]	−0.01 ± 1.0	14.6 ± 0.9 **	14.6 ± 1.2 **
Number of all eating episodes [3]	62.1 ± 2.1 **	9.0 ± 1.8 **	71.1 ± 2.3 **
Number of all snack episodes [3]	71.2 ± 2.0 **	6.0 ± 1.8 **	77.3 ± 2.3 **
Number of beverage-only episodes [3]	112.3 ± 2.4 **	−18.8 ± 2.2 **	93.5 ± 2.9 **
Length of ingestion period (h) [3]	14.1 ± 1.2 **	0.4 ± 1.0	14.6 ± 1.5 **
Reported breakfast in the 24-h dietary recall [3]	−103.8 ± 8.9 **	40.0 ± 7.3 **	−63.8 ± 10.0 **
Reported any snack in the 24-h dietary recall [3]	158.7 ± 7.1 **	45.0 ± 6.9 **	203.7 ± 9.4 **
Energy from main meals (5%)	−4.7 ± 0.4 **	5.6 ± 0.4 **	0.9 ± 0.6
Energy from snacks (5%)	30.2 ± 1.2 **	11.9 ± 1.1 **	42.1 ± 1.7 **
Energy from eating outside home (5%)	12.6 ± 0.6 **	2.1 ± 0.5 **	14.7 ± 0.8 **

[1] Data were from the Korea National Health and Nutrition Examination Surveys (KNHANES). All data except for sample size were weighted accounting for the complex study design according to the directions of the KNHANES analytical guidelines. The multiple regression models included covariates including sex, age (continuous), income (low, mid-low, mid-high, or high) and education levels (elementary school graduates, middle school graduates, high school graduates, or more than college graduate), smoking status (non-smoker, former smoker, or current smoker), the day of recalled intake (Monday–Thursday or Friday–Sunday), regular physical activity (yes or no), and body mass index (continuous); [2] Water intake from beverages (excluding plain water) and foods were estimated based on a 24-h dietary recall in the KNHANES 2008–2012. Total water intake excluding plain water was a combination of water intake from beverages (excluding plain water) intake as an independent variable; [4] All values represented βs ± standard errors (SEs) which were associated with units of measurement given in parentheses for each independent variable (for example, when the number of different kind of beverage items reported increased, water intake from beverages increased by 211 g, water intake from foods decreased by 39 g, and total water intake excluding plain water increased by 173 g); [5] *p* Values obtained from the multiple linear regression analyses indicate the significance of the association of each independent variable with all water variables (* *p* < 0.05, ** *p* < 0.01).

Independent associations of eating behaviors with contribution to water intake are listed in Table 4. The number of unique beverages consumed in the 24-h dietary recall was positively associated with water intake from beverages ($p < 0.01$), but negatively associated with water from foods ($p < 0.01$). In case of the number of non-beverage foods consumed, the reverse association with water consumed from foods was found ($p < 0.01$). Particularly, the number of different types of beverages was the most important contributor of higher intake of water from beverages. When the number of unique beverages consumed increased, water consumed from beverages increased by 211.2 ± 2.7 g. The number of beverage-only episodes and eating duration were positively related to water consumed from beverages and total water intake besides plain water ($p < 0.01$), but negatively related to water content consumed through foods ($p < 0.01$). Reported total daily energy from main meals was negatively correlated with water intake from beverages ($p < 0.01$), but positively correlated with water consumed from foods and total water ($p < 0.01$). The number of total eating episodes and snack episodes were positively related to all water intakes ($p < 0.01$). A similar trend was observed for 24-h energy intake from snacks and reporting a snack in the 24-h dietary recall. Increasing the energy consumed outside the home had positive associations with intakes of water from beverages and foods and total water intake other than plain water ($p < 0.01$). For each 5% increase in energy from snacks and eating outside the home, the 30.2 ± 1.2 g and 12.6 ± 0.6 g, respectively, increases in water intake from beverages were found.

4. Discussion

This study described total water intake from beverages and foods consumed daily and explored the significant associations of water intake with energy and dietary intakes as well as eating behaviors using 25,122 weighed dietary information from Korean adult subjects in a nationally representative sample of the KNHANES 2008–2012. These findings might help to shed light on the important contributors to water intake and aid in understanding the current status of total water intake among Korean adults.

On average, Korean adults consumed 1.1 L of total water, excluding plain water (0.4 L of water from beverages and 0.7 L of water from foods, respectively), based on the 24-h dietary recall data. Adding 1.3 L of usual plain water intake estimated from the FFQ-type question, the average amount of total water consumed daily by Koreans was 2.4 L, satisfying the AI of water intake for Koreans. This is somewhat lower than 3.1–3.2 L, the total water intake of Americans estimated from the National Health and Nutrition Examination Survey (NHANES) 2005–2006 data [2,13]. In terms of water intake including all beverages and plain water, the average was 1.7 L, similar to that of China (1.7 L) and Japan (1.5 L), whereas it was slightly lower than that of Western countries, which range from 1.9 L in Spain to 2.5 L in Germany [36]. However, it is difficult to combine plain water intake as estimated using the FFQ-type question with water intake collected from the 24-h dietary recalls, since information on the plain water intake of Koreans was collected by asking an FFQ-type question "How much water do you usually drink a day?" right after the 24-h dietary recall. In addition, Sebastian et al. reported that FFQ-type questions have limitations in that they tend to over-report dietary and energy intakes and even water intake compared to the 24-h dietary recall. Thus, they proposed that 24-h dietary recalls were more accurate for measuring water intake; therefore, continual development and improvement of the methodology are required [37].

We found that those who were younger, had higher income and education, and exercised regularly showed higher intakes of total water excluding plain water. These sociodemographic and health-related characteristics were major determinants of not only water intake but also better dietary quality among Koreans [38]. Higher water intake from beverages and usual plain water intake in current smokers were comparable to the results of previous studies [2,39,40]. There was no difference in water from beverages associated with regular physical activity, but water from foods and total water intake besides plain water were significantly higher among those who engaged in sufficient physical activity. It can be assumed that such a difference in water intake from foods results from differences in fruit and vegetable consumption, which are well-known sources of water in foods, between those who reported no physical activity and regular physical activity. Some Korean studies have reported that physically active people put more effort into reading nutrition labels and taking vitamin and mineral supplements [41]. In addition, vegetable and seafood patterns were more likely to be associated with physical activity [42]. We might conclude from previous literature that those who exercise regularly might follow a healthier diet compared with those who are not physically active.

It has been well-documented that vegetables and fruits are high-water-content foods, while oils, butter, and sugars contain the least water [43]. In other words, less high-fat intake or greater fruit and vegetable intake might be related to higher intake of water from food. Additionally, dietary energy density is inversely associated with higher consumption of fruits and vegetables [44]. This was supported by our result indicating a significantly negative association of water from foods with the energy density of all non-beverage foods. Water content of fruits and vegetables accounted for most of the water intake from foods in the Korean diet. Considering that the consumption of fruits and vegetables has a significantly positive association with water consumed from foods, adequate intake of water through foods can be achieved by higher consumption of fruit and vegetables. In our study, an increase in dietary sodium intake had a positive association with all components of water intake. Our finding was supported by the fact that an increased concentration of plasma sodium resulting from intakes of dietary salt increases fluid intake by stimulating thirst to maintain fluid homeostasis in our body [45]. In contrast, however, Kant et al. reported that dietary sodium intake was positively associated with water from foods but negatively associated with water from beverages and total water intake excluding plain water [2]. Different study populations used in both studies gave quite different results. Based on our findings, total daily energy intake from beverages in Korean adults was about 10%, which was only half of the result for Americans, who consume 20% of their daily energy from beverages [46]. The extent to which these differences in food consumption behaviors, particularly beverage-related, may cause the opposite associations between dietary sodium and intakes of total water and water consumed from beverages.

Another interesting result was observed in relation to eating behaviors and water intake. Reported snacking at the time of recall and 24-h energy from snacks were positively correlated with water intake from beverage. It is well-known that higher consumption of beverages has a significant association with increased frequency of snacking [47]. In a previous study on Korean dietary patterns, it was reported that most beverages, excluding alcoholic beverages with a meal and coffee immediately after a meal, could not be included as a part of main Korean dietary patterns. This indicated that most beverages were typically ingested not as a part of main meal but as a snack [48]. Similarly to snacking, eating outside the home was positively correlated with water consumed from beverages. This could be supported by the previous study indicating that Koreans consumed larger quantities of various kinds of beverages when eating outside the home than eating at home [32]. According to the results of existing studies, adequate water intake and healthy beverage consumption should be particularly emphasized for those who have more opportunities to snack and eat outside the home.

The present study has both limitations and strengths. Firstly, it used cross-sectional data which has limitations in identifying causal relationships between water intake and energy and dietary intakes and eating behaviors. Secondly, we adjusted for sociodemographic and health-related variables as covariates. However, we did not consider the influence of seasonal variations in water intake [49] since the KCDC does not publicly release seasonal data collected from the KNAHENS. Therefore, future research considering the seasonal effect on water intake needs to be conducted when seasonal information is available. Despite these limitations, this study is significant in that it provides the first snapshot of water intake and beverage consumption in the Korean population using large-scale data. Finally, as mentioned earlier, the necessity of nationally representative data on water intake of Koreans should be emphasized. In the US, the US Department of Agriculture and the US Department of Health and Human Services have put considerable effort into understanding all forms of water intake in the US population for a long time [37]. In line with this, since 2005–2006, the NHANES has changed the method of collection of plain water intake data from the FFQ-type question to 24-h dietary recall methods [37,50,51]. This change has allowed for more accurate estimates of total water intakes in the US. However, this is not the case with the KNHANES. While intakes of water from beverages and foods have been estimated by 24-h dietary recalls, plain water intake has continued to be measured by the FFQ-type question. Thus, total water intakes from foods and beverages quantified in our study may not include plain water intake. It was also impossible to report the association of usual plain water intake obtained from the FFQ-type question with energy, macronutrients, and other dietary constituents reported by the 24-h dietary recall. Additionally, in general, a 24-h dietary recall method is preferred as a method to obtain more valid and accurate intake data than an FFQ [52]. Therefore, additional information on plain water intake, including tap and bottled water, should be collected by the 24-h dietary recall in the KNHANES, and further study using these data needs to be conducted.

5. Conclusions

In conclusion, our study quantified total water intake and investigated the important nutritional and diet-related behavioral contributors of water intake among Korean adults. Water intake from beverages and foods was positively associated with total daily energy intake, but negatively associated with the energy density of non-beverage foods. The present study also found strong and independent associations between water intake and eating location (eating outside the home vs. at home), types of meals (main meals and snacks), and eating episodes. This additional information might help to provide more efficient strategies for nutritional education to prompt adequate water intake among people with various characteristics of dietary intakes and meal consumption behavior. Future studies using plain water intake measured by 24-h dietary recalls rather than FFQs or simple questionnaires are needed in order to answer the question "What are the best water intake guidelines for Koreans to ensure the proper role of water in the body?"

Supplementary Materials: The following are available online at www.mdpi.com/2072-6643/8/10/617/s1, Table S1: Odds ratios and 95% confidence intervals of beverage consumption according to sociodemographic and health-related characteristics in Korean adults, KNHANES 2008–2012 [1].

Acknowledgments: This study was conducted by the generous financial support of the Youlchon Foundation (Nongshim Corporation and its affiliated companies) in Korea. The funder had no role in the design, analysis, interpretation, and writing of this article. The manuscript was prepared using KNHANES 2008–2012 data obtained from the KCDC. All authors would like to thank the KCDC for the availability of the KNHANES survey data. The authors also thank Michelle Ann Arsenault for her helpful input and exceptional assistance.

Author Contributions: K.W.L. conceptualized the study, conducted the statistical analysis and drafted the manuscript. D.S. provided continuous scientific advice for the study and was involved in the manuscript preparation and revision. W.O.S. guided the manuscript development and substantially revised the paper. All authors critically reviewed and approved the final manuscript submitted for publication.

Conflicts of Interest: The authors declare that they have no competing interests.

References

1. Daniels, M.C.; Popkin, B.M. Impact of water intake on energy intake and weight status: A systematic review. *Nutr. Res.* **2010**, *68*, 505–521. [CrossRef] [PubMed]
2. Kant, A.K.; Graubard, B.I.; Atchison, E.A. Intakes of plain water, moisture in foods and beverages, and total water in the adult US population—Nutritional, meal pattern, and body weight correlates: National Health and Nutrition Examination Surveys 1999–2006. *Am. J. Clin. Nutr.* **2009**, *90*, 655–663. [CrossRef] [PubMed]
3. Häussinger, D. The role of cellular hydration in the regulation of cell function. *Biochem. J.* **1996**, *313*, 697–710. [CrossRef] [PubMed]
4. Montain, S.J.; Latzka, W.A.; Sawka, M.N. Fluid replacement recommendations for training in hot weather. *Mil. Med.* **1999**, *164*, 502–508. [PubMed]
5. Popkin, B.M.; D'Anci, K.E.; Rosenberg, I.H. Water, hydration, and health. *Nutr. Res.* **2010**, *68*, 439–458. [CrossRef] [PubMed]

6.   Korean Ministry of Health and Welfare; The Korean Nutrition Society; Korean Food and Drug Adminstration. *Dietary Reference Intakes for Koreans*; The Korean Nutrition Society: Seoul, Korea, 2015.

7.   Pan, A.; Malik, V.S.; Hao, T.; Willett, W.C.; Mozaffarian, D.; Hu, F.B. Changes in water and beverage intake and long-term weight changes: Results from three prospective cohort studies. *Int. J. Obes.* **2013**, *37*, 1378–1385. [CrossRef] [PubMed]

8.   Ilich, J.Z.; Cvijetic, S.; Baric, I.C.; Cecic, I.; Saric, M.; Crncevic-Orlic, Z.; Blanusa, M.; Korsic, M. Nutrition and lifestyle in relation to bone health and body weight in Croatian postmenopausal women. *Int. J. Food Sci. Nutr.* **2009**, *60*, 319–332. [CrossRef] [PubMed]

9.   Stookey, J.D.; Constant, F.; Popkin, B.M.; Gardner, C.D. Drinking water is associated with weight loss in overweight dieting women independent of diet and activity. *Obesity* **2008**, *16*, 2481–2488. [CrossRef] [PubMed]

10.   Pan, A.; Malik, V.S.; Schulze, M.B.; Manson, J.E.; Willett, W.C.; Hu, F.B. Plain-water intake and risk of type 2 diabetes in young and middle-aged women. *Am. J. Clin. Nutr.* **2012**, *95*, 1454–1460. [CrossRef] [PubMed]

11.   Sontrop, J.M.; Dixon, S.N.; Garg, A.X.; Buendia-Jimenez, I.; Dohein, O.; Huang, S.-H.; Clark, W.F. Association between water intake, chronic kidney disease, and cardiovascular disease: A cross-sectional analysis of NHANES data. *Am. J. Nephrol.* **2013**, *37*, 434–442. [CrossRef] [PubMed]

12.   Muñoz, C.X.; Johnson, E.C.; McKenzie, A.L.; Guelinckx, I.; Graverholt, G.; Casa, D.J.; Maresh, C.M.; Armstrong, L.E. Habitual total water intake and dimensions of mood in healthy young women. *Appetite* **2015**, *92*, 81–86. [CrossRef] [PubMed]

13.   Yang, M.; Chun, O.K. Consumptions of plain water, moisture in foods and beverages, and total water in relation to dietary micronutrient intakes and serum nutrient profiles among US adults. *Public Health Nutr.* **2015**, *18*, 1180–1186. [CrossRef] [PubMed]

14.   Nissensohn, M.; Sánchez-Villegas, A.; Ortega, R.M.; Aranceta-Bartrina, J.; Gil, Á.; González-Gross, M.; Varela-Moreiras, G.; Serra-Majem, L. Beverage consumption habits and association with total water and energy intakes in the Spanish population: Findings of the ANIBES study. *Nutrients* **2016**, *8*, 232. [CrossRef] [PubMed]

15.   Institute of Medicine, Food and Nutrition Board. *Dietary Reference Intakes for Water, Potassium, Sodium, Chloride, and Sulfate*; National Academy Press: Washington, DC, USA, 2005.

16.   European Food Safety Authority (EFSA) Panel on Dietetic Products, Nutrition, and Allergies (NDA). Scientific opinion on dietary reference values for water. *EFSA J.* **2010**, *8*, 1459.

17.   Statistics Korea. Available online: http://kostat.go.kr/portal/korea/index.action (accessed on 13 May 2016).

18.   Korea Agro-Fisheries & Food Trade Corporation. aT Food Information Statistics System. Available online: http://atfis.or.kr (accessed on 20 May 2016).

19.   Korea Health Industry Development Institute. *Food Industry Analysis Report 2014*; Korea Health Industry Development Institute: Cheongwon, Korea, 2014.

20.   Oh, S.-C.; Jang, J.-S. The effects of food-related lifestyle on carbonated beverage consumption behavior of the middle school students. *Korean J. Food Nutr.* **2014**, *27*, 1043–1050. [CrossRef]

21.   Lee, B.; Mi, K.; Kim, B.; Kim, B.; Kim, J.; Lee, I.; In, E.; Jung, S. Caffeine contained beverage intake and sleep quality of university students. *J. Korean Soc. Sch Health* **2014**, *27*, 31–38. [CrossRef]

22.   Song, H.J.; Paek, Y.J.; Choi, M.K.; Yoo, K.-B.; Kang, J.-H.; Lee, H.-J. Gender differences in the relationship between carbonated sugar-sweetened beverage intake and the likelihood of hypertension according to obesity. *Int. J. Public Health Res.* **2016**, 1–9. [CrossRef] [PubMed]

23.   Song, F.; Oh, J.; Lee, K.; Cho, M.S. The effect of coffee consumption on food group intake, nutrition intake, and metabolic syndrome of Korean adults—2010 KNHANES (V-1). *NFS J.* **2016**, *4*, 9–14. [CrossRef]

24.   Korea Centers for Disease Control and Prevention. *User Guide for the Fourth Korea National Health and Nutrition Examination Survey (KNHANES IV)*; Korea Centers for Disease Control and Prevention: Cheongwon, Korea, 2014.

25.   Ministry of Health and Welfare; Korea Centers for Disease Control and Prevention. *Korea Health Statistics 2007: Korea National Health and Nutrition Examination Survey (KNHANES IV-1)*; Korea Centers for Disease Control and Prevention: Seoul, Korea, 2008.

26.   Kweon, S.; Kim, Y.; Jang, M.-J.; Kim, Y.; Kim, K.; Choi, S.; Chun, C.; Khang, Y.-H.; Oh, K. Data resource profile: The Korea National Health and Nutrition Examination Survey (KNHANES). *Int. J. Epidemiol.* **2014**, *43*, 69–77. [CrossRef] [PubMed]

27. Korea Centers for Disease Control and Prevention. Korean National Health and Nutrition Examination Survey. Available online: http://knhanes.cdc.go.kr (accessed on 10 April 2016).

28. Popkin, B.M.; Armstrong, L.E.; Bray, G.M.; Caballero, B.; Frei, B.; Willett, W.C. A new proposed guidance system for beverage consumption in the United States. *Am. J. Clin. Nutr.* **2006**, *83*, 529–542. [PubMed]

29. Mesirow, M.S.; Welsh, J.A. Changing beverage consumption patterns have resulted in fewer liquid calories in the diets of US children: National Health and Nutrition Examination Survey 2001–2010. *J. Acad. Nutr. Diet.* **2015**, *115*, 559–566. [CrossRef] [PubMed]

30. Han, E.; Kim, T.H.; Powell, L.M. Beverage consumption and individual-level associations in South Korea. *BMC Public Health* **2013**, *13*, 195. [CrossRef] [PubMed]

31. Kim, S.D.; Moon, H.-K.; Park, J.S.; Lee, Y.C.; Shin, G.Y.; Jo, H.B.; Kim, B.S.; Kim, J.H.; Chae, Y.Z. Macromineral intake in non-alcoholic beverages for children and adolescents: Using the fourth Korea National Health and Nutrition Examination Survey (KNHANES IV, 2007–2009). *J. Nutr. Health* **2013**, *46*, 50–60. [CrossRef]

32. Lee, K.W.; Song, W.O.; Cho, M.S. Dietary quality differs by consumption of meals prepared at home vs. outside in Korean adults. *Nutr. Res. Pract.* **2016**, *10*, 294–304. [CrossRef] [PubMed]

33. Kant, A.K.; Graubard, B.I. Secular trends in patterns of self-reported food consumption of adult Americans: NHANES 1971–1975 to NHANES 1999–2002. *Am. J. Clin. Nutr.* **2006**, *84*, 1215–1223. [PubMed]

34. Kant, A.K.; Graubard, B.I. Contributors of water intake in US children and adolescents: Associations with dietary and meal characteristics: National Health and Nutrition Examination Survey 2005–2006. *Am. J. Clin. Nutr.* **2010**, *92*, 887–896. [CrossRef] [PubMed]

35. WHO Expert Consultation. Appropriate body-mass index for Asian populations and its implications for policy and intervention strategies. *Lancet* **2004**, *363*, 157–163.

36. Guelinckx, I.; Ferreira-Pêgo, C.; Moreno, L.A.; Kavouras, S.A.; Gandy, J.; Martinez, H.; Bardosono, S.; Abdollahi, M.; Nasseri, E.; Jarosz, A. Intake of water and different beverages in adults across 13 countries. *Eur. J. Clin. Nutr.* **2015**, *54*, 45–55. [CrossRef] [PubMed]

37. Sebastian, R.S.; Enns, C.W.; Goldman, J.D.; Moshfegh, A.J. Change in methodology for collection of drinking water intake in What We Eat in America/National Health and Nutrition Examination Survey: Implications for analysis. *Public Health Nutr.* **2012**, *15*, 1190–1195. [CrossRef] [PubMed]

38. Kim, K.; Hong, S.A.; Kim, M.K. Nutritional status and food insufficiency of Korean population through the life-course by education level based on 2005 National Health and Nutrition Survey. *Korean J. Nutr.* **2008**, *41*, 667–681.

39. De Castro, J.M.; Taylor, T. Smoking status relationships with the food and fluid intakes of free-living humans. *Nutrition* **2008**, *24*, 109–119. [CrossRef] [PubMed]

40. Kim, J.; Yang, Y.J. Plain water intake of Korean adults according to life style, anthropometric and dietary characteristic: The Korea National Health and Nutrition Examination Surveys 2008–2010. *Nutr. Res. Pract.* **2014**, *8*, 580–588. [CrossRef] [PubMed]

41. Kang, E.-J. Clustering of lifestyle behaviors of Korean adults using smoking, drinking, and physical activity. *Health Soc. Welf. Rev.* **2007**, *27*, 44–66.

42. Cho, Y.A.; Shin, A.; Kim, J. Dietary patterns are associated with body mass index in a Korean population. *J. Am. Diet. Assoc.* **2011**, *111*, 1182–1186. [CrossRef] [PubMed]

43. Agricultural Research Service, Food Surveys Research Group; Beltsville Human Nutrition Research Center. *The USDA Food and Nutrient Database for Dietary Studies 2011–2012*; US Department of Agriculture: Beltsville, MD, USA, 2014.

44. Azadbakht, L.; Esmaillzadeh, A. Dietary energy density is favorably associated with dietary diversity score among female university students in Isfahan. *Nutrition* **2012**, *28*, 991–995. [CrossRef] [PubMed]

45. Stachenfeld, N.S. Acute effects of sodium ingestion on thirst and cardiovascular function. *Curr. Sports Med. Rep.* **2008**, *7*, S7. [CrossRef] [PubMed]

46. Drewnowski, A.; Rehm, C.D.; Constant, F. Water and beverage consumption among adults in the United States: Cross-sectional study using data from NHANES 2005–2010. *BMC Public Health* **2013**, *13*, 1. [CrossRef] [PubMed]

47. Kant, A.K.; Graubard, B.I.; Mattes, R.D. Association of food form with self-reported 24-h energy intake and meal patterns in US adults: NHANES 2003–2008. *Am. J. Clin. Nutr.* **2012**, *96*, 044974. [CrossRef] [PubMed]

48. Kim, J.; Jo, I.; Joung, H. A rice-based traditional dietary pattern is associated with obesity in Korean adults. *J. Acad. Nutr. Diet.* **2012**, *112*, 246–253. [CrossRef] [PubMed]

49. Morimoto, T.; Shiraki, K.; Inue, T.; Yoshimura, H. Seasonal variation of water and electrolyte in serum with respect to homeostasis. *Jpn. J. Physiol.* **1969**, *19*, 801–813. [CrossRef] [PubMed]

50. National Health and Nutrition Examination Survey. 2003–2004 Data Documentation, Codebook, and Frequencies. Available online: http://wwwn.cdc.gov/nchs/nhanes/2003--2004/dr1tot_c.htm (accessed on 17 July 2016).

51. National Health and Nutrition Examination Survey. 2005–2006 Data Documentation, Codebook, and Frequencies. Available online: http://wwwn.cdc.gov/nchs/nhanes/2005--2006/dr1tot_d.htm (accessed on 17 July 2016).

52. Mons, M.; Van der Wielen, J.; Blokker, E.; Sinclair, M.; Hulshof, K.; Dangendorf, F.; Hunter, P.; Medema, G. Estimation of the consumption of cold tap water for microbiological risk assessment: An overview of studies and statistical analysis of data. *J. Water Health* **2007**, *5*, 151–170. [CrossRef] [PubMed]

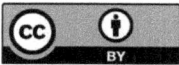

![nutrients logo] *nutrients*

MDPI

Article

Characteristics of Beverage Consumption Habits among a Large Sample of French Adults: Associations with Total Water and Energy Intakes

Fabien Szabo de Edelenyi [1], Nathalie Druesne-Pecollo [1], Nathalie Arnault [1], Rebeca González [1], Camille Buscail [1,2] and Pilar Galan [1,*]

[1] Sorbonne Paris Cité Epidemiology and Statistics Research Center (CRESS), Inserm U1153, Inra U1125, Cnam, Paris 13 University, Nutritional Epidemiology Research Team (EREN), Bobigny F93017, France; f.szabo@eren.smbh.univ-paris13.fr (F.S.d.E.); n.pecollo@eren.smbh.univ-paris13.fr (N.D.-P.); n.arnault@eren.smbh.univ-paris13.fr (N.A.); r.gonzalez@eren.smbh.univ-paris13.fr (R.G.); c.buscail@eren.smbh.univ-paris13.fr (C.B.)
[2] Public Health Department, Avicenne Hospital, Bobigny F93017, France
* Correspondence: p.galan@eren.smbh.univ-paris13.fr; Tel.: +33-148-388-976

Received: 4 July 2016; Accepted: 27 September 2016; Published: 11 October 2016

Abstract: Background: Adequate hydration is a key factor for correct functioning of both cognitive and physical processes. In France, public health recommendations about adequate total water intake (TWI) only state that fluid intake should be sufficient, with particular attention paid to hydration for seniors, especially during heatwave periods. The objective of this study was to calculate the total amount of water coming from food and beverages and to analyse characteristics of consumption in participants from a large French national cohort. Methods: TWI, as well as contribution of food and beverages to TWI was assessed among 94,939 adult participants in the Nutrinet-Santé cohort (78% women, mean age 42.9 (SE 0.04)) using three 24-h dietary records at baseline. Statistical differences in water intakes across age groups, seasons and day of the week were assessed. Results: The mean TWI was 2.3 L (Standard Error SE 4.7) for men and 2.1 L (SE 2.4) for women. A majority of the sample did comply with the European Food Safety Authority (EFSA) adequate intake recommendation, especially women. Mean total energy intake (EI) was 1884 kcal/day (SE 1.5) (2250 kcal/day (SE 3.6) for men and 1783 kcal/day (SE 1.5) for women). The contribution to the total EI from beverages was 8.3%. Water was the most consumed beverage, followed by hot beverages. The variety score, defined as the number of different categories of beverages consumed during the three 24-h records out of a maximum of 8, was positively correlated with TWI ($r = 0.4$); and with EI ($r = 0.2$), suggesting that beverage variety is an indicator of higher consumption of food and drinks. We found differences in beverage consumptions and water intakes according to age and seasonality. Conclusions: The present study gives an overview of the water intake characteristics in a large population of French adults. TWI was found to be globally in line with public health recommendations.

Keywords: nutrients; total water intake; energy intake; beverages; France

1. Introduction

Hydration status results from a tightly regulated balance between water intake and loss. It is important to equilibrate input and output because even mild dehydration can lead to a reduction of physical and cognitive performances [1,2]. A more severe dehydration status can have a very significant impact on health, especially in elderly people [3]. On the long term, some effects of hydration status on chronic diseases have been shown or suggested, with different levels of evidence [4,5].

Water requirements vary depending on environmental factors such as heat, salt intake, lifestyle (physical activity) and inter-individual variability. Water intake is fulfilled by both water contained in solid foods (20%–30%) and water from beverages and drinking water (70%–80%) [5–7].

While depending on eating and drinking habits, adaptation of the water intake to match the variation in water loss is mostly driven by thirst [8,9].

Some countries and public organizations have proposed water intake recommendations for the general public. Due to the large inter-individual variability, those recommendations struggle to give adequate reference values for total water intake. European Food Safety Authority (EFSA) proposed Dietary Reference Values (DRV) for Adequate Intake of Water (AI) for men and women of 2.5 L and 2.0 L [6].

Few data are available concerning the total amount of water coming from food or beverages and characteristics of beverage consumption in the French general population.

2. Materials and Methods

2.1. Data Collection

Data used in this study were collected using the Nutrinet-Santé cohort. The Nutrinet-Santé Study is a large web-based prospective observational cohort including adult volunteers aged 18 years or older, launched in France in May 2009 with a scheduled follow-up of 10 years. The Nutrinet-Santé study has been described in detail elsewhere [10]. The Nutrinet-Santé study was conducted according to guidelines laid down in the Declaration of Helsinki and was approved by the International Research Board of the French Institute for Health and Medical Research (IRB Inserm Paris, France No. 0000388FWA00005831) and the "Comité National Informatique et Liberté" (CNIL Paris, France No. 908450 and No. 909216). Electronic informed consent was obtained from all subjects.

At baseline, socio-demographic data including age, gender, education, income, occupational category, and household location, as well as lifestyle (smoking status, physical activity), height, weight and practice of restrictive diet were self-reported. Leisure time physical activity was assessed using the French short form of the International Physical Activity Questionnaire (IPAQ), self-administered online [11–13]. Body mass index (BMI) was assessed using self-reported height and weight.

Dietary data were also collected at baseline using three 24-h records, randomly distributed within a two-week period, including two week days and one weekend day. Participants reported all foods and beverages consumed throughout the day: breakfast, lunch, dinner and all other occasions.

In the present study, daily mean food and beverage consumptions were calculated for each participant having completed the three 24-h records, with a weighting on the type of day (week or weekend day). Identification of underreporting participants was based on the validated and published method proposed by Black [14] using Schofield equations for estimating resting metabolic rate [15]. In addition, we eliminated subjects with anomalous values for EI (men <800 or >4000 and women <500 or >3500 kcal/day) [16]. Serving sizes were estimated using purchase unit, household unit and photographs, derived from a previously validated picture booklet [17].

Participants were asked at the end of each 24-h records whether they did not forget any food intake, including snacking and beverages, and had then the possibility to add it to the records.

A total of 94,939 participants were included in this analysis.

2.2. Data Preparation and Analysis

EI and TWI were calculated through the NutriNet-Santé food composition table including more than 2000 food products [18]. Contributions of food and beverages to TWI and EI were also calculated.

Beverages have been grouped into 8 categories for further analysis: (1) hot beverages included hot tea and hot coffee; (2) milk; (3) fruit & vegetable 100% juices with no added sugar (not included nectars and mix of juice and milk); (4) caloric soft drinks (included sodas, ice tea, non-alcoholic beer or liquor, sports drinks, energy drinks, nectars and mix of juice and milk, etc.); (5) diet soft drinks (without sugar as a sweetener); (6) alcoholic drinks; (7) water (include tap water and bottled water); and (8) other beverages (included soy-based beverages, high-protein beverages). Contribution of each beverage category to the total beverage consumption was computed. A variety score defined as the number of different categories of beverages consumed during the three 24-h records out of a maximum of 8 was calculated.

Five age groups were used in the study: 18–25, 26–35, 36–50, 51–64 and 65–75 years.

In order to estimate the effect of the season on beverage consumption, nutritional data were separated according to the month of the 24 h-records: December–January–February (winter), March–April–May (spring), June–July–August (summer) and September–October–November (autumn). Beverage consumptions were also calculated separately for each day of the week in order to test whether there was a trend over a week. For this calculation, no weighting on the type of day (week or weekend day) was performed.

To investigate trends over the day, consumption occasions were aggregated into 6 periods of time, approximately corresponding to breakfast (5:30 to 10:00), mid-morning (10:00 to 12:00), lunch (12:00 to 15:00); snack (15:00 to 19:00); dinner (19:00 to 22:00); and other moments.

2.3. Statistical Analyses

Description of the population, contribution of food and beverages to total water and energy intake and beverage consumption according to time of day and day of the week were stratified by sex. Spearman partial correlations between water intake, energy intake and beverage consumption were adjusted for age, gender, body weight and physical activity level. Crude differences in TWI and beverage consumption across age groups and across seasons were assessed by sex through ANOVA-test. Pairwise comparisons of the means across groups were assessed using *T*-tests with Bonferroni correction for multiple testing. Comparisons of the means of beverage consumption across week-end days (Saturday, Sunday) and the other days of the week were assessed by sex using *T*-tests. Crude differences in beverage consumption at 6 periods of time, across age groups were assessed through ANOVA-test. Pairwise comparisons of the means were assessed using *T*-tests with Bonferroni correction for multiple testing. Partial correlations between TWI and beverage consumption in each period of time, by gender, were adjusted for age. Beverage consumption in each period was expressed as a percentage of total consumption over 24 h. All analyses were 2-tailed with a statistical significance of $p < 0.05$.

3. Results

Characteristics of the sample are presented for men and women as well as for the whole sample in Table 1. The mean age was 42.9 (0.04) (41.7 (0.05) for women and 47.3 (0.1) for men) and 78% were women; 63.7% had a post-secondary degree education level. The mean BMI was 23.8 kg/m^2, with 9.0% of participants being obese and 21.4% being overweight.

The distribution of mean total water intake (TWI) (g/day), stratified by sex is shown Figure 1. The mean TWI was 2.3 L for men and 2.1 L for women, close to the EFSA "adequate intake" (AI) recommendations for adults: 2.5 L and 2 L, respectively, though lower for men and higher for women.

The contributions of food and beverages to daily EI (kcal/day) and water intake (mL/day), by gender, are presented in Table 2. Men consumed more than two times more alcoholic drinks than women ($p < 0.0001$), while women consumed more hot beverages ($p < 0.0001$). Mean total EI was 1884 kcal/day (SE 1.5), and the relative contribution to total EI from beverages was 8.3% (9.9% in men, 7.8% in women). Furthermore, 61.9% of the TWI came from beverages and 38.1% came from food. The part of the water intake coming from the beverages was lower than the EFSA estimation (70%–80% provided by the beverages and 20%–30% coming from food).

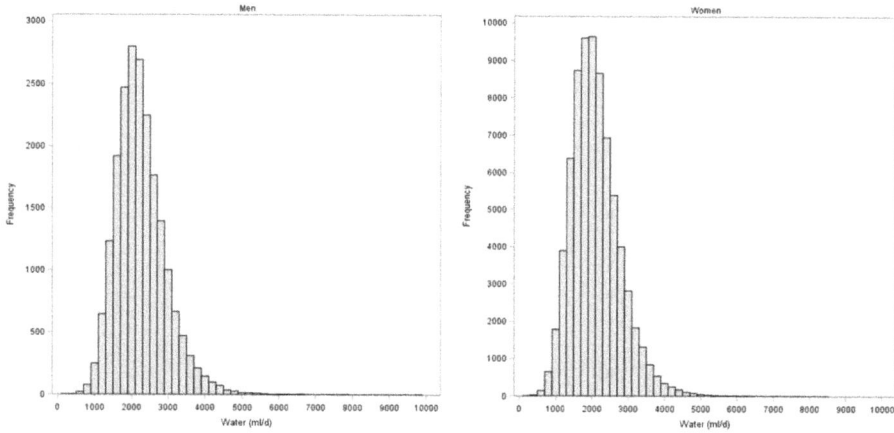

Figure 1. Frequency distribution of total water intake (mL/day) by gender.

Table 1. Statistical description for the whole sample, and by gender.

		Male	Female	Total
	Count	**20,636**	**74,303**	**94,939**
	Age (year) Means (SE)	47.3 (0.10)	41.7 (0.05)	42.9 (0.04)
Age Group	18–25 (%)	8.7	15.6	14.1
	26–35 (%)	18.0	23.0	21.9
	36–50 (%)	27.2	30.4	29.7
	51–64 (%)	33.3	26.2	27.8
	65–75 (%)	12.8	4.6	6.4
	Rate of unemployment (%)	5.0	6.5	6.1
Level of physical activity	Vigorous (%)	36.7	26.3	28.6
	Moderate (%)	32.9	38.3	37.1
	Light (%)	18.9	21.3	20.7
	Unknown (%)	11.5	14.1	13.5
Level of education	Primary (%)	23.1	17.7	18.9
	Secondary (%)	13.7	18.4	17.4
	Post-secondary (%)	63.2	63.9	63.7
Household income	<1000 €/month (%)	8.4	13.0	12.0
	1000–2000 €/month (%)	36.4	39.3	38.7
	≥2000 €/month (%)	48.3	34.6	37.6
	Unknown (%)	6.9	13.1	11.8
	Weight (kg) Means (SE)	77.4 (0.09)	63.3 (0.05)	66.4 (0.05)
	Height (cm) Means (SE)	176.5 (0.05)	164.1 (0.02)	166.8 (0.03)
	BMI (kg/m^2) Means (SE)	24.8 (0.03)	23.5 (0.02)	23.8 (0.01)
BMI class	Normal weight (%)	58.8	72.6	69.6
	Overweight (%)	32.3	18.3	21.4
	Obese (%)	8.8	9.0	9.0
	Waist Circumference * Means (SE)	90.32 (0.16)	79.92 (0.11)	82.83 (0.10)

* Subsample of individuals who had attended the clinical exam, *n* = 16,133.

Table 2. Contribution of food and beverages to total water (mL/day) and energy intake (kcal/day) for the whole sample and by gender.

		Contribution to Water Intake (mL/Day)			*p*	Contribution to Energy Intake (kcal/Day)			*p*
		Male	Female	Total		Male	Female	Total	
Count		20,636	74,303	94,939		20,636	74,303	94,939	
All food and drink	Mean (SE)	2251.0 (4.7)	2101.7 (2.4)	2134.2 (2.2)	<0.0001	2250 (3.6)	1783 (1.5)	1884 (1.5)	<0.0001
Food only	%	39.4	37.8	38.1	<0.0001	90.1	92.2	91.7	<0.0001
Beverages only	%	60.6	62.2	61.9	<0.0001	9.9	7.8	8.3	<0.0001
Hot beverages	%	14.6	19.0	18.1	<0.0001	0.3	0.4	0.4	<0.0001
Milk	%	3.6	3.5	3.5	NS	1.9	2.1	2.0	<0.0001
Fruit & vegetable juice	%	2.6	2.4	2.4	<0.0001	1.3	1.3	1.3	0.0003
Caloric soft drink	%	2.3	2.1	2.1	<0.0001	1.0	0.9	1.0	NS
Diet soft drink	%	0.7	1.1	1.0	<0.0001	0.0	0.1	0.1	<0.0001
Alcoholic drinks	%	7.3	3.1	4.0	<0.0001	5.2	2.7	3.3	<0.0001
Water	%	29.2	30.7	30.4	<0.0001	0.0	0.0	0.0	NS
Other beverages	%	0.3	0.3	0.3	NS	0.2	0.2	0.2	0.0003

NS: Not significant; SE: standard error.

Water represented almost half of the beverage consumption over 3 days period for both men and women (48.2% for women and 46.6% for men) (Figure 2). The second most popular beverage was hot beverages (respectively 30.2% and 23.5% for women and men). Alcohol was in the third position for men (13.1%) and fourth position for women (5.5%).

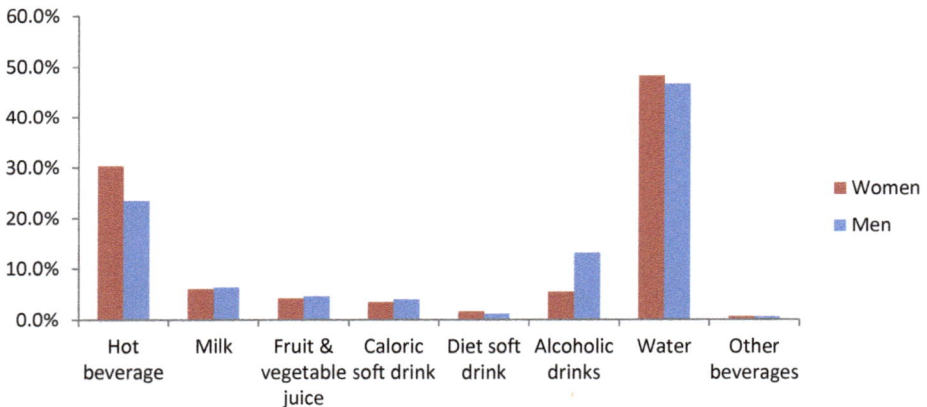

Figure 2. Percentage of the beverage consumption represented by each beverage category, separated by gender.

TWI was highly correlated with the weight of beverages and water from beverages ($r = 0.9$) and more weakly correlated with food intake ($r = 0.5$) (Table 3). Milk and alcohol drinks had moderate correlation ($r = 0.4$ and $r = 0.5$, respectively) with total energy from beverages, while for hot beverages and diet soft drinks coefficients were the lowest values. The variety of beverages was positively correlated with beverage intake (weight, energy and water intake), suggesting that a higher diversity was associated with a higher consumption of beverages.

In Table 4, we compared the water intakes and beverage consumptions across the five age groups separately for men and women. The lowest total water intake from food and beverages was found in the 18–25 years group. Elderly people (refer here to age group 65–75 years), especially men, tend also to have lower TWI than the other age groups. For both men and women, the contributions of food and beverages to the TWI were different between elderly and other adults. Elderly people had a higher water intake from food and a lower intake from beverages than the other age groups (except with (51–64) for water intake from food in men and with (18–25) for water intake from beverages in women) ($p < 0.0001$ where significant).

Consumption was generally lower in the elderly for all types of beverages, except for alcoholic drinks and hot beverages.

Consumption of alcoholic drinks for men and women adults averaged 181.3 mL/day (SE: 1.6) and 72.5 mL/day (SE: 0.4) respectively (5.2% and 2.7% of the energy intakes) and increased to 196.7 mL/day and 84.5 mL/day for elderly men and women respectively (6.3% and 3.5% of the total energy, data not shown).

In Table 5, we compared the water intakes and beverage consumptions between seasons separately for men and women. Total water intake from food and beverages was highest during the summer and lowest in the winter. Difference in TWI between summer and winter was 120 mL for men and 80 mL for women ($p < 0.0001$). Consumption of hot beverages was higher during the winter compared to the three other seasons ($p < 0.001$). Conversely, consumption of milk, caloric soft drinks, diet soft drinks, alcoholic drinks and water were higher during the spring and summer (see Table 5 for significant pairwise comparisons).

We investigated the influence of the day of the week on the beverage consumption (Figure 3).

The total amount of beverage intake (mL) was higher on Saturdays and on Sundays compared to other days of the week ($p < 0.0001$). There is a higher consumption of alcoholic drinks at weekends ($p < 0.0001$). Both men and women consumed around two times more alcoholic drinks on Saturdays than on a week day. Weekends were also associated with a lower consumption of water and hot beverages, and a higher consumption of caloric soft drink ($p < 0.0001$).

Beverage consumption according to the time of day over a timeline of 24 h was presented in Table 6. The main part of the beverage consumption was concentrated during meal times. Elderly men's and women's consumption of beverages was higher than in the other age groups during breakfast (except with group (51–64)) ($p < 0.0001$), but lower during lunch and dinner ($p < 0.0001$).

Table 3. Partial correlations between water intake, energy intake and beverage consumption, adjusted for age, gender, body weight and activity level.

	Total Water (from Food & Beverages)	Water from Beverages	Water from Food	Beverages Weight	Food Weight	Total Energy kcal	Energy from Beverages	Energy from Food
Total water (from food and beverages)		0.91 ***	0.53 ***	0.91 ***	0.54 ***	0.32 ***	0.12 ***	0.30 ***
Water from beverages	0.91 ***		0.19 ***	1.00 ***	0.22 ***	0.24 ***	0.21 ***	0.19 ***
Water from food	0.53 ***	0.19 ***		0.18 ***	0.96 ***	0.32 ***	−0.14 ***	0.38 ***
Beverages weight	0.91 ***	0.999 ***	0.18 ***		0.18 ***	0.25 ***	0.25 ***	0.18 ***
Food weight	0.54 ***	0.22 ***	0.96 ***	0.21 ***		0.51 ***	−0.12 ***	0.58 ***
Total energy kcal	0.32 ***	0.24 ***	0.32 ***	0.25 ***	0.51 ***		0.31 ***	0.95 ***
Energy from beverages	0.12 ***	0.21 ***	−0.14 ***	0.18 ***	−0.12 ***	0.31 ***		0.05 ***
Energy from food	0.30 ***	0.19 ***	0.38 ***	0.45 ***	0.58 ***	0.95 ***	0.05 ***	
(1) Hot beverages (mL)	0.46 ***	0.46 ***	0.19 ***	0.07 ***	0.19 ***	0.06 ***	−0.14 ***	0.10 ***
(2) Milk (mL)	0.03 ***	0.06 ***	−0.02 ***	0.12 ***	−0.02 ***	0.10 ***	0.42 ***	0.003
(3) Fruit & vegetable juice (mL)	0.09 ***	0.11 ***	−0.004	0.03 ***	0.003	0.12 ***	0.32 ***	0.04 ***
(4) Caloric soft drink (mL)	−0.04 ***	0.02 ***	−0.14 ***	0.06 ***	−0.10 ***	0.12 ***	0.27 ***	0.06 ***
(5) Diet soft drink (mL)	0.06 ***	0.06 ***	0.02 ***	0.17 ***	0.01 **	−0.02 ***	−0.01 **	−0.02 ***
(6) Alcoholic drinks (mL)	0.08 ***	0.15 ***	−0.10 ***		−0.09 ***	0.19 ***	0.55 ***	0.04 ***
(7) Water (mL)	0.65 ***	0.70 ***	0.15 ***	0.69 ***	0.17 ***	0.12 ***	−0.04 ***	0.15 ***
(8) Other beverages (mL)	0.06 ***	0.04 ***	0.06 ***	0.04 ***	0.06 ***	0.01 ***	0.06 ***	−0.001
Variety of beverages consumed in day (out of 8)	0.38 ***	0.43 ***	0.05 ***	0.45 ***	0.08 ***	0.25 ***	0.51 ***	0.13 ***

*** Correlation is significant at the <0.0001 level (bilateral); ** Correlation is significant at the 0.01 level (bilateral).

Table 4. Results of ANOVA test for total water intake (g/day) and beverage consumption (mL/day), by gender and by age group.

		Male								Female							
		Age Group								Age Group							
		18–25	26–35	36–50	51–64	65–75	Total	p	Pairwise Comparison	18–25	26–35	36–50	51–64	65–75	Total	p	Pairwise Comparison
		A	B	C	D	E				A	B	C	D	E			
Base		1793	3709	5614	6873	2647	20,636			11,609	17,130	22,626	19,502	3436	74,303		
Total water intake from food and beverages (mL/day)	Mean (SE)	2108.8 (16.4)	2247.3 (11.8)	2328.2 (9.7)	2269.9 (7.8)	2139.7 (11.3)	2251.0 (4.7)	<0.0001	A = E < B = D < C	1858.7 (5.9)	2073.3 (5.2)	2173.6 (4.5)	2187.8 (4.5)	2102.3 (9.9)	2101.7 (2.4)	<0.0001	A < B = E < C = D
Water from food (mL/day)	Mean (SE)	726.9 (6.4)	779.0 (4.4)	846.7 (3.7)	912.6 (3.4)	923.5 (5.2)	855.9 (1.9)	<0.0001	A < B < C < D = E	640.2 (2.2)	704.2 (1.8)	778.7 (1.6)	855.3 (1.8)	870.7 (4.2)	764.2 (0.9)	<0.0001	A < B < C < D < E
Water from beverages (mL/day)	Mean (SE)	1381.9 (14.1)	1468.3 (10.2)	1481.6 (8.4)	1357.3 (6.5)	1216.2 (9.4)	1395.1 (4.1)	<0.0001	E < D = A < B = C	1218.6 (5.0)	1369.1 (4.5)	1394.9 (3.9)	1332.5 (3.9)	1231.7 (8.3)	1337.5 (2.1)	<0.0001	A = E < D < B < C
Total beverage consumption (mL/day)	Mean (SE)	1439.7 (14.5)	1523.6 (10.4)	1531.8 (8.6)	1406.8 (4.5)	1262.7 (9.6)	1446.0 (4.1)	<0.0001	E < D = A < B = C	1260.1 (5.1)	1406.8 (4.5)	1426.5 (4.0)	1362.4 (3.9)	1261.2 (8.4)	1371.5 (2.1)	<0.0001	A = E < D < B < C
OF WHICH (mL/day)																	
Hot beverages	Mean (SE)	152.5 (5.1)	269.8 (4.5)	367.2 (4.2)	387.4 (3.4)	371.0 (5.6)	338.2 (2.1)	<0.0001	A < B < C = E; A, B, C < D	206.9 (2.5)	356.8 (2.5)	487.8 (2.5)	522.0 (2.6)	498.5 (5.8)	423.2 (1.3)	<0.0001	A < B < C = E < D
Milk	Mean (SE)	121.2 (3.5)	94.9 (2.3)	84.6 (1.8)	77.3 (1.5)	88.1 (2.6)	87.7 (0.9)	<0.0001	D < C < B < A; D < E < A	101.6 (1.2)	87.8 (1.0)	72.1 (0.8)	61.6 (0.8)	61.5 (1.9)	77.1 (0.4)	<0.0001	D = E < C < B < A
Fruit & vegetable juice	Mean (SE)	89.5 (2.7)	83.7 (1.8)	67.1 (1.3)	54.1 (1.0)	42.8 (1.4)	64.6 (0.7)	<0.0001	E < D < C < B < A	74.9 (0.9)	65.9 (0.7)	47.7 (0.5)	41.7 (0.5)	36.4 (1.1)	54.0 (0.3)	<0.0001	E < D < C < B < A
Caloric soft drink	Mean (SE)	132.4 (4.8)	82.5 (2.5)	57.4 (1.8)	29.4 (1.1)	18.2 (1.1)	54.1 (0.9)	<0.0001	E < D < C < B < A	95.0 (1.4)	55.3 (0.8)	28.0 (0.5)	17.2 (0.5)	14.4 (0.9)	41.3 (0.4)	<0.0001	E = D < C < B < A
Diet soft drink	Mean (SE)	22.3 (2.3)	32.3 (1.9)	23.0 (1.4)	7.8 (0.7)	4.5 (0.8)	17.2 (0.6)	<0.0001	E = D < C < A < B	27.1 (0.9)	36.2 (0.9)	22.6 (0.6)	11.2 (0.5)	6.5 (0.8)	22.7 (0.3)	<0.0001	E < D < C < A < B
Alcoholic drinks	Mean (SE)	129.3 (5.0)	172.1 (3.4)	167.1 (2.9)	205.4 (2.8)	196.7 (3.9)	181.3 (1.6)	<0.0001	A < B = C < D = E	57.7 (1.1)	71.8 (0.8)	71.6 (0.8)	80.8 (0.8)	84.5 (1.9)	72.5 (0.4)	<0.0001	A < B = C < D = E
Water	Mean (SE)	782.5 (12.1)	778.7 (8.3)	754.5 (7.0)	637.7 (5.5)	535.0 (7.5)	694.2 (3.4)	<0.0001	E < D < C = B = A	690.2 (4.2)	725.4 (3.6)	688.0 (3.1)	619.1 (3.0)	550.2 (6.4)	672.5 (1.7)	<0.0001	E < D < C = B = A
Other beverages	Mean (SE)	9.8 (1.2)	9.5 (1.0)	10.9 (0.7)	7.2 (0.5)	6.4 (0.8)	8.8 (0.3)	<0.0001	D < C; E < C	6.7 (0.4)	7.6 (0.3)	8.8 (0.3)	8.9 (0.3)	9.1 (0.7)	8.2 (0.1)	<0.0001	A < C, D, E, B < D

Table 5. Total water intake (g/day) and beverage consumption (mL/day), by season and by gender.

			Male						Female			
		Season				p	Pairwise Comparison	Season				p	Pairwise Comparison
		Dec–Jan–Feb A	Mar–Apr–May B	Jun–Jul–Aug C	Sep–Oct–Nov D			Dec–Jan–Feb A	Mar–Apr–May B	Jun–Jul–Aug C	Sep–Oct–Nov D		
Base		3607	9206	5518	2305			11,969	33,503	19,894	8937		
Total water intake from food and beverages (mL/day)	Mean (SE)	2196.7 (10.7)	2228.3 (7.1)	2317.6 (9.5)	2267.0 (14.1)	<0.0001	A < D; A, B, D < C	2081.2 (5.9)	2074.9 (3.6)	2154.0 (4.9)	2113.6 (7.0)	<0.0001	A = B < D < C
Water from food (mL/day)	Mean (SE)	880.2 (4.7)	831.4 (2.8)	865.6 (3.8)	892.7 (6.2)	<0.0001	B < A, C, D; C < D	774.8 (2.3)	744.0 (1.4)	782.9 (1.9)	784.3 (2.8)	<0.0001	B < A < C = D
Water from beverages (mL/day)	Mean (SE)	1316.5 (9.0)	1397.0 (6.1)	1452.0 (8.2)	1374.3 (12.0)	<0.0001	A < B = D < C	1306.3 (4.9)	1330.9 (3.1)	1371.0 (4.1)	1329.2 (5.9)	<0.0001	A < B = D < C
Total beverage consumption (mL/day)	Mean (SE)	1365.0 (9.2)	1448.4 (6.2)	1504.3 (8.4)	1423.5 (12.2)	<0.0001	A < B = D < C	1339.4 (5.0)	1365.3 (3.1)	1405.3 (4.2)	1362.5 (5.9)	<0.0001	A < B = D < C
OF WHICH (mL/day)													
Hot beverages	Mean (SE)	373.0 (5.1)	332.1 (3.0)	324.5 (3.9)	341.2 (6.2)	<0.0001	B = C = D < A	484.1 (3.6)	409.3 (2.0)	403.7 (2.5)	437.2 (3.8)	<0.0001	B = C < D < A
Milk	Mean (SE)	80.6 (2.2)	89.3 (1.4)	89.4 (1.8)	88.1 (3.0)	<0.0001	B = C = D; A < B, A < C	70.0 (1.1)	79.3 (0.7)	77.5 (0.9)	77.1 (1.3)	<0.0001	B = C = D; A < B, A < C, A < D
Fruit & vegetable juice	Mean (SE)	64.8 (1.7)	65.6 (1.0)	64.2 (1.3)	61.1 (2.0)	NS		53.1 (0.8)	54.8 (0.4)	53.7 (0.6)	52.9 (0.9)	NS	
Caloric soft drink	Mean (SE)	35.5 (1.7)	58.9 (1.4)	60.5 (1.9)	48.5 (2.4)	<0.0001	A < D < B = C	31.0 (0.8)	45.6 (0.6)	43.2 (0.7)	34.6 (0.9)	<0.0001	A = D < C < B
Diet soft drink	Mean (SE)	11.2 (1.1)	19.0 (1.0)	19.3 (1.3)	14.2 (1.5)	<0.0001	A < B, C	15.5 (0.7)	25.3 (0.5)	23.9 (0.7)	19.9 (0.9)	<0.0001	A < D < B = C
Alcoholic drinks	Mean (SE)	170.5 (3.5)	181.9 (2.4)	191.6 (3.1)	170.9 (4.5)	0.0008	A < C, D < C	71.2 (1.1)	71.1 (0.7)	76.5 (0.8)	70.5 (1.2)	<0.0001	A = B = D < C
Water	Mean (SE)	615.5 (7.3)	694.9 (5.1)	746.1 (6.9)	690.5 (10.0)	<0.0001	A < B = D < C	602.5 (3.8)	672.9 (2.5)	719.4 (3.4)	660.5 (4.7)	<0.0001	A < B = D < C
Other beverages	Mean (SE)	13.9 (1.1)	6.7 (0.4)	8.8 (0.7)	9.1 (1.0)	<0.0001	B < A, C < A, D < A	11.8 (0.5)	7.0 (0.2)	7.4 (0.3)	9.7 (0.5)	<0.0001	B = C < D < A

NS: Non significant.

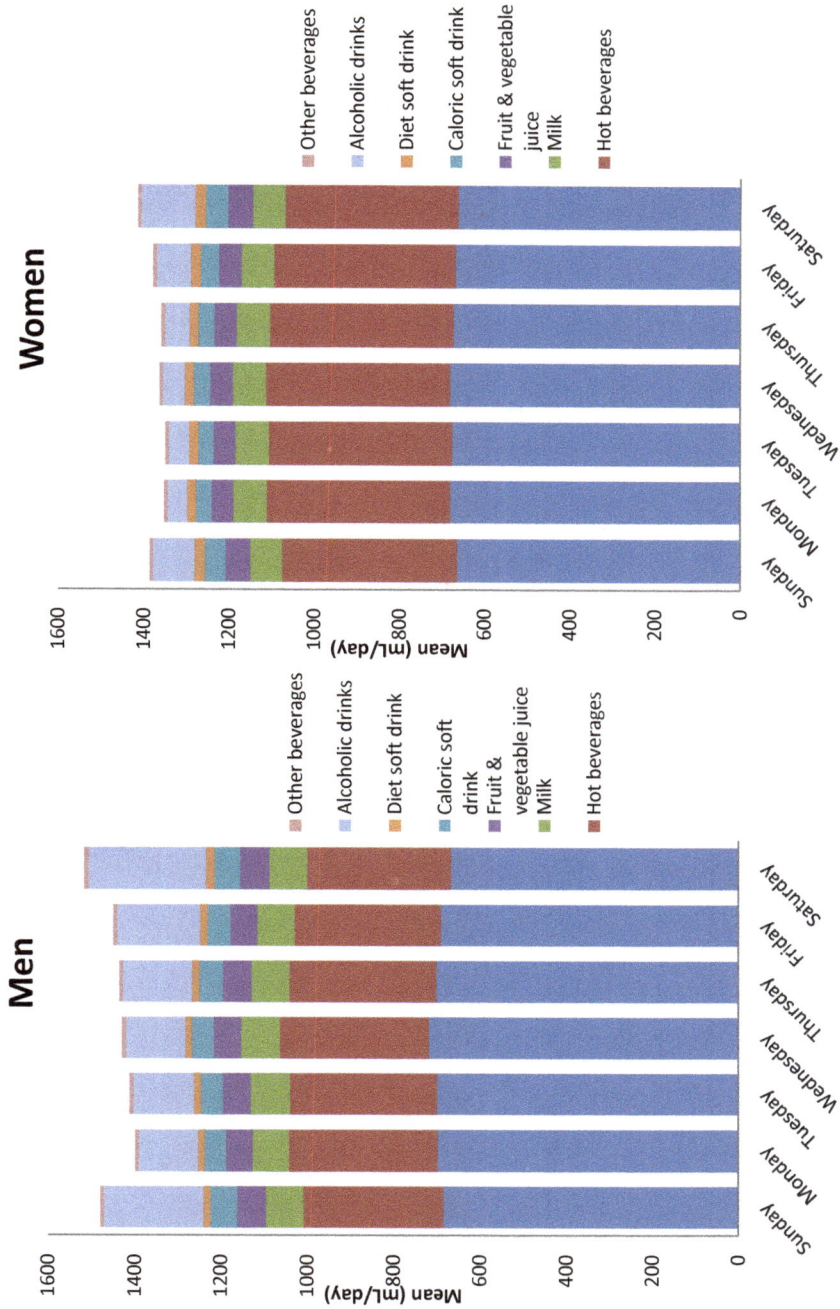

Figure 3. Amount and types of beverages consumed according to day of the week (mean mL/day), separated by gender.

Table 6. Beverage consumption according to time of day (hour interval), by gender and by age group.

Mean amount of beverages (mL/day) consumed between	Male Age Group 18-25 A	26-35 B	36-50 C	51-64 D	65-75 E	Total	p	Pairwise Comparison	Female Age Group 18-25 A	26-35 B	36-50 C	51-64 D	65-75 E	Total	p	Pairwise Comparison
	1793	3709	5614	6873	2647	20,636			11,609	17,130	22,626	19,502	3436	74,303		
Breakfast 5:30 to 10:00	251.8 (4.5)	320.3 (3.5)	384.4 (2.9)	408.3 (2.6)	405.7 (4.2)	372.1 (1.5)	<0.0001	A < B < C < D = E	246.7 (1.7)	330.3 (1.6)	405.7 (1.5)	434.4 (1.6)	445.1 (3.9)	372.8 (0.8)	<0.0001	A < B < C < D = E
Mid-morning 10:00 to 12:00	104.8 (3.3)	110.6 (2.4)	102.3 (2.1)	69.2 (1.6)	51.0 (2.1)	86.4 (1.0)	<0.0001	E < D < C = A = B	103.1 (1.2)	106.5 (1.1)	98.7 (0.9)	80.4 (1.0)	59.2 (1.9)	94.6 (0.5)	<0.0001	E < D < C < A = B
Lunch 12:00 to 15:00	378.8 (5.2)	394.3 (3.7)	392.4 (3.0)	374.0 (2.4)	346.4 (3.6)	379.5 (1.5)	<0.0001	D < B, D < C; E < A, B, C, D	334.4 (1.8)	354.6 (1.5)	341.4 (1.3)	316.7 (1.3)	291.5 (3.0)	334.6 (0.7)	<0.0001	E < D < A < C < B
Snack 15:00 to 19:00	178.3 (4.9)	173.8 (3.4)	174.1 (2.9)	151.5 (2.3)	127.9 (3.1)	161.0 (1.4)	<0.0001	E < D < A = B = C	162.0 (1.6)	184.8 (1.5)	189.6 (1.3)	181.5 (1.3)	160.2 (2.9)	180.7 (0.7)	<0.0001	A = E < B = C = D
Dinner 19:00 to 22:00	419.5 (6.0)	429.2 (4.3)	403.6 (3.2)	349.8 (2.6)	289.2 (3.6)	377.0 (1.6)	<0.0001	E < D < C = A; C, D, E < B	350.9 (2.0)	366.9 (1.7)	337.6 (1.4)	294.7 (1.4)	253.4 (3.0)	331.3 (0.8)	<0.0001	E < D < C < A < B
Night 22:00 to 5:30	107.3 (4.6)	95.2 (2.8)	75.2 (1.9)	53.6 (1.4)	42.4 (1.9)	70.2 (1.0)	<0.0001	E < D < C < B < A	63.3 (1.2)	64.0 (1.0)	53.5 (0.8)	54.9 (0.8)	52.0 (1.8)	57.8 (0.4)	<0.0001	C < A, C < B, D < A; D < B, E < A, E < B

Interestingly, we found significant positive correlations between total water intake and a consumption of beverages outside meal times, and significant negative correlations with consumption during meal times (Figure 4).

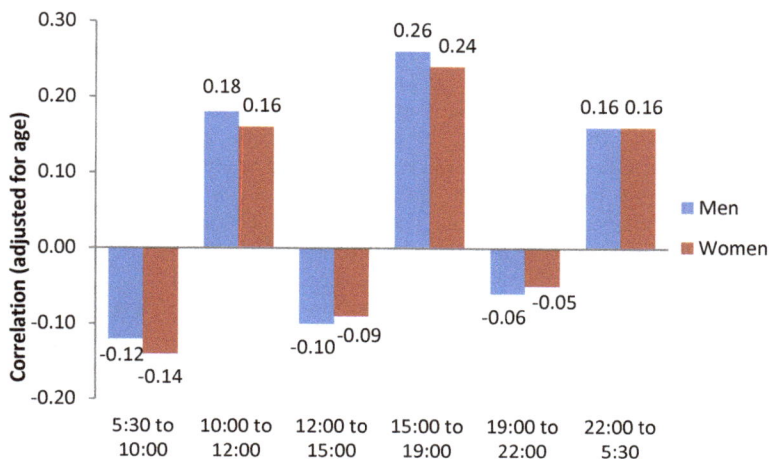

Figure 4. Partial correlations between TWI and beverage consumption in each period, by gender, adjusted for age. Beverage consumption in each period expressed as a percentage of total consumption over 24 h.

4. Discussion

In this population, TWI was in line with EFSA AI reference values [6]. We found that 61.9% of the TWI came from beverages and 38.1% came from food. The part of the water intake coming from food in our population was then higher than the EFSA estimation for European countries (70%–80% provided by the beverages and 20%–30% coming from food). Differences in percentage of TWI from food were also found in other countries, for example in Ireland (33%) [19] or in China (40%) [20], depending on dietary patterns. Importance of food in TWI should then not be neglected, especially in elderly people, for which we found that the water intake coming from food was higher than in the other age groups.

Similarly to the results found in other previous studies conducted on French adults, water was the first contributor to beverage consumption for both men and women (48.2% for women and 46.6% for men). Water represented 43%–46% of beverage consumption in Bellisle et al. [21], and 49% in Guelinckx et al. [22]. The second contributor was hot beverages (respectively 30.2% and 23.5% for women and men). Those values are comparable to the ones found in Bellisle et al. (20%) and Guelinckx et al. (25%).

The energy impact of caloric soft drinks was small in our population. For the whole sample, caloric soft drinks contributed only 1% of the total kcal. The contribution of caloric soft drinks to energetic intakes was almost equal for men and women. The elderly population had a consumption representing less than 1% of the EI. However, this consumption was higher in the youngest group (18–25 years) in which it represented 2.2% of the total kcal (data not shown). The impact of caloric soft drink consumption on weight gain [23–26], obesity [27–29] and metabolic disorders [30–33] has been shown in several studies. Large differences between countries have been observed [22] and it was interesting to investigate it in a large population of young French adults. Our results are comparable to those found previously in another smaller French population [21]. In our population, the consumption of caloric soft drinks is globally low. However, for the younger subjects, the consumption of caloric soft drinks was much higher, and this fact may be a problem in the future as excessive consumption of sugary beverages has been linked with the increasing weight of the population [34–36].

Our results suggest that in our population, alcoholic drinks had a higher impact on the total energy intake than caloric soft drinks. Alcoholic drinks contributed to 3.3% of the total energy intake (5.2% for men and 2.7% for women). The consumption of alcohol increased with age. However, the consumption of alcohol was mainly concentrated during the week-end days, which may reflect a festive consumption rather than a regular consumption.

Although we found statistically significant differences in TWI according to the seasonality, the difference of 120 g/day for men and 80 g/day for women between water intakes during winter and summer was limited compared to results of previous studies in other European countries [37,38]. However, this result can be explained by the temperate climate in France, with few extreme temperatures. In a Mediterranean country such as Greece [37], a 40% increase in total water intakes was found between winter and summer. In another study with subjects from Germany, Spain and Greece [38], the difference was 200 g/day between winter and summer.

In regard to the day of the week, it was found that the total amount of beverages consumed was higher on Sundays and Saturdays for both men and women, due to a higher consumption of alcoholic drinks during the week end. However, the higher beverages intake during the week-end may not be associated with a better hydration status due to the diuretic effect of alcohol. It should be interesting to have information from hydration biomarkers, and to study their evolution throughout the week.

We found that, in our study population, beverage consumption was concentrated during the meal times. However, in the elderly population, a higher intake was observed during breakfast compared to lunch and dinner. An original result was to find a positive correlation between TWI and consumption of beverages outside meal times. On the contrary, we found a negative correlation with consumption during meal times, especially breakfast. This negative correlation for breakfast could be due to elderly people having a lower daily water intake but a higher water intake during breakfast. This correlation pattern between TWI and time indicates that people with a higher water intake tend to consume beverages regularly throughout the day and not only concentrated during meal times. A major strength of this study is its reliance on the use of a very large population of French adults (Nutrinet-Santé study). The intakes of both food and beverages were estimated precisely using three 24-h records, randomly distributed within a two-week period, including two weekdays and one weekend day. However, our study also suffers from some limitations. For example, even if we assessed the level of physical activity using IPAQ questionnaire at baseline, the actual physical activity level during the day of the 24-h dietary records is unknown. We cannot then evaluate the impact of the physical activity level on TWI. Moreover, caution is also needed when generalizing our results, since the NutriNet-Santé study is a long-term cohort focusing on nutrition and participants are recruited on a voluntary basis, implying that they might have increased health consciousness and interest in nutritional issues as well as a healthier lifestyle.

5. Conclusions

The present study gives an overview of the characteristics of water intake in a large population of French adults. TWI was found to be globally in line with public health recommendations. However, we found significant differences in beverage consumption across age groups and seasons. Further research should be directed towards examining the association between hydration status and chronic diseases in different populations to determine the optimal level of water intake. These data will be necessary in order to formulate public health recommendations.

Author Contributions: N.A. and F.S. analysed the data. F.S. wrote the manuscript. N.D.P., R.G., C.B. and P.G. provided continuous scientific advice for the study and for the interpretation of results. These authors also critically reviewed the manuscript. All authors approved the final version of the manuscript.

Conflicts of Interest: The authors declare no conflict of interest.

References

1. Maughan, R.J. Impact of mild dehydration on wellness and on exercise performance. *Eur. J. Clin. Nutr.* **2003**, *57* (Suppl. S2), S19–S23. [CrossRef] [PubMed]
2. Watson, P.; Whale, A.; Mears, S.A.; Reyner, L.A.; Maughan, R.J. Mild hypohydration increases the frequency of driver errors during a prolonged, monotonous driving task. *Physiol. Behav.* **2015**, *147*, 313–318. [CrossRef] [PubMed]
3. Ferry, M. Strategies for ensuring good hydration in the elderly. *Nutr. Rev.* **2005**, *63*, S22–S29. [CrossRef] [PubMed]
4. Manz, F.; Wentz, A. The importance of good hydration for the prevention of chronic diseases. *Nutr. Rev.* **2005**, *63*, S2–S5. [CrossRef] [PubMed]
5. Popkin, B.M.; D'Anci, K.E.; Rosenberg, I.H. Water, hydration, and health. *Nutr. Rev.* **2010**, *68*, 439–458. [CrossRef] [PubMed]
6. Panel on Dietetic Products, Nutrition and Allergies. Scientific Opinion on Dietary reference values for Water. *EFSA J.* **2010**, *8*, 1459–1507.
7. Institute of Medicine (Panel on Dietary Reference Intakes for Electrolytes and Water). *Dietary Reference Intakes for Water, Potassium, Sodium, Chloride and Sulfate*; National Academies Press: Washington, DC, USA, 2005.
8. McKiernan, F.; Houchins, J.A.; Mattes, R.D. Relationships between human thirst, hunger, drinking, and feeding. *Physiol. Behav.* **2008**, *94*, 700–708. [CrossRef] [PubMed]
9. Perrier, E.; Demazieres, A.; Girard, N.; Pross, N.; Osbild, D.; Metzger, D.; Guelinckx, I.; Klein, A. Circadian variation and responsiveness of hydration biomarkers to changes in daily water intake. *Eur. J. Appl. Physiol.* **2013**, *113*, 2143–2151. [CrossRef] [PubMed]
10. Hercberg, S.; Castetbon, K.; Czernichow, S.; Malon, A.; Mejean, C.; Kesse, E.; Touvier, M.; Galan, P. The Nutrinet-Sante Study: A web-based prospective study on the relationship between nutrition and health and determinants of dietary patterns and nutritional status. *BMC. Public Health* **2010**, *10*, 242. [CrossRef] [PubMed]
11. Craig, C.L.; Marshall, A.L.; Sjostrom, M.; Bauman, A.E.; Booth, M.L.; Ainsworth, B.E.; Pratt, M.; Ekelund, U.; Yngve, A.; Sallis, J.F.; et al. International physical activity questionnaire: 12-country reliability and validity. *Med. Sci. Sports Exerc.* **2003**, *35*, 1381–1395. [CrossRef] [PubMed]
12. Hagstromer, M.; Oja, P.; Sjostrom, M. The International Physical Activity Questionnaire (IPAQ): A study of concurrent and construct validity. *Public Health Nutr.* **2006**, *9*, 755–762. [CrossRef] [PubMed]
13. Hallal, P.C.; Victora, C.G. Reliability and validity of the International Physical Activity Questionnaire (IPAQ). *Med. Sci. Sports Exerc.* **2004**, *36*, 556. [CrossRef] [PubMed]
14. Black, A.E. Critical evaluation of energy intake using the Goldberg cut-off for energy intake: Basal metabolic rate. A practical guide to its calculation, use and limitations. *Int. J. Obes. Relat. Metab. Disord.* **2000**, *24*, 1119–1130. [CrossRef] [PubMed]
15. Schofield, W.N. Predicting basal metabolic rate, new standards and review of previous work. *Hum. Nutr. Clin. Nutr.* **1985**, *39* (Suppl. S1), 5–41. [PubMed]
16. Willet, W. *Nutritional Epidemiology*; Issues in Analysis and Presentation of Dietary Data; Oxford University Press: New York, NY, USA, 1998.
17. Le Moullec, N.; Deheeger, M.; Preziosi, P. Validation du manuel photos utilisé pour l'enquête alimentaire de l'étude SU.VI.MAX. *Cahier de Nutrition Diététique* **2013**, *31*, 158–164. (In French)
18. Etude Nutrinet-Santé. *Table de Composition des Aliments de L'étude Nutrinet-Santé*; Economica: Paris, France, 2013. (In French)
19. O'Connor, L.; Walton, J.; Flynn, A. Water intakes and dietary sources of a nationally representative sample of Irish adults. *J. Hum. Nutr. Diet.* **2014**, *27*, 550–556. [CrossRef] [PubMed]
20. Ma, G.; Zuo, J.; Zhang, Q.; Chen, Z.; Hu, X. Water intake and its influencing factors of adults in one district of Shenzhen. *Acta Nutr. Sin.* **2011**, *33*, 253–257.
21. Bellisle, F.; Thorton, S.; Hébel, P.; Denizeau, M.; Tahiri, M. A study of fluid intake from beverages in a sample of healthy French children, adolescents and adults. *Eur. J. Clin. Nutr.* **2010**, *3*, 350–355. [CrossRef] [PubMed]
22. Guelinckx, I.; Ferreira-Pego, C.; Moreno, L.A.; Kavouras, S.A.; Gandy, J.; Martinez, H.; Bardosono, S.; Abdollahi, M.; Nasseri, E.; Jarosz, A.; et al. Intake of water and different beverages in adults across 13 countries. *Eur. J. Nutr.* **2015**, *54* (Suppl. S2), 45–55. [CrossRef] [PubMed]

23. Johnson, R.K. Children gain less weight and accumulate less fat when sugar-free, non-caloric beverages are substituted for sugar-sweetened beverages. *Evid. Based Med.* **2013**, *18*, 185–186. [CrossRef] [PubMed]

24. Malik, V.S.; Pan, A.; Willett, W.C.; Hu, F.B. Sugar-sweetened beverages and weight gain in children and adults: A systematic review and meta-analysis. *Am. J. Clin. Nutr.* **2013**, *98*, 1084–1102. [CrossRef] [PubMed]

25. Trumbo, P.R.; Rivers, C.R. Systematic review of the evidence for an association between sugar-sweetened beverage consumption and risk of obesity. *Nutr. Rev.* **2014**, *72*, 566–574. [CrossRef] [PubMed]

26. Vartanian, L.R.; Schwartz, M.B.; Brownell, K.D. Effects of soft drink consumption on nutrition and health: A systematic review and meta-analysis. *Am. J. Public Health* **2007**, *97*, 667–675. [CrossRef] [PubMed]

27. Pan, A.; Malik, V.S.; Hao, T.; Willett, W.C.; Mozaffarian, D.; Hu, F.B. Changes in water and beverage intake and long-term weight changes: Results from three prospective cohort studies. *Int. J. Obes.* **2013**, *37*, 1378–1385. [CrossRef] [PubMed]

28. Peters, J.C.; Wyatt, H.R.; Foster, G.D.; Pan, Z.; Wojtanowski, A.C.; Vander Veur, S.S.; Herring, S.J.; Brill, C.; Hill, J.O. The effects of water and non-nutritive sweetened beverages on weight loss during a 12-week weight loss treatment program. *Obesity* **2014**, *22*, 1415–1421. [CrossRef] [PubMed]

29. Tate, D.F.; Turner-McGrievy, G.; Lyons, E.; Stevens, J.; Erickson, K.; Polzien, K.; Diamond, M.; Wang, X.; Popkin, B. Replacing caloric beverages with water or diet beverages for weight loss in adults: Main results of the Choose Healthy Options Consciously Everyday (CHOICE) randomized clinical trial. *Am. J. Clin. Nutr.* **2012**, *95*, 555–563. [CrossRef] [PubMed]

30. Barrio-Lopez, M.T.; Martinez-Gonzalez, M.A.; Fernandez-Montero, A.; Beunza, J.J.; Zazpe, I.; Bes-Rastrollo, M. Prospective study of changes in sugar-sweetened beverage consumption and the incidence of the metabolic syndrome and its components: The SUN cohort. *Br. J. Nutr.* **2013**, *110*, 1722–1731. [CrossRef] [PubMed]

31. Denova-Gutierrez, E.; Talavera, J.O.; Huitron-Bravo, G.; Mendez-Hernandez, P.; Salmeron, J. Sweetened beverage consumption and increased risk of metabolic syndrome in Mexican adults. *Public Health Nutr.* **2010**, *13*, 835–842. [CrossRef] [PubMed]

32. Malik, V.S.; Popkin, B.M.; Bray, G.A.; Despres, J.P.; Willett, W.C.; Hu, F.B. Sugar-sweetened beverages and risk of metabolic syndrome and type 2 diabetes: A meta-analysis. *Diabetes Care* **2010**, *33*, 2477–2483. [CrossRef] [PubMed]

33. Yoo, S.; Nicklas, T.; Baranowski, T.; Zakeri, I.F.; Yang, S.J.; Srinivasan, S.R.; Berenson, G.S. Comparison of dietary intakes associated with metabolic syndrome risk factors in young adults: The Bogalusa Heart Study. *Am. J. Clin. Nutr.* **2004**, *80*, 841–848. [PubMed]

34. Forshee, R.A.; Anderson, P.A.; Storey, M.L. Sugar-sweetened beverages and body mass index in children and adolescents: A meta-analysis. *Am. J. Clin. Nutr.* **2008**, *87*, 1662–1671. [PubMed]

35. Hu, F.B.; Malik, V.S. Sugar-sweetened beverages and risk of obesity and type 2 diabetes: Epidemiologic evidence. *Physiol. Behav.* **2010**, *100*, 47–54. [CrossRef] [PubMed]

36. Malik, V.S.; Schulze, M.B.; Hu, F.B. Intake of sugar-sweetened beverages and weight gain: A systematic review. *Am. J. Clin. Nutr.* **2006**, *84*, 274–288. [PubMed]

37. Malisova, O.; Bountziouka, V.; Panagiotakos, D.B.; Zampelas, A.; Kapsokefalou, M. Evaluation of seasonality on total water intake, water loss and water balance in the general population in Greece. *J. Hum. Nutr. Diet.* **2013**, *26* (Suppl. S1), 90–96. [CrossRef] [PubMed]

38. Malisova, O.; Athanasatou, A.; Pepa, A.; Husemann, M.; Domnik, K.; Braun, H.; Mora-Rodriguez, R.; Ortega, J.F.; Fernandez-Elias, V.E.; Kapsokefalou, M. Water Intake and Hydration Indices in Healthy European Adults: The European Hydration Research Study (EHRS). *Nutrients* **2016**, *8*. [CrossRef] [PubMed]

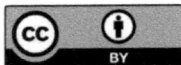

nutrients

MDPI

Article

Beverage Consumption Habits in Italian Population: Association with Total Water Intake and Energy Intake

Lorenza Mistura *, Laura D'Addezio and Aida Turrini

CREA—Consiglio per la ricerca in agricoltura e l'analisi dell'economia agraria—Centro Alimenti e Nutrizione, Via Ardeatina 546, Rome 00178, Italy; laura.daddezio@crea.gov.it (L.D.); aida.turrini@crea.gov.it (A.T.)
* Correspondence: lorenza.mistura@crea.gov.it; Tel.: +39-0651-494-571

Received: 31 July 2016; Accepted: 19 October 2016; Published: 26 October 2016

Abstract: Background: The aim of this study was to investigate total water intake (TWI) from water, beverages and foods among Italian adults and the elderly. Methods: Data of 2607 adults and the elderly, aged 18–75 years from the last national food consumption survey, INRAN-SCAI 2005-06, were used to evaluate the TWI. The INRAN-SCAI 2005-06 survey was conducted on a representative sample of 3323 individuals aged 0.1 to 97.7 years. A 3-day semi-structured diary was used for participants to record the consumption of all foods, beverages and nutritional supplements. Results: On average, TWI was 1.8 L for men and 1.7 L for women. More than 75% of women and 90% of men did not comply with the European Food Safety Authority (EFSA) Adequate Intake. The contribution of beverages to the total energy intake (EI) was 6% for the total sample. Water was the most consumed beverage, followed by alcoholic beverages for men and hot beverages for women. Conclusion: According to the present results, adults and elderly Italians do not reach the adequate intake for water as suggested by the EFSA and by the national reference level of nutrient and energy intake. Data on water consumption should also be analyzed in single socio-demographic groups in order to identify sub-groups of the population that need more attention and to plan more targeted interventions.

Keywords: total water intake; energy intake; beverages

1. Introduction

Total water intake (TWI) is essential for human health and life since it balances losses and assures adequate hydration of body tissues [1]. It is calculated that, of the total water intake consumed in a typical western diet, 20%–30% comes from food, and 70%–80% comes from beverages, but this may vary greatly among individuals depending on the diet they choose [2]. Current knowledge on water intake and its importance for the prevention of nutrition-based diseases is presented by Popkin [3]. Although good hydration is associated with reduction in urinary tract infections, hypertension, fatal coronary heart disease, various thromboembolis and cerebral infarct, all these results are not confirmed by clinical trials [3].

The role played by beverages in providing water in the diet has been recognised by international organizations such as the International Life Science Institute [4] and the European Food Safety Authority (EFSA) [2].

A recent document published by the World Federation of Hydrotherapy and Climatotherapy [5], attested and brought to the global attention the importance of water for certain body functions and the crucial role of appropriate hydration for overall health. Moreover, it represented a way to promote the inclusion of appropriate hydration as one of the goals of national and international health policies.

Drinking water during the day is of special importance for children and the elderly, the population groups that are vulnerable to dehydration. The elderly have been shown to have a higher risk of developing dehydration than younger adults. Modifications in water metabolism with aging and fluid imbalance in the frail elderly are the main factors to consider in the prevention of dehydration [6].

The EFSA Scientific Opinion on Dietary Reference Values for Water establishes that the dietary reference intake values for water should include water from drinking water (tap or bottled), all kinds of beverages, and from food moisture. The definition of adequate intakes (AI) proposed by the EFSA should be based both on observed intakes and on considerations of achievable or desirable urine osmolarity. Adequate total water intakes for females would have to be 2.0 L/day (P95 3.1 L) and for males 2.5 L/day (P95 4.0 L). The EFSA defines the same adequate intakes for the elderly as for adults [2].

The Italian Society of Human Nutrition has recently published the new reference values of adequate intake of water for the Italian population that do not vary from those defined by the EFSA [7].

Data on plain water and beverages intake are generally collected in national surveys. In order to study the patterns of beverage consumption of a population, it is not sufficient to report the average daily consumption of each beverage category. It is also essential to identify which variety of beverages are consumed and their contribution to total energy intake. In addition, the contribution of each beverage type to TWI permits an evaluation of the adequacy of drinking habits.

Methods adopted in dietary surveys differ from each other, and no standard method for the evaluation of water intake has so far been adopted [8]. This makes it difficult to compare results across and within countries.

In Italy, there are no recent studies focused on the TWI of the adult and elderly population. Recent published research regarded the consumption of energy drinks and alcohol among adolescents [9], of alcohol among adult and elderly men [10], and of caloric beverages among children and adolescents [11].

The present study aimed to investigate the TWI from plain water, beverages and foods and their contribution to overall water and energy intakes, among Italian adults and the elderly, by age group and gender. This analysis used dietary data from the INRAN-SCAI 2005-06 Study [12]. In addition, actual patterns of total daily water intake were compared with the AI recommended by the European Food Safety Authority.

2. Material and Methods

2.1. Study Population and Data Collection

The INRAN-SCAI 2005-06 survey was conducted on a representative sample of 1300 households randomly selected and stratified into the four main geographical areas of Italy (North-West, North-East, Centre, South and Islands) between October 2005 and December 2006. In total, 3323 (1501 males and 1822 females) individuals participated in the food survey, aged 0.1 to 97.7 years. A 3-day semi-structured diary was used. It is a mix of a specific format and free text where participants are able to record the consumption of all foods and beverages by meals, and nutritional supplements.

The food survey was conducted by a team of thirty well trained field workers. They met each subject three times during the survey, and carefully checked the food diaries and made specific questions to reduce errors such as misreporting and omissions (e.g., they asked if the participants took medicine and to remember to record the glass of water drunk for this purpose). In addition, to help the participants in recording the food and beverages consumed, they were given a picture booklet of the different standard portions for food and beverages.

In order to capture all the seasonal differences in intake, the sampled households were proportionally distributed among seasons (excluding Christmas and Easter periods): 25% in autumn, 25% in winter, 26% in spring and 24% in summer. In addition, the survey calendar was scheduled in order to take an adequate proportion of weekdays and weekend days at group level (78% and 22%).

Detailed information about the INRAN SCAI 2005-06 survey design, procedures, and methodologies can be found in the previous published papers [12,13].

For the present study, adults in the age range 18–75 years (*n* = 2607) were considered.

Data on nutrients intake, including water, were obtained using the updated version of the national food composition database [13]. In the case of foods and beverages that were fortified or enriched with one or more essential nutrients (including functional foods and special purpose foods), the nutrient content was retrieved at brand level from nutritional labels.

2.2. Plain Water and Beverages Consumption

Beverages were classified into eight categories: Hot beverages, including barley, coffee, tea and infusions; Milk and milk-based beverages; Fruit and vegetable juices; Caloric soft drinks, including soda and energy drinks and other sport drinks; Diet soft drinks, including beverages with sweeteners and without sugars; Alcoholic beverages (wine, beer and spirits); Water (tap and bottled); Other non-alcoholic beverages (soy based beverages and milk rice). Water added to recipes is included in the calculation of water coming from food.

2.3. Statistical Analyses

The 3-day mean of the total water intake (TWI) from the food and beverages categories previously described was evaluated for each subject. Mean values and standard errors of the food and beverages intakes were calculated for the 18–75 years old population and the sub-groups defined by gender and age classes (18–64 years and 65–75 years). Energy intake from beverage and food sources was also calculated.

The variety of beverage score was calculated as the average of the eight beverage categories on the three survey days.

To investigate the daily trend of the beverages consumption, the eating occasions were aggregated into main meals (breakfast, lunch and dinner) and snacks (morning, afternoon, after dinner).

The EFSA recommendations of water intake for each age and gender group were used to calculate the total shortfall in water consumption, and the proportion of adults who met or failed to meet the AI of water per day.

The Student's *t*-test was applied to check whether there were differences in mean consumption of the TWI, water from food, water from beverages and total beverages consumption across subgroups of subjects defined by age and gender. The Mann–Whitney Test was performed for the eight beverages categories because their intakes were non-normally distributed. A two-sided p value of 0.05 was set to denote statistical significance.

All analyses were performed using the Statistical Analysis System computer software package (SAS package version 9.01; SAS Institute Inc., Cary, NC, USA).

3. Results

The total number of adults and elderly enrolled in this survey was 2607. Women represent 54% of the sample and the elderly, in the age class 65–75 years, represent 11% for both genders. The overweight/obesity rate is 49.7% and 38.4% for males and females, respectively.

Total water intake (TWI) from all sources averages 1768.7 g/day for males and 1667.3 g/day for females (Figure 1).

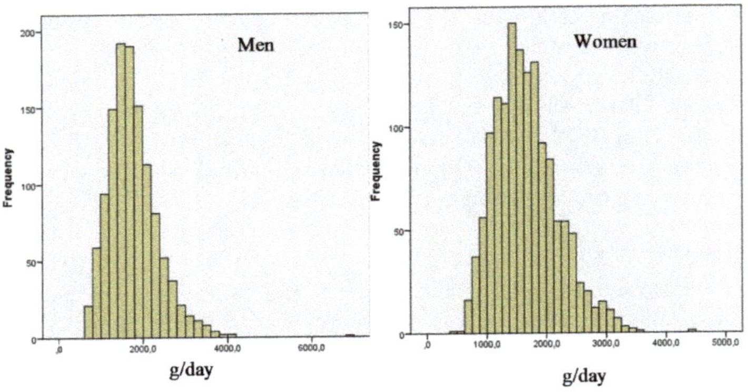

Figure 1. Frequency distribution of total water intake (g/day) over 3 days, by gender.

Beverages account for 56% of total water and 45% of the total weight of food and drink consumed (data not shown). Mean beverage consumption is 956 g/day (1015 g/day among men, 953 g/day among women). Water as a beverage is consumed by 97% of men and 99% of women and hot beverages are consumed by 95% in both genders, Figure 2.

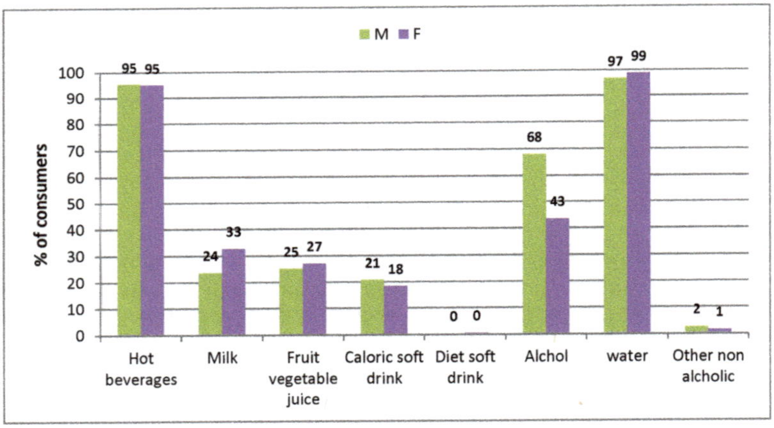

Figure 2. Popularity of beverages (% consuming over 3 days).

Among men, alcoholic drinks are the second beverage category, contributing 8.9% to the TWI with 68% of consumers, followed by milk, fruit and vegetable juices and caloric soft drinks with similar percentages of consumers (25%, 24% and 21% respectively). Diet soft drinks and other non-alcoholic beverages are consumed by very few subjects of both genders. Alcoholic beverages are the third most consumed beverage category by women (43%), with a contribution of 3.4% on the TWI. The main sources of TWI are water for both sexes followed by hot beverages in females and alcoholic beverages in males (Table 1).

Mean total energy intake (EI) is 2137 kcal/day (SE 12.2). The contribution to the total EI from beverages is 6%. Alcoholic beverages are also the category with the greatest contribution to total energy intake, 4.5% in males and 1.9% in females. Caloric soft drinks contribute only 0.4% to total energy intake for the total sample (Table 1).

Table 1. Contribution of food and beverages to total water and energy intake.

		Contribution to Water Intake (g/Day)			Contribution to Energy Intake (kcal/Day)		
		Male	Female	Total	Male	Female	Total
All food and drink	Mean (SE) *	1768 16.9	1668 14.0	1714 11.0	2381 18.5	1931 14.0	2138 12.2
Food only	%	44% 0.3%	44% 0.3%	45% 0.2%	93% 0.1%	95% 0.1%	94% 0.10%
Beverages only	%	56% 0.3%	56% 0.3%	56% 0.2%	7% 0.1%	5% 0.1%	6% 0.1%
Hot beverages	%	8% 0.2%	8% 0.2%	8% 0.1%	0% 0%	0% 0%	0% 0%
Milk	%	2% 0.1%	3% 0.1%	2% 0.1%	1% 0.1%	1% 0.1%	1% 0%
Fruit and vegetable juice	%	1% 0.1%	1% 0.1%	1% 0.1%	1% 0.0%	1% 0.0%	1% 0.0%
Caloric soft drink	%	2% 0.1%	1% 0.1%	1% 0.1%	1% 0.0%	0% 0.0%	0% 0.0%
Diet soft drink	%	0.0% 0.0%	0.0% 0.0%	0.0% 0.0%	-	-	-
Alcoholic Beverages	%	9% 0.3%	3% 0.2%	6% 0.2%	5% 0.1%	2% 0.1%	3% 0.1%
Water	%	33% 0.4%	38% 0.4%	35% 0.3%	-	-	-
Other non alcoholic beverages	%	0% 0.0%	0% 0.0%	0% 0.0%	0% 0.0%	0% 0.0%	0% 0.0%

* SE = standard error.

Table 2 presents the TWI, water intake from food and beverages, and the consumption of beverage categories. In Figure 3 the same variables are analysed by age classes in more detail. In general, water from beverages decreases with the increase of the age and the age class; 18–35 presents a significantly higher water intake from beverages than all the other classes in both genders ($p < 0.001$). Water from food significantly increases with age in both genders, and also in this case the younger age class has significantly lower intake than the others in both genders.

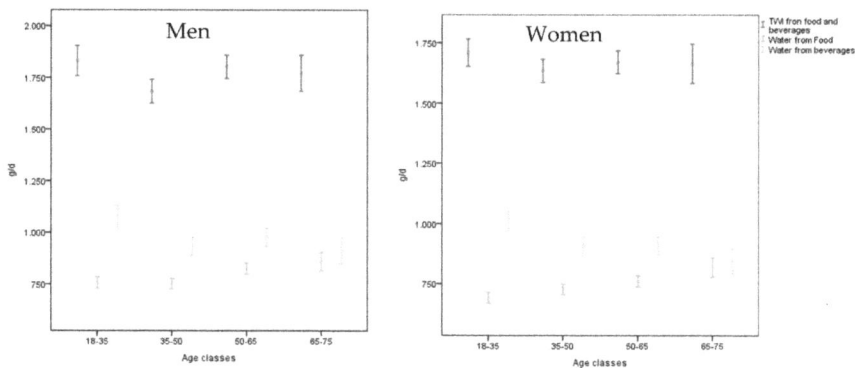

Figure 3. Mean and Confidence Interval (CI) of the Total Water Intake (TWI) from food and beverages, water from food and water from beverages by age classes and gender.

Table 2. Total water intake, water from food and beverages and beverage consumption (g/day), by gender and age group.

		Male			Female		
		18–64 (*n* = 1068)	65–75 (*n* = 134)	*p*	18–64 (*n* = 1245)	65–75 (*n* = 160)	*p*
TWI from food and beverages	Mean (SE) CI	1768 (18.2) 1732.7–1804.0	1771 (44.0) 1683.8–1857.8	n.s. *	1669 (15.0) 1639.1–1697.9	1663 (41.1) 1582.0–1744.5	n.s. *
Water from food	Mean (SE) CI	778 (7.9) 762.6–793.5	856 (22.2) 813.6–901.5	0.001 *	727 (6.6) 713.8–739.9	817 (20.6) 776.3–857.6	0.000 *
Water from beverages	Mean (SE) CI	990 (14.5) 961.7–1018.8	913 (33.2) 847.5–979.0	n.s. *	942 (12) 918.1–965.2	846 (28.6) 789.8–902.8	0.007 *
Total beverages consumption	Mean (SE) CI	1024 (14.9) 995.1–1053.5	945 (33.8) 878.4–1012.0	n.s. *	965 (12.1) 940.7–988.4	867 (29.1) 810.2–925.0	0.006 *
Hot beverages	Mean (SE)	135 (3.3)	139 (13.8)	n.s. §	138 (3.2)	129 (9)	n.s. §
Milk	Mean (SE)	38 (2.8)	39 (6.7)	n.s. §	49 (2.4)	53 (7.4)	n.s. §
Fruit vegetable juice	Mean (SE)	27 (2.3)	16 (4.8)	0.003 §	28 (1.9)	23 (4.3)	n.s. §
Caloric soft drink	Mean (SE)	33.(2.7)	7 (2.5)	0.000 §	22 (1.7)	9 (2.8)	0.000 §
Diet soft drink	Mean (SE)	1 (0.8)	0 (0.0)	n.s §	1 (0.3)	0 (0.0)	n.s. §
Alcoholic Beverages	Mean (SE)	163 (6.0)	184 (15.1)	n.s. §	58 (2.7)	66 (8.3)	n.s. §
Water	Mean (SE)	624 (12.9)	559 (31.9)	n.s. §	667 (11.1)	588 (26.4)	0.022 §
Other non alcoholic	Mean (SE)	1 (0.9)	1 (0.5)	n.s. §	2 (0.5)	0 (0.3)	n.s. §

* *t*-test comparison with a significant level 0.05; § U of the Mann–Whitney test comparison with a significant level 0.05; CI, Confidence Interval.

Among males, the mean intake of caloric soft drink and fruit and vegetable juice are significantly different by age class, even if there is a tendency to decline also in the other categories, except for alcoholic and hot beverages. Among females, the elderly drink significantly less and consume less water and caloric soft drinks than the younger participants.

The TWI correlated very highly with the weight of beverages and water from beverages ($r = 0.90$) and correlated more weakly with food weight ($r = 0.65$). Alcoholic drinks ($r = 0.28$), fruit and vegetable juice ($r = 0.17$) and caloric soft drinks ($r = 0.15$) have the highest correlation with energy intake. The mean variety score is 1.08, suggesting that adults and the elderly do not consume more than one type of beverage during the 3 days of the survey, out of the eight different beverage categories. There is a positive correlation with the TWI ($r = 0.21$) and energy intake ($r = 0.30$) (data not shown in table).

Beverage consumption has two peaks, for both gender and age classes, at lunch and dinner time. The younger males drink significantly more than older males in the evening during a nighttime snack, and the older females drink significantly less during lunch and dinner.

Finally, subjects who fulfill the EFSA AI recommendation of 2.5 L and 2.0 L are classified as criterion 1. Those who have the ratio of water/energy intake >1.0 are included as criterion 2 (it is considered as a value of 1 g of water per 1 kcal of energy intake). Those who meet both definitions (1 and 2) are classified as criterion 3. Following this analysis, the results show that more than 74% of women, and 90% of men do not comply the AI recommendation of consumption of water, as shown in Table 3.

Table 3. Combined classification for the total water intake (TWI) following established criteria.

Criteria Classification	Men (*n* = 1202)	Women (*n* = 1405)
Criterion 1: % (*n*)	10.6 (127)	23.9 (336)
Criterion 2: % (*n*)	13.3 (160)	27.0 (379)
Criterion 3 (1 and 2): % (*n*)	5.5 (66)	14.9 (210)

EFSA: European Food Safety Authority. (1) Criterion 1: TWI >2.5 L men, >2 L women (aged 14 to 75 years); (2) Criterion 2: Ratio of total water intake and total energy >1; (3) Criterion 3: Both criteria 1 and 2.

4. Discussion

This study presented an analysis of total water intake from all food and beverages conducted on a representative sample of the Italian population aged 18–75 years from the INRAN-SCAI survey. Men had a higher TWI than women of both food and beverages, however, neither group met the EFSA recommended adequate intake for adult men (2.5 L) and women (2 L).

Although AI is used as a goal for individual water intake, water needs may vary a lot due to inter-individual variation [14]. When evaluating water intakes at individual level, several additional factors need to be considered which can influence water needs: physical activity; environmental factors, such as temperature; type of work; and other dietary factors, such as sodium intake.

Of all dietary sources of water, food was the leading one. Water content of food categories varies from 90% in fruit and vegetables to less than 5% of savoury snacks and confectionary [13].

Increasing the consumption of foods rich in water may have a positive effect both on hydration status and on dietary quality, although the effect of dietary water on hydration status is very poorly investigated [15].

The second main source of dietary water of Italian adults was plain water. Drinking plain water, tap or bottled, instead of any other beverage, permits the fulfillment of hydration requirements without providing energy, but providing small amounts of calcium, sodium and magnesium. Although the TWI can be increased in many ways, the most effective would be to increase the consumption of plain water [16]. Alcoholic beverages were the second and third beverage category most consumed by males and females respectively, with a high contribution to energy intake in men. Since the water content of alcoholic beverages can sensibly vary according to the type of beverage (for example, spirits vs. beer), the effect of their consumption on water balance varies accordingly, and increasing the strength and amount of drinks can result in a loss of fluid intake, rather than an increase [15].

Similar studies on TWI were conducted in France [17], in the United States [18], in Britain [19], and more recently in Spain [8] where the values for the TWI for both genders were very close to our results—in the study conducted in Spain, 68% of the TWI came from beverages, as opposed to 56% in Italy, and consequently the contribution of all beverages to energy intake was higher (12.2 vs. 5.6%). Like in Italy, in Spain the water intake from food increased with age and the water from beverages decreased; this trend was consistent with the recent study on vulnerability to dehydration of older people [20]. In the United States the contribution of beverages to energy intake was quite higher than in Italy, going to 22% among the 20–50 years old age group, and 14% among the ≥71 years old age group [18].

The consumption of caloric soft drink was higher for younger age classes (40.8 g/day 18–35 age class) and decreased with age (6.8 g/day 65–75 age class) which, compared to the Spanish study, is very low (96.2 g/day for all samples). Consequently, the contribution to energy intake is also very low (0.4%) when compared to the Spanish [8] results (6.1%), although this data also included children and adolescents. The US results were 5.7% for 20–50 year olds, 3.5% for 51–70 year olds and 2.1% for the elderly.

According to these results, beverages including plain water were consumed only during meals, and this may suggest an underreporting, especially of plain water drunk outside the meals. This is probably due to the survey tool in which the participants had to report the water consumption during meals, and snacks between meals, and the glass of water drunk out of the standard meals may have not always been recorded. The presence of a specific question about the water consumption could help the participants to record all water drinking occasions, even those not linked to the meals. Even regarding the consumption of alcoholic beverages, an underestimation in recording the consumption occasions is likely to occur because of the belief, due to cultural reasons, that drinking is regarded as socially undesirable [21,22].

The limitations of the food consumption survey, INRAN SCAI 2005-06, are addressed by Leclercq et al. [12]. Moreover, it is well known that the self-reported dietary record produces a general underreporting of consumption [23]. This was not taken into account in the consumption estimates.

5. Conclusions

The present analysis is, to our knowledge, the first attempt to explore total water intake among Italian adults and the elderly, based on data coming from the national dietary survey. According to the present results, adults and elderly Italians do not reach the adequate intake for water suggested by the EFSA and by the national reference level of nutrient and energy intake. Therefore, data on water consumption should also be analysed in single socio-demographic groups in order to identify sub-groups of population that need more attention and to plan more targeted interventions

Acknowledgments: The current analysis included in this paper was financially supported by a Grant from the European Hydration Institute to the Canarian Science Foundation and Technology Park of the University of Las Palmas de Gran Canaria.

Author Contributions: Lorenza Mistura performed the statistical analysis and the results; Laura D'Addezio contributed to the writing of the manuscript; Aida Turrini supervised the work and commented the final version of manuscript.

Conflicts of Interest: The authors declare no conflict of interest.

References

1. Jéquier, E.; Constant, F. Water as an essential nutrient: The physiological basis of hydration. *Eur. J. Clin. Nutr.* **2010**, *64*, 115–123.
2. European Food Safety Authority (EFSA) Panel on Dietetic Products, Nutrition and Allergies. Scientific opinion on dietary reference values for water. *EFSA J.* **2010**, *8*. [CrossRef]
3. Popkin, B.M.; D'Anci, K.E.; Rosenberg, I.H. Water, hydration, and health. *Nutr. Rev.* **2010**, *68*, 439–458. [CrossRef] [PubMed]
4. International Life Sciences Institute (ILSI). Scientific Consensus Statement regarding the Importance of Hydration and Total Water Intake for Health and Disease. *J. Am. Coll. Nutr.* **2007**, *26*, 529–623.
5. World Federation of Hydrotherapy and Climatotherapy (FEMTEC). *Water and Health. How Water Protects and Improves Health Overall. HYDROLIFE Definition of a Global Framework for Hydration.* Available online: https://www.hydrationlab.it/pdf/Consensus_Paper_eng.pdf (accessed on 26 September 2016).
6. Ferry, M. Strategies for ensuring good hydration in the elderly. *Nutr. Rev.* **2005**, *63*, S22–S29. [CrossRef] [PubMed]
7. Società Italiana di Nutrizione Umana (SINU). *LARN Livelli di Assunzione di Riferimento di Nutrienti ed Energia per la Popolazione Italiana IV Revisione*; Coordinamento editoriale SINU-INRAN: Milan, Italy, 2014.
8. Nissensohn, M.; Castro-Quezada, I.; Serra-Majem, L. Beverage and water intake of healthy adults in some European countries. *Int. J. Food Sci. Nutr.* **2013**, *64*, 801–805. [CrossRef] [PubMed]
9. Flotta, D.; Micò, R.; Nobile, C.G.A.; Pileggi, C.; Bianco, A.; Pavia, M. Consumption of energy drinks, alcohol, and alcohol-mixed drinks among Italian adolescents. *Alcohol. Clin. Exp. Res.* **2014**, *38*, 1654–1661. [CrossRef] [PubMed]
10. Della Valle, E.; Stranges, S.; Trevisan, M.; Krogh, V.; Fusconi, E.; Dorn, J.M.; Farinaro, E. Drinking habits and health in Northern Italian and American men. *Nutr. Metab. Cardiovasc. Dis.* **2009**, *19*, 115–122. [CrossRef] [PubMed]
11. Losasso, C.; Cappa, V.; Neuhouser, M.L.; Giaccone, V.; Andrighetto, I.; Ricci, A. Students' consumption of beverages and snacks at school and away from school: A case study in the North East of Italy. *Front. Nutr.* **2015**, *2*. [CrossRef] [PubMed]
12. Leclercq, C.; Arcella, D.; Piccinelli, R.; Sette, S.; Le Donne, C.; Turrini, A.; INRAN-SCAI 2005-06 Study Group. The Italian National Food Consumption Survey INRAN-SCAI 2005-06: Main results in terms of food consumption. *Public Health Nutr.* **2009**, *12*, 2504–2532. [CrossRef] [PubMed]
13. Sette, S.; Le Donne, C.; Piccinelli, R.; Arcella, D.; Turrini, A.; Leclercq, C.; INRAN-SCAI 2005-06 Study Group. The third Italian National Food Consumption Survey, INRAN-SCAI 2005-06—Part 1: Nutrient intakes in Italy. *Nutr. Metab. Cardiovasc. Dis.* **2011**, *21*, 922–932. [CrossRef] [PubMed]
14. Institute of Medicine; IOM. *Dietary Reference Intakes for Water, Potassium, Sodium, Chloride and Sulfate*; The National Academies Press: Washington, DC, USA, 2004.
15. Benelam, B.; Wyness, L. Hydration and Health: A review. *Nutr. Bull.* **2010**, *35*, 3–25. [CrossRef]

16. Drewnowski, A.; Rehn, C.D.; Constant, F. Water and beverage consumption among children age 4–13 years in the United States: Analyses of 2005–2010 NHANES data. *Nutr. J.* **2013**, *12*. [CrossRef] [PubMed]
17. Bellisle, F.; Thornton, S.N.; Hébe, P.; Denizeau, M.; Tahiri, M. A study of fluid intake from beverages in a sample of healthy French children, adolescents and adults. *Eur. J. Clin. Nutr.* **2010**, *64*, 350–355. [CrossRef] [PubMed]
18. Drewnowski, A.; Rehm, C.D.; Constant, F. Water and beverage consumption among adults in the United States: Cross-sectional study using data from NHANES 2005–2010. *BMC Public Health* **2013**, *13*. [CrossRef] [PubMed]
19. Gibson, S.; Shirreffs, S.M. Beverage consumption habits "24/7" among British adults: Association with total water intake and energy intake. *Nutr. J.* **2013**, *12*. [CrossRef] [PubMed]
20. Hooper, L.; Bunn, D.; Jimoh, F.O.; Fairweather-Tait, S.J. Water-loss dehydration and aging. *Mech. Ageing Dev.* **2014**, *136*, 50–58. [CrossRef] [PubMed]
21. Del Boca, F.K.; Darkes, J. The validity of self-reports of alcohol consumption: State of the science and challenges for research. *Addiction* **2003**, *98*, 1–12. [CrossRef] [PubMed]
22. European Commission. *Special Eurobarometer 272b: Attitudes towards Alcohol*; TNS Opinion & Social: Brusssels, Belgium, 2007; pp. 40–42.
23. Krall, E.A.; Dwyer, J.T. Validity of food frequency questionnaire and food diary in short-term recall situation. *J. Am. Diet. Assoc.* **1987**, *87*, 1374–1377. [PubMed]

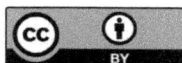

nutrients

MDPI

Article

Beverage Consumption Habits among the European Population: Association with Total Water and Energy Intakes

Mariela Nissensohn [1,2,3], Almudena Sánchez-Villegas [2,3], Pilar Galan [4], Aida Turrini [5], Nathalie Arnault [4], Lorenza Mistura [5], Adriana Ortiz-Andrellucchi [1,2,3], Fabien Szabo de Edelenyi [4], Laura D'Addezio [5] and Lluis Serra-Majem [1,2,3,*]

1   International Chair for Advanced Studies on Hydration (ICASH), University of Las Palmas de Gran Canaria, 35016 Las Palmas, Spain; marienis67@hotmail.com (M.N.); aortiza55@hotmail.com (A.O.-A.)
2   Research Institute of Biomedical and Health Sciences, University of Las Palmas de Gran Canaria, 35016 Las Palmas, Spain; almudena.sanchez@ulpgc.es
3   CIBER OBN, Biomedical Research Networking Center for Physiopathology of Obesity and Nutrition, Carlos III Health Institute, 28029 Madrid, Spain
4   Equipe de Recherche en Epidémiologie Nutritionnelle, Centre de Recherche en Epidémiologie et Statistiques, Université Paris 13, Inserm (U1153), Inra (U1125), Cnam, COMUE Sorbonne Paris Cité, F-93017 Bobigny, France; p.galan@uren.smbh.univ-paris13.fr (P.G.); n.arnault@uren.smbh.univ-paris13.fr (N.A.); f.szabo@uren.smbh.univ-paris13.fr (F.S.d.E.)
5   CREA-Consiglio per la ricerca in agricoltura e l'analisi dell'economia agraria–Centro di ricerca per gli alimenti e la nutrizione, Via Ardeatina 546, 00178 Rome, Italy; aida.turrini@crea.gov.it (A.T.); lorenza.mistura@crea.gov.it (L.M.); laura.daddezio@crea.gov.it (L.D.)
*   Correspondence: lluis.serra@ulpgc.es; Tel.: +34-928-453-475; Fax: +34-928-451-416

Received: 21 June 2016; Accepted: 7 April 2017; Published: 13 April 2017

Abstract: Background: Fluid and water intake have received limited attention in epidemiological studies. The aim of this study was to compare the average daily consumption of foods and beverages in adults of selective samples of the European Union (EU) population in order to understand the contribution of these to the total water intake (TWI), evaluate if the EU adult population consumes adequate amounts of total water (TW) according to the current guidelines, and to illustrate the real water intake in Europe. Methods: Three national European dietary surveys have been selected: Spain used the Anthropometry, Intake, and Energy Balance Study (ANIBES) population database, Italy analyzed data from the Italian National Food Consumption Survey (INRAN-SCAI 2005-06), and French data came from the NutriNet-Santé database. Mean daily consumption was used to compare between individuals. TWI was compared with European Food Safety Authority (EFSA) reference values for adult men and women. Results: On average, in Spain, TWI was 1.7 L (SE 22.9) for men and 1.6 L (SE 19.4) for women; Italy recorded 1.7 L (SE 16.9) for men and 1.7 L (SE 14.1) for women; and France recorded 2.3 L (SE 4.7) for men and 2.1 L (SE 2.4) for women. With the exception of women in France, neither men nor women consumed sufficient amounts of water according to EFSA reference values. Conclusions: This study highlights the need to formulate appropriate health and nutrition policies to increase TWI in the EU population. The future of beverage intake assessment requires the use of new instruments, techniques, and the application of the new available technologies.

Keywords: total water intake; beverages; adults; France; Italy; Spain

1. Introduction

Fluid and water intake have received limited attention in epidemiological studies. This hampers attempts to assess the adequacy of water intakes at the population level [1,2].

It is well known that adequate hydration status is associated with the preservation of physical and mental functions and that water intake is the best way to achieve hydration [3,4]. However, we have to be aware that there are other sources of liquids with similar hydration capacities, liquids with different flavors that also provide nutrients or stimulants, feed us, or are just more palatable, like milk, juices, teas, soups, beer and wine. During the last few decades, multiple types of drinks with different characteristics have been developed. Some of them are not only to satiate thirst. Soft drinks, flavored waters, or different kinds of infusions with different properties such as sedatives, digestives, antioxidants, etc. are some examples. The current selection of beverages is so broad that it is clear that there should be specific recommendations with respect to these liquids; this should include their capacity to hydrate and supply energy or other nutrients, as well as any other effects they may have on the body [5]. With this in mind, some recent studies have suggested that the variety of beverages consumed is a positive predictor of total water intake (TWI) [1,6–8].

On the other hand, in recent years, we have witnessed the emergence of obesity as a serious problem in the Western world. In fact, excessive consumption of sugary beverages has been linked to increasing weight of populations [9,10]. Unfortunately, there is little evidence to show that replacing caloric drinks with water has beneficial effects on body weight or sensitivity to insulin [11], although different studies have shown that replacing these drinks with water results in a decrease in total caloric intake [1,12]. Therefore, it seems to be prudent to encourage the consumption of drinking water instead of other caloric drinks [5].

Some countries and public organizations have proposed water intake recommendations for the general public [13–16]. They recognize that the value of adequate intake (AI) is a variable event, in which differences are due, in part, to the inter-individual variation for water needs in response to different health status, metabolism, and environmental factors, such as ambient temperature and humidity. Other individual factors, such as age, body size, and level of physical activity are involved [17]. Furthermore, water needs also depend on overall diet and the water contained in food. The European Food Safety Authority (EFSA) proposed Dietary Reference Values (DRV) for the Adequate Intake of Water per day. It included water from food and water from beverages. The range of DRVs in liters increase with age until 2.5 L and 2.0 L for 14+ year-old men and women, respectively [13].

Following the analyses of some European Union (EU) nutritional databases, the aim of this study was to compare the average daily consumption of fluids (water and other beverages) in selected samples of the EU populations in order to understand the contribution of each fluid type to total water intake. Furthermore, we will evaluate if the adult EU population consumes adequate amounts of total water according to EFSA [13] recommendations, or if those populations reached AI values defined as the ratio between TWI (g of water from food and beverages) and energy intake (EI) in kcal. This ratio suggests that water intake is inadequate when the result is less than 1. We will also explore associations between the types of beverage consumed and energy intake from the diet.

2. Materials and Methods

Three countries of the EU and their dietary surveys have been selected. Only adults ranging from 18 to 75 years were considered for the present study. The countries were chosen because of geographic proximity, similar climate and cultural characteristics, and by the method used to collect information of the food and beverage intake. Only those countries that used food records or 24-h dietary recalls were included. Food and beverage intake was recorded in each study by age and sex, as well as day and time of consumption.

2.1. Spain (ANIBES Dataset)

In Spain, the population database used was from the Anthropometry, Intake and Energy Balance Study (ANIBES), a cross-sectional study conducted using stratified multistage sampling. The representative sample of this national survey of diet and nutrition comprised 2285 healthy participants, aged 9–75 years. The sample was collected from the following geographical locations:

Northeast, Levant, Southwest, North–Central, Barcelona, Madrid, Balearic, and Canary Islands. The fieldwork for the ANIBES study was conducted from mid-September, 2013, to mid-November, 2013, with the participation of 90 interviewers allocated in 11 areas and 12 coordinators, all previously trained by the Spanish Nutrition Foundation (FEN). The survey was performed "door-to-door" following randomized routes. For better results at the main fieldwork, different informative posters about ANIBES' goals were posted in the area/neighborhood, followed by letters that were sent to all the neighbors. In addition, during the first visit by the interviewer, an informative letter from the principal investigator plus a leaflet and a set of infographics explaining the whole process were offered. Finally, the potential participant was informed about a small incentive (30 euros) for participation and a detailed final report including anthropometric data, physical activity level, and dietary/nutritional status, with an estimated value of 40–50 euros. Demographic variables collected included gender, unemployment rate, physical activity level assessed by the International Physical Activity Questionnaire (IPAQ) [18], and education level. Participants' weight, height, and waist circumference were measured, and body mass index was also calculated. Study participants were provided with a tablet device (Samsung Galaxy Tab 2 7.0, Samsung Electronics, Suwon, South Korea). If the participant declared or demonstrated that he/she was unable to use the tablet device, other possibilities were offered: photo camera plus paper or telephone interview. Participants were trained to record information by taking photos of all food and drinks consumed during three consecutive days, both at home and outside of the home. To equally represent all days of the week, study subjects participated during two weekdays and one day during the weekend. Food records were returned from the field in real-time (i.e., at the exact moment in which they were consumed), to be coded by trained coders who were supervised by dieticians. Food, beverage, energy, and nutrient intakes were calculated from food consumption records using VD-FEN 2.1 software, a Dietary Evaluation Program from the Spanish Nutrition Foundation, Spain. This software was newly developed for the ANIBES study by the FEN and is based mainly on Spanish food composition tables [19], with several expansions and updates. A food photographic atlas was used to assist in assigning gram weights to portion sizes. Details of the ANIBES study have been described in detail elsewhere [1].

2.2. Italy (INRAN-SCAI Dataset)

Data from Italy come from the national food consumption survey (INRAN-SCAI 2005-06). This cross-sectional survey was conducted on a representative sample of 1300 randomly selected households between October 2005 and December 2006. Census data were used for the multistage stratification of the sample into the four main geographical areas of Italy (North-West, North-East, Centre, South, and Islands), provinces' population size (large, medium, and small), municipalities' population size (large-medium, and small), and four strata according to household composition. In each municipality, households were randomly selected from the telephone guide. In total, 3323 (1501 males and 1822 females) individuals participated in the food survey, aged 0 to 97 years. A three-day semi-structured diary was used for participants to record the consumption of all foods, beverages, and nutritional supplements. A team of trained field workers conducted the survey, and individually met the participants who self-recorded all foods and beverages consumed, estimating portion sizes with the help of a picture booklet. Food data were coded by field workers during the data entry using a data management system developed for the purpose of the survey. Other variables collected were age, gender, education, occupation, lifestyle (smoking, physical activity, dieting). Height and weight were self-reported. Data on nutrient intake—including water—were obtained using the updated version of the Italian national food composition database [20]. The "Food Energy and Nutrient Composition Database" was used to estimate the data on energy, macro-nutrients, dietary fiber, vitamins, and minerals. Detailed information about the INRAN SCAI 2005-06 survey design, procedures, and methodologies can be found in previously published papers [7,20,21].

2.3. France (NutriNet-Santé Dataset)

French data come from the NutriNet-Santé database, a web-based observational prospective cohort including volunteers aged 18 years or older, launched in France in May 2009, with a scheduled follow up in 10 years. The study was conducted on a large sample of 94,939 participants. It aimed at determining the association of food intake, nutrients, and dietary behavior with ageing and quality of life. At baseline, socio-demographic data including age, gender, education, income, occupational category, and household location, as well as lifestyle (smoking status, physical activity), height, weight, and practice of restrictive dieting were self-reported. Leisure-time physical activity was assessed using the French short form of the International Physical Activity Questionnaire, self-administered online [22–24]. Body mass index (BMI) was assessed using self-reported height and weight. Dietary data were collected at baseline using three-day records, randomly distributed within a two-week period, including two weekdays and one day of the weekend. Participants reported all foods and beverages consumed throughout the day: breakfast, lunch, dinner, and all other occasions. Daily mean food and beverage consumptions were calculated for each participant having completed the three-day records, with a weighting on the type of day (week or weekend) so that all days of the week were equally represented. Serving sizes were estimated using purchase units, household units, and photographs, and were derived from a previously validated picture booklet. EI and TWI were calculated through the NutriNet-Santé food composition table including more than 2000 food products [25]. The NutriNet-Santé study has been described in detail elsewhere [8,26].

2.4. Statistical Analysis

Eight different categories of beverages were used to examine beverage consumption and EI for each of the three studied countries: (1) hot beverages, including hot tea and coffee; (2) milk (all types of milk without separation by fat percentage); (3) fruit and vegetable juices (including nectars, juice–milk blends, 100% fruit juices); (4) caloric soft drinks (including colas; tonic water; sodas; ginger ale; fruit-flavored drinks; iced teas in cans or bottles; sports drinks, such as isotonic drinks with mineral salts; and caffeinated energy drinks); (5) diet soft drinks (including the same beverages as in the caloric soft drinks group but with artificial sweetener); (6) alcoholic drinks, including both low-alcohol grade and high-alcohol grade groups; (7) water (including tap water and bottled water); and (8) other beverages (including soy-based beverages, non-alcoholic beer and wine, and others).

All analyses were carried out separately in men and women and across countries. Differences in demographic and anthropometric variables between Spain, France, and Italy were assessed through chi-squared test for qualitative variables and through ANOVA-test when quantitative variables were compared. The analyses were focused on the TWI of all foods and beverages by country. Description of the population and the mean daily consumption of the food and beverage intakes were calculated for the 18–75-year-old population of each country. Contributions of food and beverages to TWI and EI were calculated. In each country, pairwise comparisons of the means across groups were assessed using *t*-test. A two-sided *p*-value of 0.05 was set to denote statistical significance.

TWI was compared with the EFSA [13] Dietary Reference Values for the Adequate Intake of water for men and women, from 14 years of age onward (2.5 L and 2.0 L, respectively). Furthermore, the ratio g/kcal was applied to provide a more comprehensive estimate of the proportion from each country that fulfilled the AI recommendations. This criterion is based on the water intake per unit of energy consumed. The value suggested is 1.0 L per 1000 kcal of EI [14]. However, this value could be increased to 1.5 L/1000 kcal depending on activity level and water loss. TWI for adults should be no less than 1.0 L/1000 kcal [13]. Therefore, we used three different approaches to define water intake adequacy in order to provide a more comprehensive estimate of the proportion of participants who consume low amounts of water. The first criterion is a classification based on the AI value, defined by the EFSA as Criterion 1. The second (Criterion 2) is a ratio between TWI (water from food and beverages in grams) and EI in kcal higher than 1. The combination of both is the final criterion (Criterion 3).

3. Results

Descriptive characteristics of the three included studies are presented in Table 1. The population of the studies ranged from 18 to 75 years. The studies included 1859 participants from Spain, 94,939 from France and 2313 from Italy. There were significant differences in most demographic and anthropometric variables between countries. The rate of unemployment shows that Spain had the highest percentage of unemployed participants—data that are in line with those from the statistical office of the European Union (Eurostat) [27]. For level of education, France's males and females showed the highest University educated level.

The contribution of food and beverages to daily water intake (g/day) and EI (kcal/day) by genders are presented in Table 2. On average, in Spain, TWI for adults was 1.7 L (SE 22.9) for men and 1.6 L (SE 19.4) for women; Italy recorded 1.7 L (SE 16.9) for men and 1.7 L (SE 14.1) for women; and France recorded 2.3 L (SE 4.7) for men and 2.1 L (SE 2.4) for women. The mean daily EI for adults in Spain was 1790.8 kcal/day (SE 11.6), of which 12% was provided by beverages. For the Italian study, EI was 2137.9 (SE 12.2), and only 6% was supplied by beverages. France recorded an EI of 1884.5 (SE 1.5), of which 8% was provided by beverages.

Figure 1 provides information on the amount (in grams) of water content in food and beverages consumed by country and gender. All results are presented in g of water content, not mean intakes by volume (e.g., g of water in milk, not g of milk consumed). Water was the most consumed beverage in the three countries for both sexes, followed by the water provided by milk in Spain, water from alcoholic beverages by men from Italy, and also water from hot drinks from French men and women. Spain and France were the highest consumers of alcoholic beverages, especially by men, although consumption was similar in the three countries. Spain was also the country with the lowest consumption of water from foods. Regarding soft drinks, Italy had a lower water intake from both diet and caloric beverages.

Figure 2 represented the percentage of water consumption as a beverage category on average over the three day study period. It was represented separately from the others' beverages consumed in order to clearly highlight the differences in intake by country. The percentage of water consumption was 48% for women and 47% for men in France—the highest percentage of the three countries studied. In Spain and Italy, the higher percentage was for Spain in the female group, and was less for Italian males.

The percentages of each beverage category consumed over the assessment period by gender are presented in Figures 3 and 4. Water as a beverage category is not included in them. On average, among men, hot beverages were the most frequently consumed beverages in France, followed by milk in Spain and alcoholic drinks in Italy, with percentages of 23%, 17%, and 15%, respectively. For women, the list in decreasing order was hot beverages in France (30%) and milk in Spain (19%). For Italy, the highest percentage was also for hot beverages (9%).

Table A1 shows the percentiles of beverage consumption (gr/day) of each country among adults by sex. For both men and women, the main source was water for the three countries. Spain consumed higher amounts of milk, followed by hot beverages and alcoholic drinks for women and in the opposite order (alcoholic drinks—hot beverages) by men. For Italy, the highest values were hot drinks for both men and women, followed by alcoholic drinks for men. For France, the second-most consumed beverage was hot beverages, followed by milk for women and alcohol for men.

Table 1. Demographic and anthropometric details for included study participants from Spain (ANIBES dataset), France (NutriNet-Santé dataset) and Italy (INRAN-SCAI dataset).

			SPAIN			FRANCE			ITALY			p* Value		
			Men	Women	Total	Men	Women	Total	Men	Women	Total	Men	Women	Total
n			895	964	1859	20,636	74,303	94,939	1202	1245	2313	-	-	-
Age Group	18–64 (years)	%	89.5	88.7	88.9	87.17	95.38	93.59	88.9	88.6	88.7	0.643	0.006	0.007
	65–75 (years)	%	10.5	11.3	11.1	12.83	4.62	6.41	11.1	11.4	11.3	0.047	<0.001	<0.001
Level of education	Primary	%	26.4	27.5	27.0	23.14	17.70	18.88	34.2	37.4	35.9	<0.001	<0.001	<0.001
	Secondary	%	49.6	47.9	48.7	13.67	18.44	17.40	44.6	40.2	42.2	<0.001	<0.001	<0.001
	University	%	24.0	24.7	24.3	63.20	63.87	63.72	21.2	22.4	21.9	<0.001	<0.001	<0.001
Rate of unemployment		%	18.2	8.6	13.5	4.96	6.47	6.14	2.4	2.7	2.6	<0.001	<0.001	<0.001
Weight (kg)		Mean (SE)	82.4 (0.56)	66.8 (0.48)	74.4 (0.42)	77.4 (0.09)	63.3 (0.05)	66.4 (0.05)	78.4 (0.3)	62.7 (0.3)	69.9 (0.3)	<0.001	<0.001	<0.001
Height (cm)		Mean (SE)	174.5 (0.25)	161.2 (0.22)	167.7 (0.24)	176.5 (0.05)	164.1 (0.02)	166.8 (0.03)	175.0 (0.2)	163.0 (0.2)	169.0 (0.2)	<0.001	<0.001	<0.001
BMI (kg/m^2)		Mean (SE)	27.1 (0.18)	25.7 (0.19)	26.4 (0.13)	24.8 (0.03)	23.5 (0.02)	23.8 (0.01)	26.0 (0.1)	23.0 (0.1)	24.0 (0.1)	<0.001	<0.001	<0.001
Waist Circumference (cm)		Mean (SE)	94.0 (0.49)	83.1 (0.46)	88.4 (0.36)	90.3 (0.16)	79.9 (0.11)	82.8 (0.10)	Unrecorded	Unrecorded	Unrecorded	<0.001	<0.001	<0.001
BMI class	Healthy weight	%	36.5	47.5	42.2	58.8	72.6	69.6	50.3	71.3	61.6	<0.001	<0.001	<0.001
	Overweight	%	40.0	32.0	35.9	32.3	18.3	21.4	39.4	21.9	30.0	<0.001	<0.001	<0.001
	Obese	%	22.9	17.8	20.3	8.8	9.1	9.0	10.2	6.8	8.4	<0.001	<0.001	<0.001

p*value obtained through chi-squared test and ANOVA-test = significant (<0.001). BMI: body mass index.

Table 2. Contribution of food and beverages to total water and energy intake by gender among the populations included.

	SPAIN						FRANCE						ITALY					
	Contribution to Water Intake (g/Day)			Contribution to Energy Intake (kcal/Day)			Contribution to Water Intake (g/Day)			Contribution to Energy Intake (kcal/Day)			Contribution to Water Intake (g/Day)			Contribution to Energy Intake (kcal/Day)		
	Women	Men	Total	Women	Men	Total	Women	Men	Total	Women	Men	Total	Women	Men	Total	Women	Men	Total
All food & beverages Mean (SE)	1605.2 (19.4)	1702.9 (22.9)	1652.3 (14.9)	1653.3 (13.9)	1939.1 (17.6)	1790.8 (11.6)	2101.7 (2.4)	2251.0 (4.7)	2134.2 (2.2)	1783.0 (1.5)	2250.1 (3.6)	1884.5 (1.5)	1667.9 (14.1)	1768.6 (16.9)	1714.3 (10.9)	1929.6 (14)	2381.4 (18.5)	2137.9 (12.2)
Food only %	31.99	32.54	32.25	88.49	87.20	87.87	37.8	39.4	38.1	92.2	90.1	91.7	42.2	44.4	44.8	95.3	93.4	94.4
Beverages only %	68.61	67.46	67.75	11.51	12.80	12.13	62.2	60.6	61.9	7.8	9.9	8.3	55.8	55.5	55.7	4.7	6.6	5.6

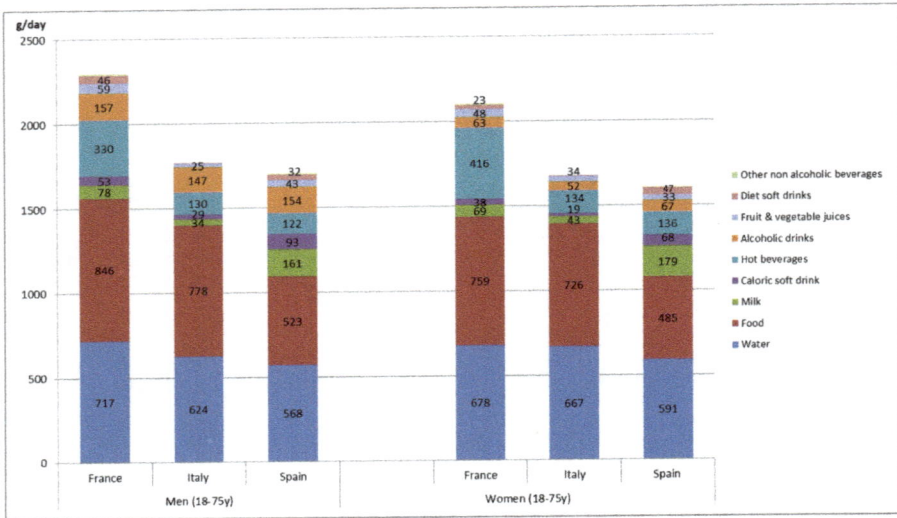

Figure 1. Daily water intake (g/day) provided by each beverage/food category according to gender among the populations included. All results are presented in g of water content in each category, not mean intakes by volume (e.g., g of water in milk, not g of milk consumed).

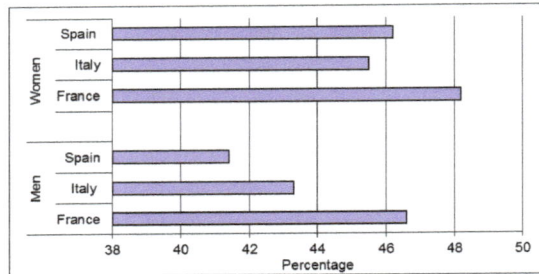

Figure 2. Percentage of water consumption in the beverage category by country and gender.

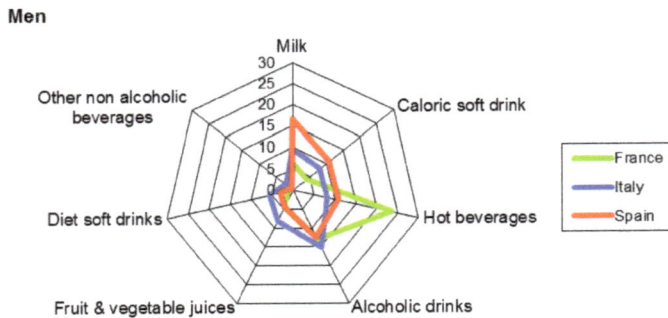

Figure 3. Percentage of each category of beverages consumed on average over the assessment period by men (18–75 years). Water as a beverage is not included in this figure.

Women

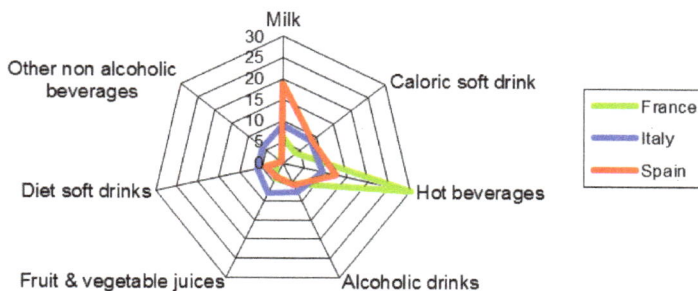

Figure 4. Percentage of each category of beverages consumed on average over the assessment period by women (18–75 years). Water as a beverage is not included in this figure.

Participants who fulfilled the EFSA AI recommendations for TWI for men and women (2.5 L and 2.0 L, respectively) were classified under Criterion 1. Participants with ratios of water/EI >1.0 were included under Criterion 2 (considering a value of 1 g of water per 1 kcal of EI). Finally, participants who met both definitions (Criterias 1 and 2) were classified under Criterion 3. Following this analysis, Table 3 shows that the group with the highest percentage of compliance with the criteria was women in France (51% fulfilled Criterion 1, 66% Criterion 2, and 46% Criterion 3). In the case of French men, no criteria exceeded 50% compliance (30% met Criterion 1, 46% Criterion 2, and 24% Criterion 3). Furthermore, Criterion 2 obtained the highest percentage of compliance obtained among the three countries. However, it is very noticeable that women achieved higher rates of compliance than men in all criteria and in all countries included in the analyses.

Table 3. Combined classification for Total Water Intake (TWI) following the established criteria.

EFSA 2.5 L Men; 2.0 L Women	Men			Women		
	Spain	Italy	France	Spain	Italy	France
n	865	1202	20636	964	1245	74,303
Criterion 1: *n* (%)	114 (13)	127 (11)	6281 (30)	216 (22)	336 (24)	38,152 (51)
Criterion 2: *n* (%)	262 (29)	160 (13)	9446 (46)	404 (42)	379 (27)	49,135 (66)
Criterion 3 (1 and 2): *n* (%)	98 (11)	66 (5)	5029 (24)	185 (19)	210 (15)	34,065 (46)

EFSA: European Food Safety Authority [13]: Criterion 1: TWI >2.5 L men, >2 L women (aged 14 to 75 years); Criterion 2: Ratio of total water/total energy intakes >1; Criterion 3: Both criteria.

4. Discussion

This study addresses the analysis of beverage intake in adults from three national European databases from France, Italy, and Spain. Fluid intake was examined using a similar methodology and the same data classification method in the three countries.

The analyses indicate that only women from France complied with the recommended value of 2.1 L (SE 2.4). Spain had the lowest water intake among the three, with 1.7 L (SE 22.9) for men and 1.6 L (SE 19.4) for women. It is evident that the insufficient consumption of water according to EFSA reference values and the high percentage of adults who did not comply with the recommendation requires more attention—not only from the scientific community, but also from the public health and education communities.

France met EFSA recommendations most closely. Similar situations have happened when the criterion applied was the ratio between TWI and total EI. However, with this same criterion, the results appear to show better compliance for the three countries. Between 50% and 80% of women and 70%–85% of men did not meet EFSA recommendations for water consumption. As we expected, TWI differed by gender in the three countries, and was always higher for women. This leads one to consider that women may tend to have healthier lifestyle patterns than men [28], or it is also possible that men are more likely to underreport fluids than women [29].

Regarding EI, the three countries recorded EIs from beverages of 12%, 8%, and 6% for Spain, France, and Italy, respectively. These percentages are very close to the 10% proposed by some international authorities [13,30], who recommended that no more than 10% of daily calorie intake should come from beverages. It is to be noted that dietary patterns are crucial in determining the percentage of calories provided by beverages. In our study, the lower percentage (6%) is derived from the higher EI (2137.9 kcal/day in Italy). In this case, although climate and cultural conditions are similar, the beverage consumption level is different; French people have a higher water intake than the others from all sources, and this can be related to a lower EI according to the major sources highlighted in Figure 1.

The compilation of the three national surveys, conducted with large samples of participants, which also kept the same classification of the beverages, is one of the most important strengths of this study. It demonstrates that water constitutes the largest proportion of total fluid intake for the three countries examined. The data of the current analysis are in line with data reported in other previously-published surveys [31].

The fact remains that there is little information regarding beverage consumption in the EU and even less that describes patterns of habitual intake. Fluid intake is part of our eating habits; it is influenced by climate and by our physiological needs, as well as by our customs. The amount of liquids consumed and our drinking patterns have consequences on our health status. Although the purpose of this study was to describe the usual profiles of water consumption and drinks in the EU, and to analyze similarities and differences in the consumption profiles of the populations of the regions studied, we are well aware that three studies are not sufficient to achieve the illustration of the status of actual water intake in Europe, nor does it reflect the possible consequences on health; this is the major limitation. However, it is enough to show the existing trend of low consumption, which is much more evident in men than it is in women and in older populations. This point deserves special attention. One important reason for this is the fact that the proportion of elderly people in the population has been greatly increasing around the world over the last decade, and these trends are expected to continue [32]. Europe is not unaware of this situation. Since the 1970s, when there were about 3.3 million people over the age of 65, this number has increased to 7.6 million in Europe, which accounts for more than 17.1% of the population. The elderly population has a high rate of chronic illness [33], and is more vulnerable to disease. The evidence of dehydration among this group is well known and documented [34,35]. Dehydration substantially increases the burden of health care in a direct way, as a disease itself, or indirectly as a comorbidity of other diseases. Therefore, this represents an important public health issue by imposing a significant economic burden [36].

On the other hand, for nutritional epidemiology, the focus of interest is based on estimating the risk of inadequate beverage intake. Methods of estimating beverage adequacy have changed over time. We have gone from estimating it from questionnaires or surveys of general food and beverages (which do not focus attention on beverage intake), to the exclusive use of questionnaires collecting information on beverage intake, which have been validated with appropriate biomarkers. However, the complexity and costs underlying the evaluation of beverage consumption do not suffice, in view of the few exclusive beverage studies that exist in the EU [37]. Current epidemiological studies that focus on beverage intake have large differences in the values obtained. A significant part of these differences are derived from the methodology used. The choice of an appropriate method is essential in order to established a precise and reliable record. The use of different methodologies leads to obtaining such disparate results that they are impossible to compare [2]. Standardization of procedures for collecting data from different studies is the first and most important step to take when such studies arise. Our experience suggests that a comparison of different methods results in a higher water intake when the food frequency questionnaires (FFQ) method for fluid intake is used [38]. Multiple-day (three or seven days) food records and 24-h dietary recalls have been used successfully [39,40]. These seem to improve the assessment of water throughout the day, and can be very useful in nutrition surveys. In fact, in this analysis, we have been forced to discard some studies that could potentially have been included in the current work due to the high differences in the results caused by the use of different methodologies.

The interpretation of these results should be carefully considered for a number of reasons. First, the number of studies that were eligible for inclusion in this analysis was small, which limited the possibility of showing the real pattern of fluid consumption in Europe. Furthermore, although the statistical analysis was the same for the three countries included, the difference in the recruitment and sampling of the studies could explain some of the obtained results. For example, the higher level of University Education found in the French population [8,26] was because the sample included mostly volunteers; that is, more educated people for research [41]. Second, the studies were cross-sectional in design, which provides evidence for associations, but not causal relationships. Furthermore, it is well-known that intake assessed by self-reports is subject to random and systematic reporting errors, which may introduce bias into the estimate of water consumption. However, according to the scientific literature [42], these kinds of records continue to be the chosen dietary assessment methods for epidemiological studies.

5. Conclusions

This study attempts to show actual water consumption in some EU countries. It highlights the need to formulate appropriate health and nutrition policies in order to increase TWI in these populations.

Without a doubt, Europe needs a collective effort to contribute to standardizing the assessment of beverage intakes, as well as to minimize the use of inappropriate dietary instruments. The future of beverage intake assessment requires the use of new instruments and techniques, the application of available new technologies, and an open discussion regarding the clarity and transparency of the procedures required.

Acknowledgments: The current analyses included in this paper were financially supported by a grant from the former European Hydration Institute, now International Chair for Advanced Studies on Hydration (ICASH) to the Canarian Science Foundation and Technology Park of the University of Las Palmas de Gran Canaria. The ANIBES study was supported by Coca-Cola Iberia through an agreement with the Spanish Nutrition Foundation (FEN) who assisted with technical advice. The INRAN-SCAI Study was funded by the Italian Ministry of Agriculture, project 'Qualità Alimentare'. The NutriNet-Santé study is supported by the French Ministry of Health (DGS), the Institut de Veille Sanitaire (IVS), the Institut National de Prévention et d'Education pour la Santé (INPES), the Institut National de la Santé et de la Recherche Médicale (Inserm), the Institut National de la Rechereche Agronomique (Inra), the Conservatoire National des Arts et Métiers (CNAM), and the Paris 13 University. The funding sponsors had no role in the design of the study, the collection, analysis, or interpretation of the data, writing of the manuscript, or in the decision to publish the results.

Author Contributions: M.N. and L.S.M. drafted and wrote the manuscript. The Research team for the Hydration European Database Study (EHYDAS) A.S.V., P.G., A.T., N.A., L.M., A.O.Á., F.S.E. and L.D. analyzed the data and also contributed to writing the manuscript. They provided continuous scientific advice for the study and for interpretation of the results. All authors approved the final version of the manuscript.

Conflicts of Interest: The authors declare no conflicts of interest.

Appendix A

Table A1. Percentiles of beverage consumption (g/day) among adults by sex.

Adults 18–75 Years	Spain Total n	P25	P50	P75	Spain Women n	P25	P50	P75	Spain Men n	P25	P50	P75	Italy Total n	P25	P50	P75	Italy Women n	P25	P50	P75	Italy Men n	P25	P50	P75	France Total n	P25	P50	P75	France Women n	P25	P50	P75	France Men n	P25	P50	P75
Hot bev. (g/day)	1655	33.3	100.0	183.3	857	46.7	108.3	193.3	798	26.7	90.0	171.7	2313	60.0	113.6	180.0	1245	60.0	115.0	180.0	1068	60.0	110.0	180.0	94,939	150.0	339.3	567.8	74,303	160.7	353.6	594.6	20,636	116.4	294.4	475.0
Milk (g/day)	1655	90.0	173.3	266.7	857	101.7	183.3	273.3	798	70.0	155.0	258.3	2313	0.0	0.0	50.0	1245	0.0	0.0	83.3	1068	0.0	0.0	0.0	94,939	0.0	0.0	123.8	74,303	0.0	0.0	120.0	20,636	0.0	0.0	139.3
Juices (g/day)	1655	0.0	0.0	66.7	857	0.0	0.0	66.7	798	0.0	0.0	66.7	2313	0.0	0.0	2.0	1245	0.0	0.0	2.0	1068	0.0	0.0	2.0	94,939	0.0	0.0	96.4	74,303	0.0	0.0	90.8	20,636	0.0	0.0	120.0
Caloric soft bev. (g/day)	1655	0.0	0.0	133.3	857	0.0	0.0	110.0	798	0.0	0.0	166.7	2313	0.0	0.0	0.0	1245	0.0	0.0	0.0	1068	0.0	0.0	0.0	94,939	0.0	0.0	42.8	74,303	0.0	0.0	42.9	20,636	0.0	0.0	53.6
Diet soft bev.(g/day)	1655	0.0	0.0	0.0	857	0.0	0.0	0.0	798	0.0	0.0	0.0	2313	0.0	0.0	0.0	1245	0.0	0.0	0.0	1068	0.0	0.0	0.0	94,939	0.0	0.0	0.0	74,303	0.0	0.0	0.0	20,636	0.0	0.0	0.0
Alcohol (g/day)	1655	0.0	0.0	140.0	857	0.0	0.0	85.0	798	0.0	44.2	220.0	2313	0.0	0.0	0.0	1245	0.0	0.0	93.3	1068	0.0	110.0	255.7	94,939	0.0	35.7	132.2	74,303	0.0	21.6	100.4	20,636	0.0	112.2	265.7
Water (g/day)	1655	200.0	450.0	863.3	857	250.0	456.7	873.3	798	166.7	450.0	850.0	2313	373.3	586.7	853.3	1245	400.0	600.0	853.3	1068	320.0	586.7	826.7	94,939	354.3	591.4	907.2	74,303	354.3	589.3	900.0	20,636	653.6	604.3	932.2
Other non-alcohol bev. (g/day)	1655	0.0	0.0	0.0	857	0.0	0.0	0.0	798	0.0	0.0	0.0	2313	0.0	0.0	0.0	1245	0.0	0.0	0.0	1068	0.0	0.0	0.0	94,939	0.0	0.0	0.0	74,303	0.0	0.0	0.0	20,636	0.0	0.0	0.0

References

1. Nissensohn, M.; Sánchez-Villegas, A.; Ortega, R.M.; Aranceta-Bartrina, J.; Gil, A.; González-Gross, M.; Varela-Moreiras, G.; Serra-Majem, L. Beverage Consumption Habits and Association with Total Water and Energy Intakes in the Spanish Population: Findings of the ANIBES Study. *Nutrients* **2016**, *8*, 232. [CrossRef] [PubMed]
2. Nissensohn, M.; Castro-Quezada, I.; Serra-Majem, L. Beverage and water intake of healthy adults in some European countries. *Int. J. Food Sci. Nutr.* **2013**, *64*, 801–805. [CrossRef] [PubMed]
3. Lieberman, H.R. Hydration and cognition: A critical review and recommendations for future research. *J. Am. Coll. Nutr.* **2007**, *26* (Suppl. 5), 555S–561S. [CrossRef] [PubMed]
4. Murray, B. Hydration and physical performance. *J. Am. Coll. Nutr.* **2007**, *26* (Suppl. 5), 542S–548S. [CrossRef] [PubMed]
5. Rosado, C.I.; Villarino Marín, A.L.; Martínez, J.A.; Cabrerizo, L.; Gargallo, M.; Lorenzo, H.; Quiles, J.; Planas, M.; Polanco, I.; Romero de Ávila, D.; et al. On behalf of the Spanish Federation of Nutrition, Food and Dietetics (FESNAD). Importance of water in the hydration of the Spanish population: Document FESNAD 2010. *Nutr. Hosp.* **2011**, *26*, 27–36.
6. Gibson, S.; Shirreffs, S.M. Beverage consumption habits "24/7" among British adults: Association with total water intake and energy intake. *Nutr. J.* **2013**, *10*, 9. [CrossRef] [PubMed]
7. Mistura, L.; D'Addezio, L.; Turrini, A. Beverage consumption habits in Italian population: Association with total water intake and energy intake. *Nutrients* **2016**, *8*, 674. [CrossRef] [PubMed]
8. Szabo de Edelenyi, F.; Druesne-Pecollo, N.; Arnault, N.; Gonzáles, R.; Buscail, C.; Galan, P. Characteristics of beverage consumption habits among a large sample of French adults: Associations with total water and energy intakes. *Nutrients* **2016**, *8*, 627. [CrossRef] [PubMed]
9. Forshee, R.A.; Anderson, P.A.; Storey, M.L. Sugar-sweetened beverages and body mass index in children and adolescents: A meta-analysis. *Am. J. Clin. Nutr.* **2008**, *87*, 1662–1671. [PubMed]
10. Hu, F.B.; Malik, V.S. Sugar-sweetened beverages and risk of obesity and type 2 diabetes: Epidemiologic evidence. *Physiol. Behav.* **2010**, *100*, 47–54. [CrossRef] [PubMed]
11. Muckelbauer, R.; Libuda, L.; Clausen, K.; Toschke, A.M.; Reinehr, T.; Kersting, M. Promotion and provision of drinking water in schools for overweight prevention: Randomized, controlled cluster trial. *Pediatrics* **2009**, *123*, e661–e667. [CrossRef] [PubMed]
12. Dennis, E.A.; Flack, K.D.; Davy, B.M. Beverage consumption and adult weight management: A review. *Eat. Behav.* **2009**, *10*, 237–246. [CrossRef] [PubMed]
13. EFSA Panel on Dietetic Products, Nutrition, and Allergies (NDA): Scientific Opinion on Dietary reference values for water. *EFSA J.* **2010**, *8*, 1459.
14. Institute of Medicine, Panel on Dietary Reference Intakes for Electrolytes and Water: Dietary Reference Intakes for Water, Potassium, Sodium, Chloride and Sulfate. Food and Nutrition Board. Washington DC: The National Academies Press. 2005. Available online: http://www.nap.edu/openbook.php?isbn=0309091691 (accessed on 16 May 2016).
15. WHO (World Health Organisation). *Nutrients in Drinking Water*; WHO: Geneva, Switzerland, 2005.
16. National Health and Medical Research Council (NHMRC). Nutrients-Water. Available online: https://www.nrv.gov.au/nutrients/water (accessed on 17 July 2016).
17. Jéquier, E.; Constant, F. Water as an essential nutrient: The physiological basis of hydration. *Eur. J. Clin. Nutr.* **2012**, *64*, 115–123. [CrossRef] [PubMed]
18. Roman-Viñas, B.; Serra-Majem, L.; Hagströmer, M.; Ribas-Barba, L.; Sjöström, M.; Segura-Cardona, R. International physical activity questionnaire: Reliability and validity in a Spanish population. *Eur. J. Sport Sci.* **2010**, *10*, 297–304. [CrossRef]
19. Moreiras, O.; Carbajal, A.; Cabrera, L.; Cuadrado, C. *Tablas de Composición de Alimentos/Guía de Prácticas*, 16th ed.; Ediciones Pirámide: Madrid, Spain, 2013.
20. Sette, S.; Le Donne, C.; Piccinelli, R.; Arcella, D.; Turrini, A.; Leclercq, C.; On behalf of the INRAN-SCAI 2005-06 Study Group. The third Italian National Food Consumption Survey, INRAN-SCAI 2005-06—Part 1: Nutrient intakes in Italy. *Nutr. Metab. Cardiovasc. Dis.* **2011**, *21*, 922–932. [CrossRef] [PubMed]

21. Leclercq, C.; Arcella, D.; Piccinelli, R.; Sette, S.; Le Donne, C.; Turrini, A.; INRAN-SCAI 2005-06 Study Group. The Italian National Food Consumption Survey INRAN-SCAI 222 2005-06: Main results in terms of food consumption. *Public Health Nutr.* **2009**, *12*, 2504–2532. [CrossRef] [PubMed]

22. Craig, C.L.; Marshall, A.L.; Sjostrom, M.; Bauman, A.E.; Booth, M.L.; Ainsworth, B.E.; Pratt, M.; Ekelund, U.; Yngve, A.; Sallis, J.F.; et al. International physical activity questionnaire: 12-country reliability and validity. *Med. Sci. Sports Exerc.* **2003**, *35*, 1381–1395. [CrossRef] [PubMed]

23. Hagstromer, M.; Oja, P.; Sjostrom, M. The International Physical Activity Questionnaire (IPAQ): A study of concurrent and construct validity. *Public Health Nutr.* **2006**, *9*, 755–762. [CrossRef] [PubMed]

24. Hallal, P.C.; Victora, C.G. Reliability and validity of the International Physical Activity Questionnaire (IPAQ). *Med. Sci. Sports Exerc.* **2004**, *36*, 556. [CrossRef] [PubMed]

25. Etude Nutrinet-Santé. *Table de Composition des Aliments de L'étude Nutrinet-Santé*; Economica: Paris, France, 2013. (In French)

26. Hercberg, S.; Castetbon, K.; Czernichow, S.; Malon, A.; Mejean, C.; Kesse, E.; Touvier, M.; Galan, P. The Nutrinet-Sante Study: A web-based prospective study on the relationship between nutrition and healthand determinants of dietary patterns and nutritional status. *BMC Public Health* **2010**, *10*, 242. [CrossRef] [PubMed]

27. Statistical office of the European Union: Eurostat. Available online: http://ec.europa.eu/eurostat (accessed on 2 February 2017).

28. Ferreira-Pego, C.; Babio, N.; Fenandez-Alvira, J.M.; Iglesia, I.; Moreno, L.A.; Salas-Salvado, J. Fluid intake from beverages in Spanish adults; cross-sectional study. *Nutr. Hosp.* **2014**, *29*, 1171–1178. [PubMed]

29. Muckelbauer, R.; Sarganas, G.; Grüneis, A.; Müller-Nordhom, J. Association between water consumption and body weight outcomes: a systematic review. *Am. J. Clin. Nutr.* **2014**, *22*, 2462–2475. [CrossRef] [PubMed]

30. WHO/FAO (World Health Organization/Food and Agriculture Organization of the United Nations). *Diet, Nutrition and the Prevention of Chronic Diseases*; Report No. 916; World Health Organization: Geneva, Switzerland, 2002.

31. Guelinckx, I.; Ferreira-Pêgo, C.; Moreno, L.A.; Kavouras, S.A.; Gandy, J.; Martinez, H.; Bardosono, S.; Abdollahi, M.; Nasseri, E.; Jarosz, A.; et al. Intake of water and different beverages in adults across 13 countries. *Eur. J. Nutr.* **2015**, *54*, 45–55. [CrossRef] [PubMed]

32. WHO (World Health Organization). *Health and Ageing*; World Health Organization: Geneva, Switzerland, 2002.

33. Wakefield, B.J.; Mentes, J.; Holman, J.E.; Culp, K. Risk factors and outcomes associated with hospital admission for dehydration. *Rehabil. Nurs.* **2008**, *33*, 233–241. [CrossRef] [PubMed]

34. Hong, X.; Janet, B.; Campbell, E.S. Economical, Burden of Dehydration among elderly hospitalized patients. *Am. J. Health Syst. Pharm.* **2004**, *61*, 2534–2540.

35. Warren, J.L.; Bacon, W.E.; Haris, T.; Mcbean, A.M.; Foley, D.J.; Phillips, C. The burden and outcomes associated with dehydration among US elderly, 1991. *Am. J. Public Health* **1994**, *84*, 1265–1269. [CrossRef] [PubMed]

36. Frangeskou, M.; Lopez-Valcarcel, B.; Serra-Majem, L. Dehydration in the Elderly: A Review Focused on Economic Burden. *J. Nutr. Health Aging* **2015**, *19*, 619–627. [CrossRef] [PubMed]

37. Serra-Majem, L. Dietary assessment of micronutrient intakes: A European perspective. *Br. J. Nutr.* **2009**, *101*, S2–S5. [CrossRef] [PubMed]

38. Serra-Majem, L.; Santana-Armas, J.F.; Ribas, L.; Salmona, E.; Ramon, J.M.; Colom, J.; Salleras, L. A comparison of five questionnaires to assess alcohol consumption in a Mediterranean population. *Public Health Nutr.* **2002**, *5*, 589–594. [CrossRef] [PubMed]

39. Armstrong, B.K.; White, E.; Saracci, R. Monographs in Epidemiology and Biostatistics. In *Principles of Exposure Measurement in Epidemiology*; Oxford University Press: New York, NY, USA, 1994.

40. Kwan, M.L.; Kushi, L.H.; Song, J.; Timperi, A.W.; Boynton, A.M.; Johnson, K.M.; Standley, J.; Kristal, A.R. A practical method for collecting food record data in a prospective cohort study of breast cancer survivors. *Am. J. Epidemiol.* **2010**, *172*, 1315–1323. [CrossRef] [PubMed] ·

41. Nappo, S.A.; Iafrate, G.B.; Sanchez, Z.M. Motives for participating in a clinical research trial: A pilot study in Brazil. *BMC Public Health* **2013**, *13*, 19. [CrossRef]

42. Willett, W.C. *Nutritional Epidemiology*, 2nd ed.; Oxford University Press: New York, NY, USA, 1998.

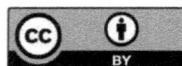

nutrients

MDPI

Article

Contribution of Water from Food and Fluids to Total Water Intake: Analysis of a French and UK Population Surveys

Isabelle Guelinckx [1], Gabriel Tavoularis [2], Jürgen König [3], Clémentine Morin [1], Hakam Gharbi [1] and Joan Gandy [4,5,*]

1   Hydration and Health Department, Danone Research, Palaiseau 91767, France; isabelle.guelinckx@danone.com (I.G.); clementine.morin@danone.com (C.M.); hakam.gharbi@danone.com (H.G.)
2   CREDOC (Centre de Recherche pour l'Etude et l'Observation des Conditions de Vie), Paris 75013, France; tavoularis@credoc.fr
3   Department of Nutritional Sciences, Faculty of Life Sciences, University of Vienna, Vienna 1090, Austria; juergen.koenig@univie.ac.at
4   British Dietetic Association, Birmingham B3 3HT, UK
5   School of Life and Medical Services, University of Hertfordshire, Hatfield AL10 9EU, UK
*   Correspondence: joan.gandy@btinternet.com; Tel.: +44-795-142-2767

Received: 30 July 2016; Accepted: 27 September 2016; Published: 14 October 2016

Abstract: Little has been published on the contribution of food moisture (FM) to total water intake (TWI); therefore, the European Food Safety Authority assumed FM to contribute 20%–30% to TWI. The aim of the present analysis was to estimate and compare TWI, the percentage of water from FM and from fluids in population samples of France and UK. Data from 2 national nutrition surveys (Enquête Comportements et Consommations Alimentaires en France (CCAF) 2013 and the National Diet and Nutrition Survey (NDNS) 2008/2009–2011/2012) were analyzed for TWI and the contribution of water from FM and fluids. Children and adults TWI were significantly lower in France than in the UK. The contribution of water from foods was lower in the UK than in France (27% vs. 36%). As TWI increased, the proportion of water from fluids increased, suggesting that low drinkers did not compensate by increasing intake of water-rich foods. In addition, 80%–90% of the variance in TWI was explained by differences in water intake from fluids. More data on the contribution of FM to TWI is needed to develop more robust dietary recommendations on TWI and guidance on fluid intake for the general public.

Keywords: total water intake; fluid intake; food moisture; adequate intake

---

1. Introduction

With increasing recognition of the relationship and understanding of the mechanism between water and beverage intake, hydration and health [1–4], it is important to develop evidence-based recommendations and guidelines for water intake. Recommendations, such as those published by the European Food Safety Authority (EFSA) on adequate intakes (AIs) of total water intake (TWI) [5], form the basis of public health strategies, intervention programs and food based dietary guidelines. Recommendations on the AI of total water are based partly (e.g., EFSA) [5], or wholly on population survey intake data (e.g., Institute of Medicine (IOM)) [6]. It is important to emphasize that these recommendations are for TWI, i.e., water from fluids (drinking water and water from all other beverages) and water from foods (food moisture (FM)).

The water content of foods is highly variable. For example, cucumber and lettuce are approximately 96% water, whole, boiled chicken eggs are 75% water, while digestive (semi-sweet)

biscuits contain only 2.8% water [7–10]. Clearly, the type and quantities of foods eaten will determine the contribution of FM in the overall diet to total water intake. Many factors influence the selection of foods including food availability, climate, cultural factors, health and economical status, age, psychosocial factors, religious factors and agricultural practices [11]. As a consequence, the amount of water obtained from food will vary between individuals and countries. For example, in China, food contributes 40% of TWI [12] while the IOM in USA estimated, when making its recommendations on AI of TWI, that, in adults, food contributed only 19% [6]. This was confirmed by a later analysis of the National Health and Nutrition Examination Surveys (NHANES) that estimated FM to be 19% in adults (NHANES 1999–2006) [13]. More recently, analyses of NHANES 2005–2010 have estimated FM to be 17%–25% in adults and 25%–30% in children aged 4–13 years [14,15]. In Mexico, FM has been estimated to be higher at 34.5% in children and adolescents aged 1–18 years [16] despite high intake of beverages by children in Mexico [17].

While data on the water content of foods are usually available in food composition tables and databases, the overall contribution of water in foods to TWI is seldom reported. In a recent survey of population nutrition and diet surveys in Europe, only one country reported calculating FM [18]. As a consequence of this lack of data, the EFSA assumed that the contribution of FM to TWI was 20%–30% when formulating their recommendations on AI of total water.

Dietary recommendations must be easily understood by the general public enabling them to know what they should eat and/or drink. Dietary reference values, such as EFSA's scientific opinion on TWI, need to be put into a clear and readily understandable format such as food based dietary guidelines (FBDG), e.g., the German three-dimensional food pyramid [19], or the UK's Eatwell Guide [20]. For TWI, it has to be considered that estimating water from food is difficult, if not impossible, for members of the general public. Therefore, FBDG should specify quantities of fluids (water and other beverages). Publications reporting on the mean water content of the population's food would facilitate more accurate FBDG on water intake. However, not only the mean but also the variability of the ratio of water from FM to water from fluid across the population should be analyzed in order to identify those food and fluids promoting adherence to the AI of water. It is possible that foods rich in FM may ensure adherence to AI of TWI. In addition, publications of observed intake of TWI would benefit the development of future recommendations.

Therefore, the aim of the present analysis was to estimate and compare TWI and the contribution of water from FM and fluids to TWI in two population surveys (France and UK). In addition, it aimed to compare the ratio of water from FM and Fluids according to deciles of TWI and adherence to EFSA AIs for TWI.

2. Materials and Methods

Data from two nationally representative population surveys were accessed and analyzed; the French nutrition survey (called Enquête Comportements et Consommations Alimentaires en France (CCAF) 2013 translated as the Survey of Nutritional Behavior and Intakes in France) and the UK's National Diet and Nutrition Survey (NDNS) 4 Year Rolling Programme 2008/2009–2011/2012.

2.1. The French Nutritional Survey (CCAF 2013)

The French survey was a descriptive, cross-sectional study conducted in 2012–2013 by the Research Centre for the Study of Life Conditions (CREDOC). This is a non-profit government organization that studies living and lifestyle conditions in France and periodically collects data about intake of food, energy, macro- and micronutrients of the French population.

The details of participant recruitment are consistent with the CREDOC methodology [21]. A quota method, taking into account age, socioeconomic level, region, town size and household size was used to recruit, through face-to-face interviews, a nationally representative sample of 2000 French households. The final sample for this analysis consisted of 901 children aged 3–18 years and 1062 adults aged 19 years and over. The data collection was conducted between October 2012 and

July 2013. To control for seasonal differences in intake, the study was carried out in four successive phases (October–December, January–March, April–mid-June, mid-June–July), during each of which approximately a quarter of the participants were included.

A seven-day diary was used to assess all dietary intake (fluids and solids). The participants received written instructions on how to complete the seven-day food and fluid diary. The diary was used to record information on all eating and drinking occasions throughout the day and for individual eating occasions. The circumstances of intake (time and location) were noted. Respondents completed the food diary with the aid of a validated photographic booklet [22], which presented various common foods and beverages in different portion sizes. Investigators ensured completeness of the seven-day diary through face-to-face interviews. The water content of reported intakes was obtained from a recognized French food composition table [23].

2.2. The UK Nutritional Survey (NDNS 2008/2009–2011/2012)

The NDNS is a survey of the health and diet of a nationally representative sample of adults and children in the UK. The present survey was funded by Public Health England (Department of Health) and the Food Standards Agency and conducted by NatCen Social Research, MRC Human Nutrition Research (HNR) and the University College London Medical School. It was conducted as a 4 year rolling programme from 2008/2009 to 2011/2012 [24] and all seasons were sampled.

One adult (aged 19 years and over) and one child (aged 1.5–18 years) were randomly selected from individual households. A sample was taken from a list of all addresses in the UK and clustered into Primary Sampling Units (PSUs) based on small geographical areas, which were randomly selected from postcode sectors. A sample of 21,573 addresses was then randomly selected from the PSUs, which had also been randomly selected. A total sample of 4156 individuals aged 1.5 and over (including 386 young children aged 1.5–2 years, 1687 children aged 3–18 years and 2083 adults aged 19 years and over) completed three or four dietary recording days for years 1–4 combined. To ensure comparability between age groups of both surveys, data from children aged less than four years was excluded in the NDNS sample. Some individuals later agreed to be interviewed by a nurse with fewer agreeing to give blood or urine samples. The data were weighted to minimize selection bias. All relevant research ethics and governance committees approved the survey.

Subjects were asked to complete a four-day estimated food diary with a randomly selected start date, which facilitated sampling across all days of the week. An interviewer visited the household to explain how to keep the four-day food diary. Interviewers visited or phoned the household on day two or three to check the ongoing diary completion and visited to review and collect the diary no more than three days after the final recording day. Photograph atlases were provided to aid estimation of portion sizes. Parents or carers assisted children aged 11 years and younger with completion of the diary. A trained nurse measured height and weight on a subsequent visit.

Completed diaries were coded and entered into HNR's dietary assessment system (DINO, Diet In Nutrients Out) that used food composition data from the Department of Health's NDNS Nutrient Database to estimate dietary intake of foods, including water and beverages and nutrients, including energy and water. Computerized raw data files and documentation from this survey were obtained under license from the UK Data Archive [25].

The food groups considered as fluids are shown in supplementary materials Table S1. Soup was categorized as a food and milk as fluid.

2.3. Statistical Analysis

The SAS 9.2 software (SAS Institute Inc., Cary, NY, USA) was used for statistical analysis. The data of TWI were normally distributed. Continuous variables are presented as mean and standard deviation as appropriate and dichotomous variables as frequency and percentage. The number and proportion of participants with an inadequate TWI was calculated by comparing TWI to the age and gender specific AI of TWI set by EFSA [5], which are shown in Table 1. General linear models were used to identify the variation in TWI due to water from fluids or FM.

Table 1. Dietary reference intakes (adequate intakes) for total water set by the European Food Safety Authority (EFSA) [5].

Age and Physiological Classes		Total Water Adequate Intake
Infants	0–6 months	680 mL/day through milk
	6–12 months	800–1000 mL/day
Children	1–2 years	1100–1200 mL/day
	2–3 years	1300 mL/day
	4–8 years	1600 mL/day
	9–13 years Boys	2100 mL/day
	Girls	1900 mL/day
	>14 years	Same as adults
Adults	Men	2500 mL/day
	Women	2000 mL/day
Pregnant women		+300 mL/day vs. adults
Lactating women		+600–700 mL/day vs. adults
Elderly		Same as adults

Before analyzing the four waves of NDNS as one sample, a statistical comparison between the waves was performed. A significant difference in TWI between waves was observed only among subjects aged 11–18 years ($p = 0.006$), and not among subjects aged 4–10 years, 19–64 years and $\geq$65 years. Since the difference in TWI between consecutive waves was on average 63 mL/day and not consistent across age groups, aggregating the four waves for analysis was considered appropriate.

Students' *t*-test was used for comparative statistics; a *p*-value < 0.05 was considered significant. These data were normally distributed and are reported as mean (SD). Data of water intake were not normally distributed and are reported as median (interquartile ranges (IQR)).

3. Results

There were significant differences in demographic data for the two countries as shown in Table 2. French children were significantly lighter ($p = 0.002$ and 0.001 for males and females, respectively); however, French children had significantly higher energy intakes ($p = 0.0007$ and < 0.0001 for males and females respectively). Similarly, UK adults were significantly heavier than French adults despite reporting significantly lower energy intakes.

Table 2. Demographics of the both survey samples.

	CCAF 2013		NDNS 2008/2009–2011/2012		*p*-Values	
	France		UK			
	Males	Females	Males	Females	Males	Females
4–18 years						
Sample size	478	423	859	828		
Weight (kg)	41 ± 17	41 ± 17	45 ± 13	44 ± 14	0.0002	0.0001
Height (m)	146 ± 23	144 ± 21	148 ± 15	145 ± 14	0.1407	0.5264
Energy Intake (kcal/day)	1906 ± 598	1636 ± 478	1802 ± 303	1540 ± 244	0.007	<0.0001
≥19 years						
Sample size	426	636	901	1182		
Weight (kg)	78 ± 14	65 ± 12	85 ± 20	72 ± 20	<0.0001	<0.0001
Height (m)	175 ± 8	163 ± 6	175 ± 10	161 ± 8	0.3374	0.0002
Energy Intake (kcal/day)	2229 ± 523	1832 ± 399	2109 ± 851	1588 ± 591	0.0018	<0.0001

Data are presented as mean ± standard deviation. Abbreviations: CCAF Enquête Comportements et Consommations Alimentaires en France, NDNS National Diet and Nutrition Survey.

3.1. Contribution of Water from Food Moisture and Fluids to Total Water Intake According to Country, Gender and Age Groups

TWI was significantly higher in males compared with females in France (p = 0.0055) and the UK (p < 0.0001) as shown in Table 3. Mean TWI in French children was significantly lower than UK children (p = 0.019). The contribution of water from fluids was consistently higher in the UK than in France, overall (73% vs. 64%) and for each age and gender category. In France, males had a higher proportion of water coming from fluids; however, in the UK, there was little difference between the genders for all age groups. Water intake from fluids and food moisture were significantly higher in UK adults than in French adults (both p < 0.0001).

Table 3. Contribution of water from food and fluids to total water intake (TWI) according to country, gender and age groups.

		N	TWI (mL/Day) *	Water from Fluids (mL/Day) *	% TWI	Water from Food (mL/Day) *	% TWI
CCAF 2013—France							
4–10 years	Males	252	1254 (1074–1519)	738 (616–912)	61%	483 (405–606)	39%
	Females	194	1213 (1016–1519)	752 (585–948)	64%	450 (372–549)	36%
11–18 years	Males	226	1510 (1255–1818)	951 (740–1182)	62%	560 (473–689)	38%
	Females	229	1382 (1143–1649)	846 (676–1055)	64%	520 (394–617)	36%
19–64 years	Males	324	1922 (1559–2273)	1188 (921–1573)	65%	671 (538–814)	35%
	Females	492	1763 (1437–2143)	1139 (840–1458)	66%	597 (488–745)	34%
≥65 years	Males	102	1929 (1699–2325)	1115 (874–1420)	59%	810 (664–972)	41%
	Females	144	1921 (1633–2373)	1130 (882–1460)	61%	782 (638–923)	39%
4–18 years	total	901	1358 (1114–1645)	825 (650–1055)	65%	508 (402–611)	35%
≥19 years	Males	426	1923 (1591–2281)	1186 (916–1532)	62%	697 (569–858)	38%
≥19 years	Females	636	1796 (1479–2199)	1135 (847–1458)	65%	631 (508–795)	35%
NDNS 2008/2009–2011/2012—UK							
4–10 years	Males	414	1253 (1045–1509)	837 (664–1056)	67%	418 (343–502)	33%
	Females	389	1225 (1016–1470)	789 (627–994)	67%	411 (328–508)	33%
11–18 years	Males	445	1588 (1289–1978)	1110 (860–1486)	72%	463 (367–570)	28%
	Females	439	1348 (1083–1678)	934 (699–1249)	72%	392 (316–482)	28%
19–64 years	Males	710	2415 (1890–3018)	1793 (1306–2369)	76%	573 (457–732)	24%
	Females	945	2060 (1692–2578)	1522 (1150–1981)	75%	536 (413–656)	25%
≥65 years	Males	191	2260 (1796–2703)	1645 (1200–2026)	72%	628 (503–764)	28%
	Females	237	2002 (1692–2468)	1466 (1170–1840)	72%	567 (460–665)	28%
4–18 years	total	1687	1352 (1102–1686)	920 (692–121)	67%	416 (337–522)	33%
≥19 years	Males	901	2386 (1875–2968)	1745 (1292–2289)	76%	591 (469–739)	24%
≥19 years	Females	1182	2050 (1692–2559)	1510 (1153–1921)	72%	542 (425–658)	28%

* Data presented as median (25th–75th percentile); Abbreviations: CCAF Enquête Comportements et Consommations Alimentaires en France, NDNS National Diet and Nutrition Survey, TWI total water intake.

3.2. Contribution of Water from Food Moisture and Fluids to TWI According to Deciles of Total Water Intake

Figure 1 shows TWI and the proportion of water from food and fluids split into deciles for male adults. In both countries, as TWI increased, the proportion of water from fluids increased accordingly. The finding was consistent in the female adults (supplementary materials Figure S1) and children (supplementary materials Figure S2).

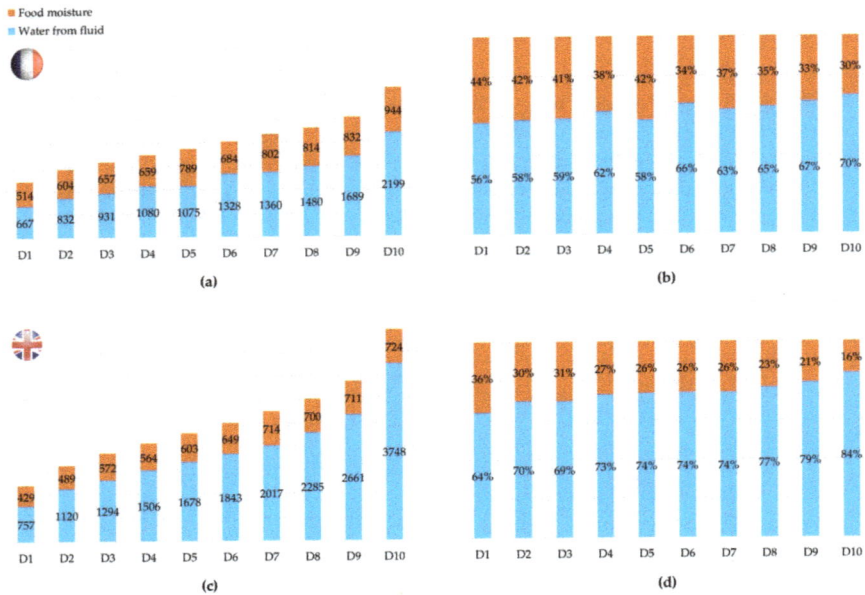

Figure 1. Volume and contribution to total water intake of water from fluid and food moisture in the male adult sample of the French 2013 survey called Enquête Comportements et Consommations Alimentaires en France (CCAF) (**a,b**) and the UK surveys called National Diet and Nutrition Survey (NDNS) 2008/2009–2011/2012 (**c,d**).

Figure 2 shows the relationship between TWI and water from food or fluids in adults (male and female) in France (a) and the UK (b). There was a higher correlation between TWI and water from fluids than between TWI and water from FM for adults in France ($R^2 = 0.8002$ vs. $R^2 = 0.3098$) and the UK ($R^2 = 0.9088$ vs. $R^2 = 0.2203$). These regressions suggested that 80%–90% of the variance in TWI was explained by differences in water intake from fluids. In children, the variance in TWI was explained by differences in water from fluids and to a lesser extent with water from foods ($R^2 = 0.7612$ vs. $R^2 = 0.4766$ in France and $R^2 = 0.8868$ vs. $R^2 = 0.2699$ in the UK; supplementary materials Figure S3).

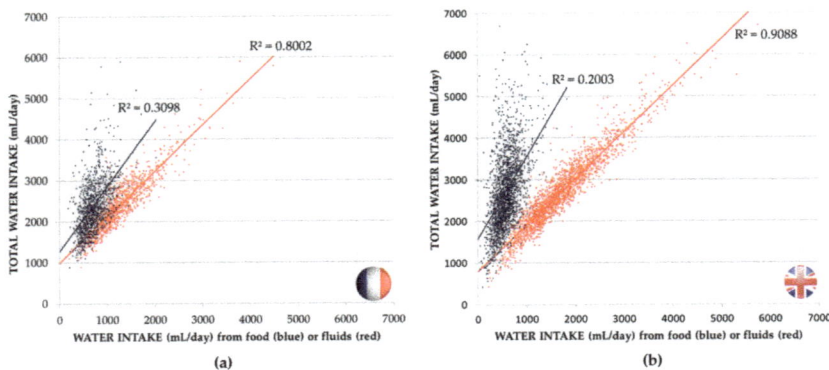

Figure 2. Water from food moisture (in **blue**) or total fluid intake (in **red**) as a function of total water intake in the adult sample of the French CCAF 2013 survey (**a**) and the UK NDNS 2008/2009–2011/2012 surveys (**b**).

3.3. Contribution of Water from Food Moisture and Fluids to TWI According to Adherence to EFSA Adequate Intake

In both countries, most children (88%–90%) had TWI below the EFSA recommendations for AI (Table 4). Fewer adults achieved the EFSA recommendations in France than in the UK; women were consistently more likely to have adequate intakes than men. In France, those who achieved the recommendations drank more than those who did not: children drank about 629 mL more and adults 804–884 mL more, representing a 6% to 7% higher contribution of water from fluids than from food. In the UK, there was a mean difference of 920–986 mL in water from fluids between those who achieved the recommendations and those who did not. This represented a 10% higher contribution of water from fluids to TWI than from food.

Table 4. Contribution of water from food moisture and water from fluids to total water intake of children (3–18 years), male and female adults (≥19 years) in France and UK according to intakes above or below the EFSA adequate intake (AI) of total water [5].

			TWI	Water from Fluids		Water from Food	
		N (%)	mL/Day *	mL/Day *	% TWI	mL/Day *	% TWI
CCAF 2013—France							
Children	<AI	811 (91%)	1310 (1082–1528)	786 (629–985)	62%	498 (398–593)	38%
	≥AI	85 (9%)	2079 (1849–2276)	1450 (1233–1641)	68%	627 (505–800)	32%
Male adults	<AI	435 (84%)	1832 (1534–2144)	1102 (879–1371)	62%	675 (546–810)	38%
	≥AI	82 (16%)	2752 (2609–3100)	1928 (1680–2195)	68%	870 (731–1093)	32%
Female adults	<AI	361 (64%)	1592 (1338–1776)	950 (754–1131)	61%	574 (473–714)	39%
	≥AI	199 (36%)	2384 (2167–2689)	1585 (1405–1964)	69%	778 (607–960)	31%
NDNS 2008/2009–2011/2012—UK							
Children	<AI	1477 (88%)	1288 (1056–1526)	864 (675–1093)	68%	404 (329–502)	32%
	≥AI	210 (12%)	2186 (1893–2665)	1688 (1349–2161)	78%	520 (405–637)	22%
Male adults	<AI	495 (56%)	1922 (1586–2204)	1326 (1089–1615)	71%	528 (422–658)	29%
	≥AI	406 (44%)	3086 (2794–3579)	2377 (2072–2883)	79%	682 (540–834)	21%
Female adults	<AI	538 (47%)	1661 (1396–1831)	1141 (907–1301)	69%	477 (374–580)	31%
	≥AI	644 (53%)	2493 (2227–2932)	1894 (1648–2312)	77%	606 (483–710)	23%

* Data presented as median (25th–75th percentile); Abbreviations: AI adequate intake, CCAF Enquête Comportements et Consommations Alimentaires en France, NDNS National Diet and Nutrition Survey, TWI total water intake.

4. Discussion

Given the increasing interest in water intake and health, it is important that population studies be designed and executed with due consideration of the methodological issues inherent in recording fluids. In addition to reporting, detailed information on TWI and its sources is essential. Therefore, this study aimed to analyze and report the contribution of water from fluids and food moisture to TWI in two nationally representative surveys. Independently of gender, adults (≥19 years) in the French survey had lower TWI intakes compared with UK adults. This finding is mirrored in studies of total fluid intake (TFI) with French adults having lower intakes compared with those in the UK [26]. The TWI observed in the 2008/2009–2011/2012 NDNS is comparable to the analysis of the 2002/2001 NDNS data, which showed that adult men had a TWI of 2.53 ± 0.86 L/day and women a TWI of 2.03 ± 0.71 [27]. The TWI of children was comparable to analyses of other TFI data sets that also showed lower TFI in French children compared with the UK [28]. The TWI for French children was comparable to data from another French national survey (INCA) conducted in 2006/2007 [29]. Data on TWI in children in the UK from other analyses have not been published to date.

Regardless of the difference in TWI between both surveys, many children and adults in both countries had TWI below the EFSA (2010) AIs. This was especially true for children, nearly 90% of whom had a TWI lower than the AI. However, the median intakes for UK adults were close to the recommendations. The French results are similar to those of Vieux et al. who reported that 89%–93% in children aged 4–13 years had intakes less than EFSA's AIs [29]. No comparable studies are available on TWI for the UK, although Iglesia et al. [28] and Gandy [30] have reported that 30%–56% of children and adolescents did not achieve the AIs when estimating TFI alone. Despite these differences, the present study and previous analyses show that the observed median intake of the sample is lower than the age- and gender-specific AI. However, when making such comparisons, it is important to consider the purpose of the AIs and how they were developed, and to only draw generalizable conclusions. The AIs are partly based on population intakes and are designed for population comparisons not for use in individuals. It is also important to note that, in the absence of hydration biomarkers, an intake below AI does not automatically equate to underhydration or dehydration. However, there is increasing evidence that, in children, dehydration and an increased fluid intake may impact cognitive and physical performance, and overall well-being [31–33]. Therefore, it would seem prudent to include biomarkers in future surveys in order to establish if those with reported low TWIs are at risk of mental and/or health issues.

There are undoubtedly many reasons for the differences in TWI between French and UK adults including climate, physical activity, assessment method and psychosocial factors. It is doubtful that these differences could be explained by climate, as while Northern France has a climate similar to the UK, the south is generally hotter than the UK. Likewise, since activity levels are low in both samples, they are unlikely to be explained by differences in physical activity levels. In addition, differences in methodologies may have contributed to these differences, even though both surveys used food diaries. Social factors are likely to explain some, if not most, of the variation. Dietary intake patterns vary between the countries. For example, Bellisle et al. estimated that, in France, 80%–87% of TFI was drunk *during* meals [34], and similarly Vieux et al. estimated that nearly 70% of all fluids are being consumed during three principle meals [29]. In the UK, the opposite was observed in a fluid specific survey; up to 70% of beverages were consumed *outside* of meals [30], when there are obviously more opportunities to consume fluids.

The importance of fluid intake to obtain a higher TWI was confirmed in the present analysis when looking at the contribution of FM to TWI. Indeed, the regression analyses demonstrated that differences in TWI were predominately due to differences in the amount of water from fluids. This was confirmed by the analysis of the ratio of FM and water from fluids by deciles of TWI; as the contribution of water from fluids to TWI increased 13%–20% between the first and tenth deciles in male adults in France and UK, respectively. However, the volume of this increase appeared more important (e.g., difference in male adults 1532 mL in France and 2991 mL in the UK). This analysis also suggests that participants with a low water intake from fluids did not compensate by having a higher intake of FM.

The mean percentage contribution of water from FM to TWI in the UK sample was consistently lower due to more fluids being consumed than among the French sample—27% and 36%, respectively. Similar values have been reported from earlier surveys in France: using data from the 2002/2003 CCAF survey Bellisle et al. estimated FM to be 36%–38% in French children and 36%–41% in French adults [34]. Similarly, Vieux et al. estimated FM to be 40% of TWI in French children aged 4–13 years [29]. In the UK, no specific data on FM have been reported for children; however, values of 23%–32% for all age groups (1.5–64 years) [35] and 25% in adults [27] have been reported, values in line with those in the present analysis. In other European countries, FM levels of 33%–38% have been reported in German children [36] and 32% for 9–75 year olds in Spain [37]. O'Connor has reported a FM of 33% for adults in the Republic of Ireland [38]. Therefore, the current analysis and the existing literature seem to confirm the EFSA's assumption that FM contributes for 20%–30% to TWI. However, this ratio may not be applicable to all European countries [5]. It would be beneficial if future national food surveys record and report both TWI and the contribution of water from FM and fluids. More primary data published on this topic will enable the development of robust dietary recommendations on TWI. Moreover, further exploration of the contribution of specific foods, especially high water content foods such as fruit and vegetables, to total FM may yield additional insight into these country differences, as would an exploration of social differences between countries regarding drinking and eating behavior.

The present analysis has several strengths. Both surveys used an estimated food diary, a method that is considered to be the most robust available dietary assessment method [39]. Using surveys with the same assessment method was a selection criterion since different methods could create a bias in the results. For example, fluids can be underestimated when intake is assess with a 24 h recall and, consequently, this could bias the ratio of water from FM/water from fluids [40]. The collection of data across all seasons in both surveys will have minimized seasonal variations in food choices e.g., variation in type and quality of fruit and vegetables or fluids consumed. Such variations would have influenced the findings in this study due to variations in FM.

However, some limitations in the present analysis must be acknowledged besides those inherent in dietary surveys. While both surveys are considered representative of the respective country's populations, the sampling methods were slightly different. The data from the UK is a summary of four years of a rolling program as opposed to France's one year survey, which is repeated on a three-year basis. This resulted in significantly different sample sizes, with over twice as many subjects being surveyed in the UK compared with France. Additionally, in France, a seven-day diary was used while a four-day diary was used in the UK. However the four-day diary used by NDNS was validated against the previously used seven-day diary, and, therefore, is considered as representative and comparable [41]. Any dietary survey is subject to potential errors inherent in the methodology, for example underreporting. In this analysis, energy intake was lower than in the UK than in France, despite UK children and adults being heavier. Interestingly, TWI and its sources were lower in France, clearly demonstrating the need for methodologies validated for specific nutrients.

5. Conclusions

The findings, together with the current literature, indicated that TWI and the contribution of water from FM and fluids were variable between countries. Also within one country, TWI as well as the contribution of water from FM varied greatly. More publications of primary data analysis from more countries on this topic are needed to develop more robust dietary recommendations on TWI and FBDG, preferably on fluid intake in addition to TWI. Water from fluids was shown to be the main driver of TWI. Encouraging the consumption of fluids, especially drinks that do not contribute to total energy intake such as water, seems therefor appropriate to increase TWI to the levels recommended by EFSA.

Supplementary Materials: The following are available online at http://www.mdpi.com/2072-6643/8/10/630/s1, Figure S1: Volume and contribution to total water intake of water from fluid and FM in the female adult sample of the French CCAF 2013 survey (a,b) and the UK NDNS (c,d) 2008/2009–2011/2012 surveys, Figure S2: Volume and contribution to total water intake of water from fluid and food moisture in the children's sample of the French CCAF 2013 survey (a,b) and the UK NDNS (c,d) 2008/2009–2011/2012 surveys, Figure S3: Water from food moisture (in blue) or total fluid intake (in red) as a function of total water intake in the children's sample (4–18 years) of the French CCAF 2013 survey (a) and the UK NDNS 2008/2009–2011/2012 surveys (b), Table S1: the categorization and codes of fluids used in analysis of the CCAF survey and NDNS survey.

Acknowledgments: CREDOC received funding for data access and data analysis, and J.G. for paper redaction from Danone Research. The costs to publish in open access were covered by Danone Research.

Author Contributions: J.G., I.G., H.G., C.M. and G.T. conceived and designed the experiments; G.T. analyzed the data; all authors contributed to data interpretation; and all authors contributed to the manuscript.

Conflicts of Interest: I.G., H.G., and C.M. are full-time employees of Danone Research. G.T. has received research funding of Danone Research. J.G. is a member of the fluid intake expert group of Danone Research. J.K. has no conflict of interest to declare.

References

1. Clark, W.F.; Sontrop, J.M.; Huang, S.H.; Moist, L.; Bouby, N.; Bankir, L. Hydration and chronic kidney disease progression: A critical review of the evidence. *Am. J. Nephrol.* **2016**, *43*, 281–292. [CrossRef] [PubMed]
2. Guelinckx, I.; Vecchio, M.; Perrier, E.T.; Lemetais, G. Fluid intake and vasopressin: Connecting the dots. *Ann. Nutr. Metab.* **2016**, *68*, 6–11. [CrossRef] [PubMed]
3. Melander, O. Vasopressin, from regulator to disease predictor for diabetes and cardiometabolic risk. *Ann. Nutr. Metab.* **2016**, *68*, 24–28. [CrossRef] [PubMed]
4. Popkin, B.M.; D'Anci, K.E.; Rosenberg, I.H. Water, hydration, and health. *Nutr. Rev.* **2010**, *68*, 439–458. [CrossRef] [PubMed]
5. EFSA Panel on Dietetic Products Nutrition and Allergies (NDA). Scientific opinion on dietary reference values for water. *EFSA J.* **2010**, *8*, 1459.
6. Institute of Medicine, Food and Nutrition Board. *Dietary Reference Intakes for Water, Potassium, Sodium, Chloride and Sulfate*; National Academies Press: Washington, DC, USA, 2004.
7. Food Composition and Diet Team, Public Health Directorate. Nutrient Analysis of Fish and Fish Products. 2013. Available online: https://www.gov.uk/government/publications/nutrient-analysis-of-fish (accessed on 10 July 2016).
8. Department of Health/Food Standards Agency. Nutrient Analysis of Biscuits, Buns, Cakes and Pastries—Summary Report. 2011. Available online: https://www.gov.uk/government/publications/nutrient-analysis-survey-of-biscuits-buns-cakes-and-pastries (accessed on 10 July 2016).
9. Food Composition and Diet Team, Public Health Directorate. Nutrient Analysis of Fruit and Vegetables. 2013. Available online: https://www.gov.uk/government/publications/nutrient-analysis-of-fruit-and-vegetables (accessed on 10 July 2016).
10. Food Composition and Diet Team, Public Health Directorate. Nutrient Analysis of Eggs. 2013. Available online: https://www.gov.uk/government/publications/nutrient-analysis-of-eggs (accessed on 10 July 2016).
11. Mela, D.J. Food choice and intake: The human factor. *Proc. Nutr. Soc.* **1999**, *58*, 513–521. [CrossRef] [PubMed]
12. Zhang, Q.; Hu, X.; Zou, S.; Zou, J.; Pan, Q.; Liu, C.; Pan, H.; Ma, G. Water intake of adults in four cities of China in summer. *Chin. J. Prev. Med.* **2011**, *45*, 677–682.
13. Kant, A.K.; Graubard, B.I.; Atchison, E.A. Intakes of plain water, moisture in foods and beverages, and total water in the adult US population—Nutritional, meal pattern, and body weight correlates: National health and nutrition examination surveys 1999–2006. *Am. J. Clin. Nutr.* **2009**, *90*, 655–663. [CrossRef] [PubMed]
14. Drewnowski, A.; Rehm, C.D.; Constant, F. Water and beverage consumption among adults in the United States: Cross-sectional study using data from NHANES 2005–2010. *BMC Public Health* **2013**, *13*, 1068. [CrossRef] [PubMed]
15. Drewnowski, A.; Rehm, C.D.; Constant, F. Water and beverage consumption among children age 4–13 years in the United States: Analyses of 2005–2010 NHANES data. *Nutr. J.* **2013**, *12*, 85. [CrossRef] [PubMed]
16. Piernas, C.; Barquera, S.; Popkin, B.M. Current patterns of water and beverage consumption among Mexican children and adolescents aged 1–18 years: Analysis of the mexican national health and nutrition survey 2012. *Public Health Nutr.* **2014**, *17*, 2166–2175. [CrossRef] [PubMed]
17. Guelinckx, I.; Iglesia-Altaba, I.; Bottin, J.H.; De Miguel-Etayo, P.; Gonzalez-Gil, E.M.; Salas-Salvado, J.; Kavouras, S.A.; Gandy, J.; Martinez, H.; Bardosono, S.; et al. Intake of water and beverages of children and adolescents in 13 countries. *Eur. J. Nutr.* **2015**, *54*, S69–S79. [CrossRef] [PubMed]
18. Gandy, J.; Le Bellego, L.; Konig, J.; Piekarz, A.; Tavoularis, G.; Tennant, D.R. Recording of fluid, beverage and water intakes at the population level in Europe. *Br. J. Nutr.* **2016**, *116*, 677–682. [CrossRef] [PubMed]
19. German Nutrition Society. Dreidimensionale DGE-Lebensmittelpyramide. Available online: https://www.dge.de/ernaehrungspraxis/vollwertige-ernaehrung/lebensmittelpyramide/ (accessed on 10 July 2016).
20. Public Health England; Welsh Government Food Standards Scotland; The Food Standards Agency Northern Ireland. *Eatwell Guide*; Public Health England: London, UK, 2016.
21. Hebel, P. *Comportements et Consommations Alimentaires en France*; Lavoisier: Paris, France, 2012.
22. Hercberg, S.; Deheeger, M.; Preziosi, P. *Su-vi-Max. Portions Alimentaires. Manuel Photos pour l'Estimation des Quantités*; Poly Technica: Paris, France, 1994.

23. French Agency for Food, Environmental and Occupational Health Safety. French Food Composition Table. Table Ciqual 2012. Available online: http://www.ansespro.fr/TableCIQUAL/ (accessed on 16 November 2015).

24. Bates, B.; Lennox, A.; Prentice, A.; Bates, C.; Page, P.; Nicholson, S.; Swan, G. *National Diet and Nutrition Survey Results from Years 1, 2, 3 and 4 (Combined) of the Rolling Programme (2008/2009–2011/2012)*; Public Health England Publications: London, UK, 2014.

25. University of Essex. UK Data Archive. Available online: http://www.data-archive.ac.uk (accessed on 15 November 2015).

26. Ferreira-Pego, C.; Guelinckx, I.; Moreno, L.A.; Kavouras, S.A.; Gandy, J.; Martinez, H.; Bardosono, S.; Abdollahi, M.; Nasseri, E.; Jarosz, A.; et al. Total fluid intake and its determinants: Cross-sectional surveys among adults in 13 countries worldwide. *Eur. J. Nutr.* **2015**, *54*, 35–43. [CrossRef] [PubMed]

27. Gibson, S.; Shirreffs, S.M. Beverage consumption habits "24/7" among British adults: Association with total water intake and energy intake. *Nutr. J.* **2013**, *12*, 9. [CrossRef] [PubMed]

28. Iglesia, I.; Guelinckx, I.; De Miguel-Etayo, P.M.; Gonzalez-Gil, E.M.; Salas-Salvado, J.; Kavouras, S.A.; Gandy, J.; Martinez, H.; Bardosono, S.; Abdollahi, M.; et al. Total fluid intake of children and adolescents: Cross-sectional surveys in 13 countries worldwide. *Eur. J. Nutr.* **2015**, *54*, 57–67. [CrossRef] [PubMed]

29. Vieux, F.; Maillot, M.; Constant, F.; Drewnowski, A. Water and beverage consumption among children aged 4–13 years in France: Analyses of INCA 2 (Etude Nationale des Consommations Alimentaires 2006–2007) data. *Public Health Nutr.* **2016**, *19*, 2305–2314. [CrossRef] [PubMed]

30. Gandy, J. First findings of the United Kingdom fluid intake study. *Nutr. Today* **2012**, *47*, S14–S16. [CrossRef]

31. Bar-David, Y. The effect of voluntary dehydration on cognitive functions of elementaty school children. *Acta Paediatr.* **2005**, *94*, 1667–1673. [CrossRef] [PubMed]

32. Kavouras, S.A.; Arnaoutis, G.; Makrillos, M.; Garagouni, C.; Nikolaou, E.; Chira, O.; Ellinikaki, E.; Sidossis, L.S. Educational intervention on water intake improves hydration status and enhances exercise performance in athletic youth. *Scand. J. Med. Sci. Sports* **2011**, *22*, 684–689. [CrossRef] [PubMed]

33. Landau, D.; Tovbin, D.; Shalev, H. Pediatric urolithiasis in southern Israel: The role of uricosuria. *Pediatr. Nephrol.* **2000**, *14*, 1105–1110. [CrossRef] [PubMed]

34. Bellisle, F.; Thornton, S.N.; Hebel, P.; Denizeau, M.; Tahiri, M. A study of fluid intake from beverages in a sample of healthy French children, adolescents and adults. *Eur. J. Clin. Nutr.* **2010**, *64*, 350–355. [CrossRef] [PubMed]

35. Ng, S.W.; Ni, M.C.; Jebb, S.A.; Popkin, B.M. Patterns and trends of beverage consumption among children and adults in Great Britain, 1986–2009. *Br. J. Nutr.* **2012**, *108*, 536–551. [CrossRef] [PubMed]

36. Sichert-Hellert, W.; Kersting, M.; Manz, F. Fifteen year trends in water intake in German children and adolescents: Results of the donald study. Dortmund nutritional and anthropometric longitudinally designed study. *Acta Paediatr.* **2001**, *90*, 732–737. [CrossRef] [PubMed]

37. Nissensohn, M.; Sanchez-Villegas, A.; Ortega, R.M.; Aranceta-Bartrina, J.; Gil, A.; Gonzalez-Gross, M.; Varela-Moreiras, G.; Serra-Majem, L. Beverage consumption habits and association with total water and energy intakes in the Spanish population: Findings of the anibes study. *Nutrients* **2016**, *8*, 232. [CrossRef] [PubMed]

38. O'Connor, L.; Walton, J.; Flynn, A. Water intakes and dietary sources of a nationally representative sample of Irish adults. *J. Hum. Nutr. Dietet.* **2014**, *27*, 550–556. [CrossRef] [PubMed]

39. Nelson, M.; Bingham, S. Assessment of food consumption and nutrient intake. In *Design Concepts in Nutritional Epidemiology*; Margetts, B., Nelson, M., Eds.; Oxford University Press: Oxford, UK, 1997; pp. 153–191.

40. Bardosono, S.; Monrozier, R.; Permadhi, I.; Manikam, N.; Rohan, R.; Guelinckx, I. Total fluid intake assessed with a seven-dayfluid record versus a 24 h dietary recall: A cross-over study in Indonesian adolescents and adults. *Eur. J. Nutr.* **2015**, *54*, 17–25. [CrossRef] [PubMed]

41. Henderson, L.; Gregory, J.; Swan, G. *National Diet and Nutrition Survey: Adults Aged 19 to 64 Years*; TSO: London, UK, 2002; Volume 1.

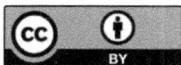

nutrients

MDPI

Article

Water and Beverage Consumption: Analysis of the Australian 2011–2012 National Nutrition and Physical Activity Survey

Zhixian Sui *, Miaobing Zheng, Man Zhang and Anna Rangan

Charles Perkins Centre, School of Life and Environmental Sciences, The University of Sydney,
Camperdown 2006, NSW, Australia; miaobing.zheng@sydney.edu.au (M.Z.);
mzha7338@uni.sydney.edu.au (M.Z.); anna.rangan@sydney.edu.au (A.R.)
* Correspondence: zhixian.sui@sydney.edu.au; Tel.: +61-2-8627-4751

Received: 16 August 2016; Accepted: 21 October 2016; Published: 26 October 2016

Abstract: Background: Water consumption as a vital component of the human diet is under-researched in dietary surveys and nutrition studies. Aim: To assess total water and fluid intakes and examine demographic, anthropometric, and dietary factors associated with water consumption in the Australian population. Methods: Dietary intake data from the 2011 to 2012 National Nutrition and Physical Activity Survey were used. Usual water, fluid and food and nutrient intakes were estimated from two days of dietary recalls. Total water includes plain drinking water and moisture from all food and beverage sources; total fluids include plain drinking water and other beverages, but not food moisture. Results: The mean (SD) daily total water intakes for children and adolescents aged 2–18 years were 1.7 (0.6) L for males and 1.5 (0.4) L for females, and for adults aged 19 years and over were 2.6 (0.9) L for males and 2.3 (0.7) L for females. The majority of the population failed to meet the Adequate Intake (AI) values for total water intake (82%) and total fluids intake (78%) with the elderly at highest risk (90%–95%). The contributions of plain drinking water, other beverages and food moisture to total water intake were 44%, 27%, and 29%, respectively, among children and adolescents, and 37%, 37% and 25% among adults. The main sources of other beverages were full-fat plain milk and regular soft drinks for children and adolescents, and tea, coffee, and alcoholic drinks for adults. For adults, higher total water intake was associated with lower percent energy from fat, saturated fat, and free sugars, lower sodium and energy-dense nutrient poor food intakes but higher dietary fibre, fruit, vegetable, caffeine, and alcohol intakes. No associations were found between total water consumption and body mass index (BMI) for adults and BMI z-score for children and adolescents. Conclusion: Reported water consumption was below recommendations. Higher water intakes were suggestive of better diet quality.

Keywords: water intake; dietary pattern; drinking water; diet quality; adults; children

1. Introduction

Water is an essential nutrient required for most of the body's functions. Evidence suggests that severe dehydration is associated with various clinical conditions, including impaired mental and physical performance, hypertension, urolithiasis, stroke, and certain cancers [1,2]. Even mild dehydration has been shown to impair cognitive functioning, alertness, and exercise capacity [3–5]. Despite the consistent evidence linking low water consumption and adverse health outcomes, water intake estimation in free-living populations with ad libitum access to water is lacking.

Recommended intakes for water have been set by a number of organizations although there is no single level of water intake that would ensure adequate hydration and optimal health in all environmental conditions. Requirements vary widely according to environmental conditions, physical activity, dietary intake and individual metabolism. The World Health Organization (WHO) guidelines [6] recommend 2.9 L per day for males and 2.2 L for females to maintain hydration, assuming average sedentary adults under average conditions. In reality, there is substantial scientific evidence relating to differences in water intake across gender, age, anthropometric, and socio-economic subgroups [7–10].

In Australia, the recommended Adequate Intake (AI) for total water (both fluids and food moisture) and total fluids (excluding food moisture) are set by the National Health and Medical Research Council (NHMRC) and are derived from the median intake estimates from the National Nutrition Survey [2]. The AIs for total water intake (including food moisture) for adults is 3.4 L for males, 2.8 L for females and 1.4–2.2 L for children/adolescents depending on age and gender [2]. The AIs for total fluids are set at 2.6 L for adult males, 2.1 L for adult females, and 1.0–1.9 L for children/adolescents.

The Australian Dietary Guidelines (ADG) encourage water as the fluid of choice and as a general guide for fluids, suggest about 4–5 cups of fluids a day for children up to 8 years, about 6–8 cups for adolescents, 8 cups for women (9 cups in pregnancy and lactation) and 10 cups for men [11]. There is currently little available data on water and fluid intake, beverage sources of intake, and whether recommendations are being met in the Australian population. Although many commonly consumed fluids provide water, they may also be acidic such as low-joule soft drink or contain added sugar, alcohol or caffeine. Recent evidence from the U.S. suggests that plain drinking water consumption is associated with better diet quality [12], and substituting water for sugary beverages is associated with reduced energy consumption and improved body weight management in both children/adolescents and adults [13,14]. However, knowledge of the role of water consumption on diet quality in the Australian population remains limited.

The present study aimed to assess total water and fluid intakes in a nationally representative sample of the Australian population and to examine demographic, anthropometric, and dietary correlates of total water consumption. The secondary aim was to examine the relationship between plain drinking water consumption and dietary factors. These findings will provide fundamental information for future guidelines and may assist further research in the area of water consumption and diet quality, demographic features, and specific health outcomes.

2. Materials and Methods

2.1. Respondents and Water Intake Data Collection

The present study analysed data from the National Nutrition and Physical Activity Survey (NNPAS) 2011–2012, undertaken by the Australian Bureau of Statistics (ABS). The survey was conducted between May 2011 and June 2012, in adults and children/adolescents aged two years and over. Ethics approval for the survey was granted by the Australian Government Department of Health and Ageing Departmental Ethics Committee in 2011. Further details about the scope and the methodology of the survey are available from the NNPAS Users Guide [15]. A total of 12,153 respondents were interviewed face-to-face for the collection of dietary intake data using an Automated Multiple-Pass 24-h recall [15] and a second 24-h recall was collected from 7735 respondents via a telephone interview. Respondents were specifically probed regarding water intake and other beverages. After each 24-h recall the respondents were asked additional questions about the intake and main source of plain drinking water. This systematic process has been validated to be effective in maximizing the respondents' ability to recall and report foods eaten in the previous 24 h [15]. For children under 15 years of age, parents/guardians were used as proxies. Where permission was granted by a parent/guardian, adolescents aged 15–17 years old were interviewed in person. If permission was not granted, questions were answered by an adult [15]. The validity of proxy report for children's 24-h dietary intake data collection has been reported previously [16]. A food composition database, AUSNUT 2011–2013, developed specifically for NNPAS 2011–2012, was used to estimate water, fluid, food moisture, foods, beverages, and nutrient intakes [17].

2.2. Water, Moisture, and Food Sources

In this study, intake of total water was defined as plain drinking water plus other beverages, and food moisture, in line with the descriptions in the Nutrition Reference Values for Australia and New Zealand [2]. Plain drinking water included tap water (domestic tap, tank or rain water) and bottled water (packaged with- and without fortified water). Other beverages included moisture obtained from tea (regular, decaffeinated and herbal tea), coffee (regular, decaffeinated and coffee beverage), fruit/vegetable juice (freshly and commercially prepared, fortified fruit juice), fruit drinks (ready to drink, prepared from concentrated and dry powder), regular/diet cordial, regular/diet soft drinks, energy/sport drinks, full/reduced fat milk, flavoured milk, milk substitute, alcoholic drinks, and other flavoured and non-flavoured beverage drinks. Water used to dilute concentrated drinks was categorized according to the beverage type. Milk added to tea, coffee, and breakfast cereal was separated and categorized according to milk type.

2.3. Anthropometry, Demographic, and Other Characters

Respondents' weight, height, and waist circumference (WC) were objectively measured. Body Mass Index (BMI) for adults was calculated as weight (kg) divided by height squared (m^2). BMI z-scores for children/adolescents were calculated using World Health Organization age-and gender-specific growth charts [18]. Age groups were categorized based on the NNPAS age categories (2–3, 4–8, 9–13, 14–18, 19–30, 31–50, 51–70, and 70+ years) and socio-economic quintiles were based on the Socio-Economic Index of Disadvantage for Areas (SEIFA), where the first SEIFA quintile indicates the most disadvantaged areas [19]. Lifestyle factors including total minutes of physical activity during the past week and total sleep duration the day prior to the interview were self-reported at the time of interview.

2.4. Dietary Factors

The term "core food groups" as used in this study refers to grains, vegetables, fruits, dairy products, and meat and alternatives, as described in the Australian Guide to Healthy Eating (AGHE) [11,20]. To assess consumption of all foods within a food group, all individually recorded food items and foods as part of a mixed dish were included. The individual food components from a mixed dish were estimated using the AUSNUT 2011–2013 recipe file [17] and were classified under their respective core food group. Discretionary foods (solid) such as cakes, biscuits, confectionary, deep-fried fast foods, and processed meat, and discretionary beverages such as soft drinks, fruit drinks and alcoholic drinks are defined as "foods high in saturated fat and/or added sugars, added salt or alcohol and low in fibre" and were categorized accordingly [19].

2.5. Misreporting

Misreporting has been identified in the NNPAS 2011–2012 survey, with 16%–26% of the respondents classified as under-reporting total energy intake [19]. To enable a more accurate interpretation of dietary data, it has been suggested that analysis be conducted with and without potential under- and over-reporters [21–23]. Plausible reporters were identified based on the Goldberg cut-off (energy intake: basal metabolic rate 0.92–2.17 for usual intake from 2 days' data) [24]. The Goldberg cut-offs have been validated for use with data from 24-h recalls [25]. In this paper, only the results from plausible-reporters are presented.

2.6. Statistical Analysis

Statistical analyses were performed using SPSS for Windows 22.0 software (IBM Corp. Released 2013. IBM SPSS Statistics for Windows, Version 22.0., Armonk, NY, USA). Respondent's usual intakes of plain drinking water, other beverages, food moisture, core food groups, and discretionary foods/beverages from the two 24-h recalls were analysed using the Multiple Source Method [26] (presented in Tables 1, 2 and 4 and Figure 1). Only the first day of recall was used to examine proportions of contributions to total water intake (Table 3 and Figure 2). Descriptive statistics were used to report the total water intake according to different characteristics. Children/adolescents and adults were analysed separately and also by gender due to the different recommended intakes [2]. Data were presented as the per capita mean and standard deviation (SD), median and the 25th and 75th percentiles, or as a percentage (%). Total water intake was categorized into quartiles to assess respondents' characteristics and dietary intakes. Chi-square tests and ANOVA analysis were used to assess the differences between proportions and to compare mean differences in consumption and linear trends where appropriate. Median differences were compared using Kruskal-Wallis tests. Multiple linear regression methods were used to examine the relationship between usual plain drinking water intake and covariates including gender, age, socio-economic status, and dietary factors, adjusted for total energy intake and physical activity level. For all tests, a *p*-value of < 0.05 was considered statically significant.

3. Results

3.1. Total Water Intake

Data presented in Table 1 show total water intake in children/adolescents and adults, by gender and age groups. Per capita total water intakes for children/adolescents were 1.7 L and 1.5 L for boys and girls, respectively, and for adults were 2.6 L and 2.3 L for males and females, respectively. Total water intake increased with older age in children/adolescents (ANOVA trend *p* < 0.001) but declined for adults (*p* < 0.001). Large variation was observed in the inter-quartile ranges for fluids intake particularly for adolescent boys and adult males.

Total water intake and total fluids intake were compared to age and gender specific AI values (Figure 1). Overall, about 18% of the respondents met AI for total water, and 22% met AI for total fluids. These proportions did not vary significantly between age groups for children/adolescents, but declined with increasing age in adults (*p* < 0.001) with only 5% of men and 10% of women aged over 71 years meeting the AI.

Table 2 presents the demographic, anthropometric, lifestyle, and dietary characteristics by quartile of total water intake. Age, gender, season of interview, country of birth and socioeconomic status were significantly associated with total water intake among children/adolescents and/or adults, and were thus adjusted for in subsequent analysis.

Among children/adolescents, total water intake was positively associated with waist circumference, but not BMI z-score. Children/adolescents reporting higher total water intake had greater intakes of energy, protein (as percent energy, %E), dietary fibre (%E), and fruit (g/Mj) and dairy products (g/Mj) but lower total fat (%E), saturated fat (%E), free sugar (%E), sodium (mg/Mj), and discretionary foods (g/Mj).

Among adults, being born in non-English speaking countries and categorized in the lowest socio-economic quintile were associated with lower total water intake. No BMI gradient for total water intake was observed. Adults reporting higher total water intake also reported higher intakes of energy, dietary fibre (%E) and caffeine (mg/Mj) but lower intakes of total fat (%E), saturated fat (%E), total carbohydrates (%E), free sugar (%E), sodium (mg/Mj). Higher food densities of vegetable, fruits, dairy products, and alcoholic drinks but lower densities of grains and discretionary foods/beverages were also reported by those with higher total water intakes.

3.2. Sources of Water

The contributions from different sources to total water intake are presented in Table 3. Plain drinking water, mostly obtained from tap water, was the most common source of total water intake, but children/adolescents and adults reported different choices of other beverages.

Among children/adolescents the contributions of plain drinking water, other beverages, and food moisture to total water intake were 44.1%, 26.9%, and 29.0%, with full-fat plain milk being the most common other beverage followed by regular soft drinks and fruit juice. Analysis of different sources of total water intake by age indicated that older children/adolescents reported a higher proportion of total water from tea/coffee, soft/sports drinks, and alcoholic drinks but a lower proportion from juice, fruit drinks/cordials and milk.

Among adults, the proportions of plain drinking water, other beverages, and food moisture to total water intake were 37.4%, 25.2%, and 37.4%. Apart from plain drinking water, tea, coffee, and alcoholic drinks were the largest contributors to total water intake, with older adults reporting larger proportions of total water intake from tea, coffee, reduced fat and skim milk, and food moisture compared with younger adults.

Figure 2 summarises the principal sources of total water intake by gender. Among children/ adolescents, girls reported higher proportions from plain drinking water and food moisture compared to boys. Boys reported larger proportions of soft/sports drinks, fruit drinks/cordials, and alcoholic drinks than girls. Among adults, females were more likely than males to consume plain drinking water and tea/coffee, whereas males consumed higher proportions of soft/sports drinks, fruit drinks/cordials, and alcoholic drinks than females. Notably, adult males reported higher intakes of other beverages (39.4% total water intake) than plain drinking water (34.7%) ($p < 0.001$).

Table 1. Total water and total fluids intakes (L) by gender and age groups.

Children/Adolescents		Age (Years)	2–18	2–3	4–8	9–13	14–18	p-Value *
Males		n	1017	159	295	294	269	
	Total water	AI		1.4	1.6	2.2	2.7	
		Mean (SD)	1.7 (0.6)	1.2 (0.4)	1.5 (0.4)	1.7 (0.5)	2.1 (0.6)	<0.001
		Median (IQR)	1.6 (1.3–2.0)	1.2 (1.0–1.4)	1.4 (1.2–1.7)	1.7 (1.4–2.0)	2.0 (1.6–2.5)	<0.001
	Total fluids	AI		1.0	1.2	1.6	1.9	
		Mean (SD)	1.2 (0.5)	0.9 (0.3)	1.0 (0.4)	1.3 (0.4)	1.6 (0.6)	<0.001
		Median (IQR)	1.1 (0.9–1.5)	0.8 (0.6–1.1)	1.0 (0.8–1.2)	1.2 (1–1.5)	1.5 (1.1–1.9)	<0.001
	Food moisture	Mean (SD)	0.4 (0.2)	0.4 (0.1)	0.4 (0.1)	0.5 (0.1)	0.5 (0.2)	<0.001
		Median (IQR)	0.4 (0.3–0.5)	0.3 (0.3–0.4)	0.4 (0.3–0.5)	0.4 (0.4–0.6)	0.5 (0.4–0.6)	<0.001
Females		n	953	160	276	295	222	
	Total water	AI		1.4	1.6	1.9	2.2	
		Mean (SD)	1.5 (0.4)	1.1 (0.3)	1.3 (0.3)	1.3 (0.3)	1.7 (0.5)	<0.001
		Median (IQR)	1.4 (1.1–1.7)	1.1 (0.9–1.3)	1.2 (1.1–1.5)	1.6 (1.3–1.8)	1.7 (1.4–2)	<0.001
	Total fluids	AI		1.0	1.2	1.4	1.6	
		Mean (SD)	1.0 (0.4)	0.8 (0.3)	0.9 (0.3)	1.1 (0.4)	1.3 (0.4)	<0.001
		Median (IQR)	1.0 (0.8–1.3)	0.7 (0.6–0.9)	0.8 (0.7–1.1)	1.1 (0.9–1.3)	1.2 (1.0–1.5)	<0.001
	Food moisture	Mean (SD)	0.4 (0.1)	0.4 (0.1)	0.4 (0.1)	0.5 (0.1)	0.5 (0.2)	<0.001
		Median (IQR)	0.4 (0.3–0.5)	0.4 (0.3–0.4)	0.4 (0.3–0.5)	0.4 (0.4–0.5)	0.4 (0.3–0.5)	<0.001

Adults		Age (Years)	19+	19–30	31–50	51–70	71+	p-Value
Males		n	2999	553	1160	925	361	
	Total water	AI	3.4	3.4	3.4	3.4	3.4	
		Mean (SD)	2.6 (0.9)	2.8 (1.0)	2.7 (0.9)	2.5 (0.8)	2.2 (0.6)	<0.001
		Median (IQR)	2.4 (2.0–3.0)	2.6 (2.1–3.3)	2.5 (2.1–3.1)	2.4 (2–2.9)	2.1 (1.8–2.5)	<0.001
	Total fluids	AI	2.6	2.6	2.6	2.6	2.6	
		Mean (SD)	2.0 (0.8)	2.2 (0.9)	2.1 (0.8)	1.9 (0.7)	1.6 (0.5)	<0.001
		Median (IQR)	1.8 (1.4–2.4)	2.0 (1.6–2.7)	2.0 (1.6–2.5)	1.8 (1.4–2.3)	1.5 (1.2–1.8)	<0.001
	Food moisture	Mean (SD)	0.6 (0.2)	0.6 (0.2)	0.6 (0.2)	0.6 (0.2)	0.6 (0.2)	ns
		Median (IQR)	0.6 (0.4–0.7)	0.5 (0.5–0.7)	0.5 (0.4–0.7)	0.6 (0.5–0.7)	0.6 (0.5–0.7)	ns
Females		n	3233	548	1189	1024	472	
	Total water	AI	2.8	2.8	2.8	2.8	2.8	
		Mean (SD)	2.3 (0.7)	2.2 (0.7)	2.4 (0.7)	2.3 (0.7)	2.0 (0.6)	<0.001
		Median (IQR)	2.2 (1.8–2.7)	2.1 (1.8–2.6)	2.3 (1.9–2.7)	2.2 (1.8–2.7)	2.0 (1.6–2.3)	<0.001
	Total fluids	AI	2.1	2.1	2.1	2.1	2.1	
		Mean (SD)	1.8 (0.6)	1.7 (0.6)	1.9 (0.7)	1.8 (0.6)	1.5 (0.5)	<0.001
		Median (IQR)	1.7 (1.3–2.1)	1.6 (1.3–2.1)	1.8 (1.4–2.2)	1.7 (1.3–2.1)	1.4 (1.1–1.8)	<0.001
	Food moisture	Mean (SD)	0.5 (0.2)	0.5 (0.2)	0.5 (0.2)	0.5 (0.2)	0.5 (0.2)	ns
		Median (IQR)	0.5 (0.4–0.6)	0.5 (0.4–0.6)	0.5 (0.4–0.6)	0.5 (0.4–0.6)	0.5 (0.4–0.6)	ns

* p-value for trends analysis (ANOVA) for means; Kruskal-Wallis tests for medians; ns: not statistically significant; AI: Adequate Intake (L/day); IQR: 25th–75th percentile; SD: Standard Deviation.

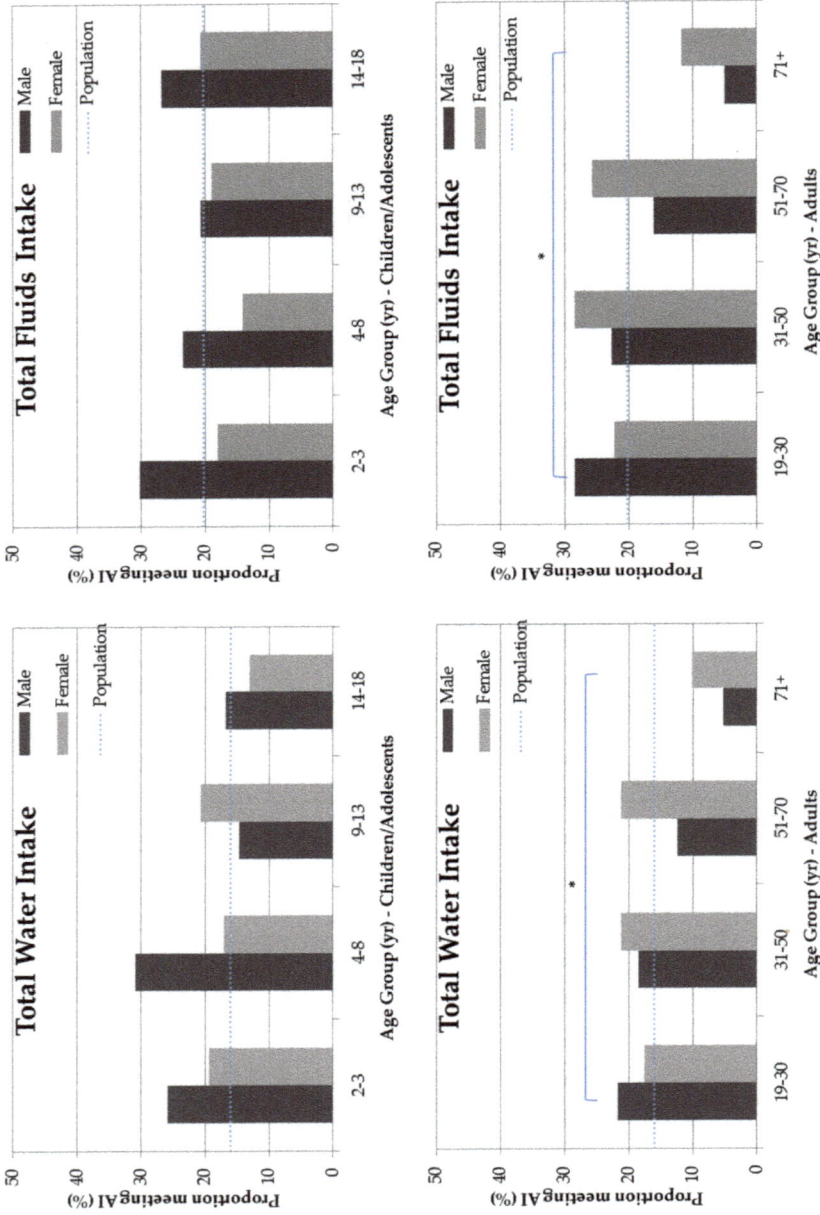

Figure 1. The proportion of the respondents (%) meeting the adequate intake (AI) for total water intake and total fluids intake. * significant trend with age (ANOVA) ($p < 0.001$).

Table 2. Anthropometric, demographic, and lifestyle characteristics by quartile of total water intakes in children/adolescents and adults.

Quartiles	Children/Adolescents					Adults				
	Q1 (<1.2)	Q2 (1.2-1.5)	Q3 (1.5-1.8)	Q4 (>1.8)	p-Value *	Q1 (<1.9)	Q2 (1.9-2.3)	Q3 (2.3-2.8)	Q4 (>2.8)	p-Value *
Mean total water intake (L)	1.0 (0.1)	1.3 (0.1)	1.7 (0.1)	2.3 (0.4)	<0.001	1.6 (0.2)	2.1 (0.1)	2.5 (0.1)	3.5 (0.7)	<0.001
Demographic										
Age (year)	5.7 (3.9)	8.4 (4.5)	10.3 (4.4)	12.9 (3.4)	<0.001	52.1 (19.4)	49.8 (17.5)	48.3 (16.6)	44.9 (15.3)	<0.001
Male (%)	39.1	50.2	51.7	65.4	<0.001	37.0	44.0	50.4	61.0	<0.001
Interviewed in summer (%)	25.4	24.6	26.8	32.7	<0.001	25.0	28.7	28.8	29.3	<0.001
Born in NE countries (%) +	5.3	5.5	6.5	6.3	ns	19.8	17.1	16.0	13.2	<0.001
Lowest SES quintile (%)	16.6	17.3	16.6	14.8	ns	21.0	16.6	16.8	16.5	0.01
Highest SES quintile (%)	24.1	25.8	28	26	ns	22.7	24.6	25.2	24.0	ns
Anthropometric^										
BMI (z-score for children, kg/m² for adults)	0.5 (1.2)	0.4 (1.2)	0.5 (1.1)	0.7 (1.1)	ns	27.1 (0.4)	27.7 (0.4)	27.3 (0.4)	27.5 (0.4)	ns
Waist circumference (cm)	63.9 (0.8)	64.7 (0.8)	64.8 (0.7)	67.3 (0.8)	<0.001	99.9 (4.2)	100.8 (4.2)	97.9 (4.1)	100.3 (4.2)	ns
Lifestyle^										
Physical activity in last week (min)	104.2 (26.3)	213.1 (20.1)	260.2 (11.5)	252.3 (14.1)	ns	199.7 (18)	231.5 (17.9)	251.3 (17.8)	290.1 (18.2)	<0.001
Sleep duration (min)	581.4 (10.8)	593.2 (8.3)	590.4 (7.5)	583.6 (7.6)	ns	479.1 (4.8)	477.2 (4.8)	473.3 (4.8)	465.9 (4.9)	0.001
Currently smoking (%)	-	-	-	-	-	14.3	14.4	14.1	14.3	ns
Nutrients^										
Water density (L/Mj)	0.15 (0.1)	0.19 (0.1)	0.22 (0.1)	0.27 (0.1)	<0.001	0.20 (0.1)	0.25 (0.04)	0.29 (0.1)	0.36 (0.2)	0.001
Energy (Mj)	7.2 (0.2)	7.8 (0.2)	8.3 (0.2)	9.2 (0.2)	<0.001	8.5 (0.1)	9.2 (0.1)	9.6 (0.1)	10.4 (0.1)	<0.001
Protein (%E)	15.9 (0.4)	15.7 (0.4)	16.6 (0.4)	16.7 (0.4)	0.001	17.6 (0.3)	17.7 (0.3)	17.9 (0.3)	18.0 (0.3)	ns
Total fat (%E)	32.4 (0.7)	31.5 (0.6)	31.1 (0.6)	30.3 (0.7)	0.002	32.7 (0.4)	31.8 (0.4)	31.2 (0.4)	29.9 (0.4)	<0.001
Saturated fat (%E)	14.1 (0.4)	14.1 (0.4)	13.7 (0.4)	13.4 (0.4)	0.03	13.3 (0.2)	12.7 (0.2)	12.2 (0.2)	11.7 (0.2)	<0.001
Total carbohydrates (%E)	49.1 (0.8)	50.2 (0.7)	49.5 (0.7)	49.8 (0.8)	ns	43.8 (0.5)	43.4 (0.5)	42.7 (0.5)	41.4 (0.5)	<0.001
Free sugar (%E)	11.9 (2.3)	11.4 (1.8)	10.4 (1.5)	10.3 (1.3)	<0.001	9.5 (1.0)	9.0 (0.9)	8.5 (0.9)	8.2 (0.7)	<0.001
Dietary fibre (%E)	1.9 (0.1)	2.0 (0.1)	2.1 (0.1)	2.2 (0.1)	<0.001	2.0 (0.1)	2.2 (0.1)	2.2 (0.1)	2.3 (0.1)	<0.001
Sodium (mg/Mj)	298.4 (10.3)	285.6 (9.4)	279.4 (9.4)	292 (10.3)	0.04	286.2 (6)	279.1 (6)	276.7 (6)	268.4 (6.1)	0.001
Caffeine (mg/Mj)	2.2 (0.4)	1.9 (0.4)	2.0 (0.4)	2.3 (0.4)	ns	17.0 (1.0)	19.6 (1)	22.0 (1)	23.1 (1.0)	<0.001
Food groups^										
Grains (g/Mj)	22.8 (0.9)	21.7 (0.8)	22.4 (0.8)	22.6 (0.9)	ns	20.8 (0.5)	20.4 (0.4)	20.4 (0.4)	19.7 (0.5)	0.02
Vegetable (g/Mj)	16.4 (0.8)	15.3 (0.7)	16.2 (0.7)	16.4 (0.8)	ns	20.8 (0.5)	21.2 (0.5)	21.9 (0.5)	21.9 (0.5)	0.005
Fruits (g/Mj)	21.8 (1.4)	24 (1.3)	24 (1.3)	24.9 (1.4)	0.03	17.7 (0.7)	19.2 (0.7)	19.4 (0.7)	20.2 (0.7)	<0.001
Dairy products (g/Mj)	30.4 (2.0)	31 (1.8)	32.9 (1.8)	34.7 (2.0)	0.02	25.3 (0.8)	26.4 (0.8)	26.9 (0.8)	26.7 (0.8)	0.048
Meat and alternatives (g/Mj)	12.4 (0.6)	11.6 (0.5)	12.1 (0.5)	12.3 (0.6)	ns	15.1 (0.3)	14.8 (0.3)	14.9 (0.3)	15 (0.3)	ns
Discretionary foods (g/Mj)	23.2 (0.9)	21.7 (0.8)	19.8 (0.8)	20.4 (0.9)	<0.001	18.4 (0.4)	17.3 (0.4)	16.3 (0.4)	16.1 (0.4)	<0.001
Discretionary beverages (g/Mj)	26.7 (2.2)	26.5 (2)	24.1 (2)	25.8 (2.2)	ns	21.7 (0.9)	20.6 (0.9)	19.4 (0.9)	18.1 (1.0)	<0.001
Alcoholic drinks (g/Mj)	-	-	-	-	-	14.7 (1.7)	18.7 (1.7)	22.3 (1.7)	34.3 (1.7)	<0.001

* Trends analysis (ANOVA) for p-values for mean; Chi-square tests for p-values for proportion; + Born in non-English speaking countries; ^ Adjusted for age, gender, whether born in non-English speaking countries, and season of interview; ns: not statistically significant; %E: percentage energy.

Table 3. Proportion of contribution by sources of total water intake (%) by age group (year).

Children/Adolescents	2-18	2-3	4-8	9-13	14-18	p-Value *	Adults	19+	19-30	31-50	51-70	71+	p-Value
Plain drinking water	44.1	39.1	45.1	44.2	44.4	ns	**Plain drinking water**	37.4	43.9	38.7	32.0	29.5	<0.001
Tap water	42.0	38.1	42.7	42.0	42.3	ns	Tap water	33.7	39.4	34.7	28.9	28.1	<0.001
Bottled water	2.1	1.0	2.4	2.2	2.1	ns	Bottled water	3.8	4.5	4.0	3.1	1.3	<0.001
Tea/coffee	1.4	0.2	0.4	0.7	3.3	<0.001	**Tea/coffee**	16.2	8.1	16.0	21.2	24.2	<0.001
Tea	0.9	0.2	0.4	0.6	1.6	<0.001	Tea	8.2	4.3	7.2	11.2	14.7	<0.001
Coffee	0.5	<0.1	<0.1	0.1	1.6	<0.001	Coffee	7.9	3.8	8.8	10.1	9.5	<0.001
Juices	3.1	3.6	3.4	2.9	2.9	<0.001	**Juices**	1.7	2.0	1.6	1.5	1.6	<0.001
Fruit Juice	3.1	3.5	3.4	2.9	2.9	<0.001	Fruit Juice	1.6	2.0	1.5	1.4	1.4	<0.001
Vegetable Juice	<0.1	<0.1	<0.1	<0.1	<0.1	ns	Vegetable Juice	0.1	<0.1	<0.1	0.1	0.2	ns
Milk	10.1	17.4	10.0	9.9	8.5	<0.001	**Milk**	4.8	5.0	4.5	4.8	6.4	<0.001
Plain Milk (Full Fat)	6.3	14.1	6.7	5.8	4.4	<0.001	Plain Milk (Full Fat)	2.1	2.5	1.9	1.9	2.4	ns
Plain Milk (Reduced Milk)	1.7	2.3	1.8	1.8	1.4	ns	Plain Milk (Reduced Milk)	1.5	1.1	1.4	1.7	2.5	<0.001
Plain Milk (Skim)	0.4	0.4	0.4	0.5	0.2	ns	Plain Milk (Skim)	0.6	0.4	0.5	0.7	1.0	<0.001
Flavoured Milk	1.7	0.5	1.2	1.7	2.5	<0.001	Flavoured Milk	0.7	1.0	0.8	0.5	0.4	<0.001
Milk substitute	<0.1	<0.1	<0.1	<0.1	<0.1	ns	Milk substitute	<0.1	<0.1	<0.1	<0.1	<0.1	<0.001
Soft/sports drinks	6.6	0.9	3.1	6.8	10.6	<0.001	**Soft/sports drinks**	5.5	7.8	5.8	4.0	1.9	<0.001
Regular Soft Drinks	5.4	0.9	2.9	5.4	8.4	<0.001	Regular Soft Drinks	3.2	5.1	3.2	2.1	1.2	<0.001
Diet Soft Drinks	0.8	<0.1	0.2	1.0	1.4	<0.001	Diet Soft Drinks	1.8	1.7	2.1	1.9	0.6	<0.001
Energy & Sports Drinks	0.4	<0.1	<0.1	0.3	0.9	<0.001	Energy & Sports Drinks	0.4	1.0	0.5	0.1	<0.1	<0.001
Fruit drinks/cordials	5.3	6.7	5.8	5.8	3.9	ns	**Fruit drinks/cordials**	2.3	4.1	2.1	1.6	1.9	<0.001
Fruit Drinks	2.4	3.2	2.7	2.4	2	ns	Fruit Drinks	1.0	1.8	0.8	0.6	1.1	<0.001
Regular Cordial	2.1	2.3	2.4	2.5	1.5	ns	Regular Cordial	0.9	1.8	1.0	0.6	0.6	<0.001
Diet Cordial	0.3	0.8	0.3	0.2	0.1	ns	Diet Cordial	0.2	0.2	0.2	0.2	<0.1	ns
Others	0.5	0.3	0.3	0.8	0.4	ns	Others	0.2	0.3	0.1	0.1	0.1	ns
Alcoholic Drinks	0.4	<0.1	<0.1	<0.1	1.2	<0.001	**Alcoholic Drinks**	7.0	6.1	7.1	8.3	5.1	<0.001
Food moisture	29.0	32.1	32.1	29.8	25.1	ns	Food moisture	25.2	23.8	24.2	26.6	29.4	0.02

* Chi-square tests for proportion; ns: not statistically significant.

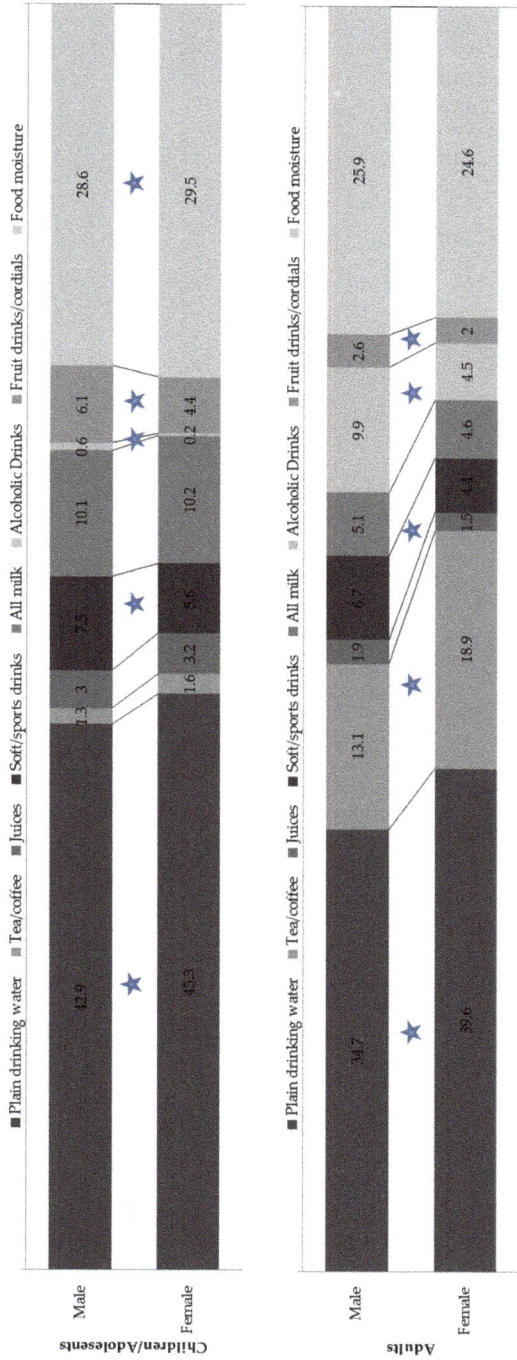

Figure 2. Proportion of contribution by sources of total water intake (%) by gender (Star indicates a significant difference ($p < 0.05$) between genders).

3.3. Plain Drinking Water

Among children/adolescents, plain drinking water intake was associated with being female, older age, and lower consumption of dairy products and discretionary beverages/foods (Table 4). Among adults, plain drinking water intake was higher in females and those of higher socio-economic status, but decreased with age. Plain drinking water was also associated with higher consumption of fruit, but lower consumption of grains, dairy products and discretionary foods/beverages. Analyses were adjusted for energy intake, physical activity, country of birth, season of interview, BMI z-score for children/adolescents, and BMI for adults (Table 4).

Table 4. Association of plain drinking water intake with dietary covariates.

Plain Drinking Water Intake (mL)		Children/Adolescents			Adults		
		β	SE	*p*-Value	β	SE	*p*-Value
Gender (Ref. Male)		−63.3	19.1	<0.001	−10.2	16.5	0.01
Age (year)		37.3	3.7	<0.001	−8.9	0.4	<0.001
BMI *		2.6	0.7	ns	3.3	0.9	ns
SEIFA (Ref. 1st quintile)	2nd quintile	−0.7	30.0	ns	44.3	22.5	0.04
	3rd quintile	62.7	29.4	ns	49.5	22.5	0.03
	4th quintile	38.9	30.0	ns	92.9	23.4	<0.001
	5th quintile	32.1	28.1	ns	69.2	21.8	0.002
Grain (100 g)		−11.0	3.8	ns	−34.3	9.1	<0.001
Vegetables (100 g)		−10.0	20.0	ns	−11.7	9.4	ns
Fruit (100 g)		−6.1	3.9	ns	27.1	6.3	<0.001
Dairy products (100 g)		−30.8	9.8	0.002	−31.2	4.9	<0.001
Meat and alternatives (100 g)		19.1	5.4	ns	13.6	13.7	ns
Discretionary beverages (100 g)		−74.8	9.0	<0.001	−34.7	4.1	<0.001
Discretionary foods (100 g)		−46.4	14.2	0.001	−64.3	10.5	<0.001
Alcoholic drinks (100 g)					−4.0	2.1	ns

Note: β indicates the change of plain drinking water in mL per unit change of the covariates, adjusted for total energy intake, physical activity, whether born in non-English speaking countries, and season of interview; * BMI z-score for children/adolescents, and BMI for adults; SE: Standard Error; ns: not statistically significant.

4. Discussion

These analyses based on a representative sample of Australian population showed estimated total water intakes to be 1.5–1.7 L for children/adolescents, and 2.3–2.6 L for adults. Plain drinking water was the most commonly consumed beverage type for Australian children/adolescents and adults, in line with Dietary Guideline recommendations. Full-fat plain milk and regular soft drinks were the main contributors to other beverages for children/adolescents, and tea, coffee, and alcoholic drinks for adults. Total water intake was higher in males than females, and in older age groups in children/adolescents and younger age groups in adults. Plain water intake was higher in females than males, and was inversely associated with the consumption of dairy products and discretionary foods/beverages in adults.

Our data can be compared to similar national nutrition surveys from the US and European countries. In the US National Health and Nutrition Examination Survey (NHANES) 2005–2012, per capita total water intake for children/adolescents was 1.6–1.7 L, similar to our findings, and 2.2–3.5 L for adults with large gender and age variations [7,8]. Total water intake in French children aged 4–13 years was 1.3 L [27], and adults reported 2.1–2.5 L in the Irish national survey in 2008–2010 [10]. These surveys used 24-h recalls or food records to estimate water intake.

The amounts of total water intake and total fluids intake were compared to AI values by gender and age group and showed that the majority of the respondents failed to meet the recommended total water intake (82%) and total fluids intake (78%). The Australian Nutrition Reference Values acknowledge that there is no single level of water intake that would ensure adequate hydration and optimal health for the whole population. Thus, the total water and total fluids AI values were based on the median intake from the National Nutrition Survey 1995 and were set at the level of the highest median intake from any of the four age categories for each gender [28] and therefore represent only crude guidelines.

The sub-group that was least likely to meet the AI values were older adults aged over 70 years (5% for males and 10% for females). The average shortfall was 1.2 L for males and 0.8 L for females. Older adults are at risk of dehydration due to decreased perception of thirst, inadequate fluid intake, a decline in kidney function and increased use of diuretics and laxatives in this age group. The outcomes of dehydration in the elderly are serious and include cognitive impairment, functional decline, falls or stroke [11], and close monitoring of water consumption in this age group is warranted [29].

We found that season of interview, physical activity level, socio-economic status, and gender were associated with total water intake, in agreement with other research [7,8,10]. Our findings also showed that BMI in adults or BMI z-score in children/adolescents was not associated with total water intake or plain drinking water intake. Similar observations were reported in the US, where BMI was associated with beverage intake but not plain drinking water in adults aged 20 years and over [9].

Higher total water consumption was associated with better diet quality, indicated by higher intakes of dietary fibre, fruit and vegetables, and lower intakes of fat, saturated fat, free sugars, sodium and discretionary foods. In addition, higher consumption of plain drinking water, which comprised more than one-third of total water intake, was also associated with lower consumption of discretionary choices, confirming that promoting water intake could be a useful public health strategy. As the majority of plain drinking water was consumed as tap water (95% in children/adolescents, 90% in adults), which is fluoridated in Australia, additional benefits are conferred for the development of strong teeth and bones.

Food moisture is an important source of total water intake in the population, accounting for about 30% of total water intake in children/adolescents and 25% in adults. The water content of food is one of the major determinants of dietary energy density. Dietary energy density has been positively associated with obesity, diabetes and inversely associated with dietary quality [30,31]. Although Australia has not developed a specific recommendation for the optimal dietary water-to-energy ratio, this substantial contribution of food moisture suggests that assessing fluid intake without considering food intake would provide misleading results.

Our results highlight the high consumption of sugar-sweetened beverages consumption by children/adolescents, especially adolescents, where soft/sports drinks contribute to over 10% of total water intakes (approximately 14% of total fluids intake). Our analysis shows that these beverages replace milk and juice in the older age groups. Sugar-sweetened beverages have been shown to have a detrimental impact on health [32–34]. The effects of increased consumption of certain beverages on health outcomes have been well documented. Past studies have focused on the contribution of beverages to energy and nutrient intakes [9,35], and examined the potential beneficial outcomes of replacing sugar-sweetened beverages with plain water or more nutrient-dense options such as milk [13,32,36]. Our results show that there is considerable room for further improvement in fluid intakes of Australian children/adolescents. Among adults, the major sources of other beverages were tea and coffee, followed by alcohol. Tea and coffee are suitable alternatives to plain drinking water but the caffeine content may have unwanted stimulant effects in susceptible people [11,37,38].

The present analysis had several limitations. First, our results are derived from cross-sectional data and causal relationships cannot be inferred. Second, recall bias is a serious limitation in the collection of dietary intake data and under-reporting or selective reporting of discretionary foods and beverages is common. The recall of water intake is particularly challenging using self-report methods but a number of additional questions were asked during the interview to encourage best possible estimates. Third, biomarkers of hydration status were not available to assess hydration status in this population as these methods tend to be expensive and time-consuming [39]. However, ongoing research suggests that urinary biomarkers such as 24-h urine volume and osmolality are strongly correlated with total fluid intake in normal daily living conditions and may be useful in future studies of fluid intake [40]. Lastly, proxy recall for younger children may be an additional source of error. Despite these limitations, these data have a number of advantages as they represent a large, nationally representative data source that forms the basis for dietary surveillance in Australia. In addition, we used "usual intake" data based on two days of recall rather than one day only, which may result in slightly lower estimated intakes [15,41].

5. Conclusions

This study provides valuable new data on the consumption of water and other beverages in a sample representative of the Australian population. Reported water consumption was below recommendations, particularly for the elderly population who may be at higher risk of inadequate hydration. Additionally, our results showed that higher intakes of plain drinking water were associated with positive dietary features, thus making water an optimal beverage choice. Given the interest in understanding the association of water intake with a variety of health outcomes, these findings provide fundamental information to develop effective health promotion policies and campaigns for the Australian population.

Acknowledgments: Australian Bureau of Statistics for the 2011–2012 NNPAS.

Author Contributions: M.Z. and A.R. formulated the research question, suggested statistical analysis and provided critical input into the manuscript. Z.S. and M.Z. conducted the statistical analysis. Z.S. drafted the initial manuscript. All authors revised, edited and approved the manuscript.

Conflicts of Interest: The authors declare no conflict of interest.

References

1. Institute of Medicine. *DRI, Dietary Reference Intakes for Water, Potassium, Sodium, Chloride, and Sulfate;* National Academy Press: Washington, DC, USA, 2005.
2. National Health and Medical Research Council. Nutrients-Water. Available online: https://www.nrv.gov.au/nutrients/water (accessed on 17 July 2016).
3. Jequier, E.; Constant, F. Water as an essential nutrient: The physiological basis of hydration. *Eur. J. Clin. Nutr.* **2010**, *64*, 115–123. [CrossRef] [PubMed]
4. Armstrong, L.E. Challenges of linking chronic dehydration and fluid consumption to health outcomes. *Nutr. Rev.* **2012**, *70*, S121–S127. [CrossRef] [PubMed]
5. Masento, N.A.; Golightly, M.; Field, D.T.; Butler, L.T.; van Reekum, C.M. Effects of hydration status on cognitive performance and mood. *Br. J. Nutr.* **2014**, *111*, 1841–1852. [CrossRef] [PubMed]
6. World Health Organization. Water for Health-Who Guidelines for Drinking-Water Quality. Available online: http://www.who.int/water_sanitation_health/WHS_WWD2010_guidelines_2010_6_en.pdf?ua=1 (accessed on 18 July 2016).
7. Drewnowski, A.; Rehm, C.D.; Constant, F. Water and beverage consumption among adults in the United States: Cross-sectional study using data from NHANES 2005–2010. *BMC Public Health* **2013**, *13*. [CrossRef] [PubMed]
8. Drewnowski, A.; Rehm, C.D.; Constant, F. Water and beverage consumption among children age 4–13 years in the United States: Analyses of 2005–2010 NHANES data. *Nutr. J.* **2013**, *12*. [CrossRef] [PubMed]
9. Kant, A.K.; Graubard, B.I.; Atchison, E.A. Intakes of plain water, moisture in foods and beverages, and total water in the adult us population—Nutritional, meal pattern, and body weight correlates: National health and nutrition examination surveys 1999–2006. *Am. J. Clin. Nutr.* **2009**, *90*, 655–663. [CrossRef] [PubMed]
10. O'Connor, L.; Walton, J.; Flynn, A. Water intakes and dietary sources of a nationally representative sample of Irish adults. *J. Hum. Nutr. Diet.* **2014**, *27*, 550–556. [CrossRef] [PubMed]
11. National Health and Medical Research Council. *Eat for Health-Educator Guide;* National health and Medical Research Council: Canberra, Australia, 2013.
12. An, R.; McCaffrey, J. Plain water consumption in relation to energy intake and diet quality among us adults, 2005–2012. *J. Hum. Nutr. Diet.* **2016**, *29*, 624–632. [CrossRef] [PubMed]
13. Zheng, M.B.; Rangan, A.; Olsen, N.J.; Andersen, L.B.; Wedderkopp, N.; Kristensen, P.; Grontved, A.; Ried-Larsen, M.; Lempert, S.M.; Allman-Farinelli, M.; et al. Substituting sugar-sweetened beverages with water or milk is inversely associated with body fatness development from childhood to adolescence. *Nutrition* **2015**, *31*, 38–44. [CrossRef] [PubMed]

14. Stookey, J.D.; Constant, F.; Gardner, C.D.; Popkin, B.M. Replacing sweetened caloric beverages with drinking water is associated with lower energy intake. *Obesity (Silver Spring)* **2007**, *15*, 3013–3022. [CrossRef] [PubMed]

15. Australian Bureau of Statistics. *Australian Health Survey: User's Guide, 2011–2013*; Australian Government Publishing Service; Australian Bureau of Statistics: Canberra, Australia, 2013.

16. Bornhorst, C.; Bel-Serrat, S.; Pigeot, I.; Huybrechts, I.; Ottavaere, C.; Sioen, I.; de Henauw, S.; Mouratidou, T.; Mesana, M.I.; Westerterp, K.; et al. Validity of 24-h recalls in (pre-)school aged children: Comparison of proxy-reported energy intakes with measured energy expenditure. *Clin. Nutr.* **2014**, *33*, 79–84. [CrossRef] [PubMed]

17. Food Standards Australia New Zealand. *Australian Food, Supplement and Nutrient Database (Ausnut)*; Food Standards Australia New Zealand: Canberra, Australia, 2014.

18. World Health Organization. *Length/Height-for-Age, Weight-for-Age, Weight-for-Length, Weight-for-Height and Body Mass Index-for-Age: Methods and Development*; World Health Organization: Geneva, Switzerland, 2006.

19. Australian Bureau of Statistics. *Australian Health Survey: Nutrition First Results-Foods and Nutrients, 2011–2012*; Australian Bureau of Statistics: Canberra, Australia, 2014.

20. National Health and Medical Research Council. *Australian Guide to Healthy Eating*; National Health and Medical Research Council: Canberra, Australia, 2013.

21. Rangan, A.; Allman-Farinelli, M.; Donohoe, E.; Gill, T. Misreporting of energy intake in the 2007 Australian children's survey: Differences in the reporting of food types between plausible, under- and over-reporters of energy intake. *J. Hum. Nutr. Diet.* **2014**, *27*, 450–458. [CrossRef] [PubMed]

22. Gemming, L.; Jiang, Y.; Swinburn, B.; Utter, J.; Mhurchu, C.N. Under-reporting remains a key limitation of self-reported dietary intake: An analysis of the 2008/2009 New Zealand adult nutrition survey. *Eur. J. Clin. Nutr.* **2014**, *68*, 259–264. [CrossRef] [PubMed]

23. Vanrullen, I.B.; Volatier, J.L.; Bertaut, A.; Dufour, A.; Dallongeville, J. Characteristics of energy intake under-reporting in french adults. *Br. J. Nutr.* **2014**, *111*, 1292–1302. [CrossRef] [PubMed]

24. Black, A.E. The sensitivity and specificity of the goldberg cut-off for EI:BMR for identifying diet reports of poor validity. *Eur. J. Clin. Nutr.* **2000**, *54*, 395–404. [CrossRef] [PubMed]

25. Rennie, K.L.; Coward, A.; Jebb, S.A. Estimating under-reporting of energy intake in dietary surveys using an individualised method. *Br. J. Nutr.* **2007**, *97*, 1169–1176. [CrossRef] [PubMed]

26. Harttig, U.; Haubrock, J.; Knuppel, S.; Boeing, H.; Consortium, E. The MSM program: Web-based statistics package for estimating usual dietary intake using the multiple source method. *Eur. J. Clin. Nutr.* **2011**, *65* (Suppl. 1), S87–S91. [CrossRef] [PubMed]

27. Vieux, F.; Maillot, M.; Constant, F.; Drewnowski, A. Water and beverage consumption among children aged 4–13 years in France: Analyses of INCA 2 (etude individuelle nationale des consommations alimentaires 2006–2007) data. *Public Health Nutr.* **2016**, *19*, 2305–2314. [CrossRef] [PubMed]

28. National Health and Medical Research Council. Nutrient Reference Values for Australia and New Zealand. Available online: https://www.nrv.gov.au/ (accessed on 15 June 2016).

29. Frangeskou, M.; Lopez-Valcarcel, B.; Serra-Majem, L. Dehydration in the elderly: A review focused on economic burden. *J. Nutr. Health Aging* **2015**, *19*, 619–627. [CrossRef] [PubMed]

30. Wang, J.; Luben, R.; Khaw, K.T.; Bingham, S.; Wareham, N.J.; Forouhi, N.G. Dietary energy density predicts the risk of incident type 2 diabetes: The European prospective investigation of cancer (EPIC)-NORFOLK study. *Diabetes Care* **2008**, *31*, 2120–2125. [CrossRef] [PubMed]

31. Mendoza, J.A.; Drewnowski, A.; Christakis, D.A. Dietary energy density is associated with obesity and the metabolic syndrome in US Adults. *Diabetes Care* **2007**, *30*, 974–979. [CrossRef] [PubMed]

32. Millar, L.; Rowland, B.; Nichols, M.; Swinburn, B.; Bennett, C.; Skouteris, H.; Allender, S. Relationship between raised BMI and sugar sweetened beverage and high fat food consumption among children. *Obesity (Silver Spring)* **2014**, *22*, E96–E103. [CrossRef] [PubMed]

33. Jayalath, V.H.; de Souza, R.J.; Ha, V.; Mirrahimi, A.; Blanco-Mejia, S.; di Buono, M.; Jenkins, A.L.; Leiter, L.A.; Wolever, T.M.; Beyene, J.; et al. Sugar-sweetened beverage consumption and incident hypertension: A systematic review and meta-analysis of prospective cohorts. *Am. J. Clin. Nutr.* **2015**, *102*, 914–921. [CrossRef] [PubMed]

34. Keller, A.; Bucher, D.T.S. Sugar-sweetened beverages and obesity among children and adolescents: A review of systematic literature reviews. *Child. Obes.* **2015**, *11*, 338–346. [CrossRef] [PubMed]

35. An, R. Plain water and sugar-sweetened beverage consumption in relation to energy and nutrient intake at full-service restaurants. *Nutrients* **2016**, *8*. [CrossRef] [PubMed]

36. Zheng, M.; Rangan, A.; Allman-Farinelli, M.; Rohde, J.F.; Olsen, N.J.; Heitmann, B.L. Replacing sugary drinks with milk is inversely associated with weight gain among young obesity-predisposed children. *Br. J. Nutr.* **2015**, *114*, 1448–1455. [CrossRef] [PubMed]

37. Ali, A.; O'Donnell, J.M.; Starck, C.; Rutherfurd-Markwick, K.J. The effect of caffeine ingestion during evening exercise on subsequent sleep quality in females. *Int. J. Sports Med.* **2015**, *36*, 433–439. [CrossRef] [PubMed]

38. Owens, J.A.; Mindell, J.; Baylor, A. Effect of energy drink and caffeinated beverage consumption on sleep, mood, and performance in children and adolescents. *Nutr. Rev.* **2014**, *72* (Suppl. 1), 65–71. [CrossRef] [PubMed]

39. Perrier, E.; Vergne, S.; Klein, A.; Poupin, M.; Rondeau, P.; le Bellego, L.; Armstrong, L.E.; Lang, F.; Stookey, J.; Tack, I. Hydration biomarkers in free-living adults with different levels of habitual fluid consumption. *Br. J. Nutr.* **2013**, *109*, 1678–1687. [CrossRef] [PubMed]

40. Perrier, E.; Rondeau, P.; Poupin, M.; le Bellego, L.; Armstrong, L.E.; Lang, F.; Stookey, J.; Tack, I.; Vergne, S.; Klein, A. Relation between urinary hydration biomarkers and total fluid intake in healthy adults. *Eur. J. Clin. Nutr.* **2013**, *67*, 939–943. [CrossRef] [PubMed]

41. Tooze, J.A.; Midthune, D.; Dodd, K.W.; Freedman, L.S.; Krebs-Smith, S.M.; Subar, A.F.; Guenther, P.M.; Carroll, R.J.; Kipnis, V. A new statistical method for estimating the usual intake of episodically consumed foods with application to their distribution. *J. Am. Diet. Assoc.* **2006**, *106*, 1575–1587. [CrossRef] [PubMed]

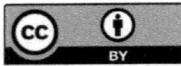

nutrients

MDPI

Article

Drinking Water Intake Is Associated with Higher Diet Quality among French Adults

Rozenn Gazan [1,2,†], Juliette Sondey [1,†], Matthieu Maillot [1,*], Isabelle Guelinckx [3] and Anne Lluch [4]

1   MS-Nutrition, Faculté de médecine La Timone, AMU, Marseille 13005, France;
    rozenn.gazan@ms-nutrition.com (R.G.); juliette.sondey@ms-nutrition.com (J.S.)
2   Aix Marseille Univ, INSERM, INRA, NORT, Marseille 13005, France
3   Hydration & Health Department, Danone Research, Palaiseau 91120, France;
    Isabelle.GUELINCKX@danone.com
4   Danone Research, Palaiseau 91120, France; Anne.LLUCH@danone.com
*   Correspondence: matthieu.maillot@ms-nutrition.com; Tel.: +33-491-324-594
†   These authors contributed equally to this work.

Received: 28 July 2016; Accepted: 27 October 2016; Published: 31 October 2016

Abstract: This study aimed to examine the association between drinking water intake and diet quality, and to analyse the adherence of French men and women to the European Food Safety Authority 2010 Adequate Intake (EFSA AI). A representative sample of French adults ($\geq$18) from the Individual and National Survey on Food Consumption (INCA2) was classified, by sex, into small, medium, and large drinking water consumers. Diet quality was assessed with several nutritional indices (mean adequacy ratio (MAR), mean excess ratio (MER), probability of adequate intakes (PANDiet), and solid energy density (SED)). Of the total sample, 72% of men and 46% of women were below the EFSA AI. This percentage of non-adherence decreased from the small to the large drinking water consumers (from 95% to 34% in men and from 81% to 9% in women). For both sexes, drinking water intake was associated with higher diet quality (greater MAR and PANDiet). This association remained significant independently of socio-economic status for women only. Low drinking water consumers did not compensate with other sources (beverages and food moisture) and a high drinking water intake was not a guarantee for reaching the EFSA AI, meaning that increasing consumption of water should be encouraged in France.

Keywords: total water intake; drinking water intake; diet quality; nutritional index

1. Introduction

Water is not only an essential nutrient for bodily and mental functions [1–3], it is starting to be identified as one of the key elements for chronic disease prevention [4–8]. In separate cohorts, lower total fluid intake [8], lower plain water intake [4], and lower 24 h urine volume [7] were all associated with increased risk for chronic kidney disease, and low water intake has also been associated with new-onset hyperglycaemia [6].

The adequate intake (AI) for total water intake (TWI) proposed by the European Food Safety Authority (EFSA) is 2.5 L/day for adult males and 2.0 L/day for adult females [9]. This dietary reference intake is less restrictive than the AI established by the US Institute of Medicine (IOM) at 3.7 L/day for men and 2.7 L/day for women [10].

Sources of TWI are fluid intake (sum of drinking water and all other beverages), food moisture, and metabolic water (derived from oxidation of macronutrients). Despite a general consensus on the major role of fluids [3], the quantitative contribution of the different sources to the TWI is lacking evidence. Based on observed fluid intake data from the National Health and Nutrition

Examination Survey (NHANES) III, the IOM reported that 81% of TWI came from fluids and 19% from foods [10]. The assumption made by EFSA is that fluids contribute 70%–80% of TWI and food moisture 20%–30% [9]. A limited number of studies in Europe reported contributions of fluids to TWI ranging from 67% in Ireland up to 75% in the UK [11–14]. These ratios were means established in a population sample, and possibly masked a large variability depending on fluid intake. Documenting the contributions of water from fluids and from food moisture could be essential when translating the AI for TWI into an easy-to-understand and practical dietary guideline on fluid intake for the general population.

In France, studies describing TWI using a representative sample of the population are scarce. Drinking water was found to be the main source of fluids in all age groups [15] with existing variations between tap water and bottled water intakes [13]. A multi-country fluid intake survey confirmed that France was characterised by a high contribution of drinking water to total fluid intake [16]. However, a study based on national population-based data of 2005–2007 estimated a TWI at 2285 mL/day for French adults aged 18–79 years old [13], suggesting that a part of the French population is at risk of inadequate intake. Considering that in 2006–2007 about 90% of children aged four to 13 years in France failed to meet the EFSA water intake recommendations [17], it seemed opportune to investigate adherence to EFSA guidelines among French adults.

Addressing the complex delineation of the role of fluids in a healthy diet, the US-led publication the Beverage Guidance Panel suggested that the consumption of water and other beverages with no or few calories should take precedence over the consumption of beverages with more calories [18]. Further studies conducted on the US population found that an elevated consumption of drinking water—tap water and bottled water—was associated with higher nutritional quality, defined either by a healthier dietary pattern (i.e., greater consumption of vegetables, low-fat dairy products, and/or whole grains) [19], a higher food variety [20], the Healthy Eating Index (HEI) [20,21], a better micronutrient adequacy [22], or reduced energy intakes [20,21]. An elevated consumption of drinking water was also associated with higher levels of physical activity [22,23]. However, in France, there is a paucity of studies describing drinking water patterns in light of socio-demographic determinants and a complete lack of research on the association between drinking water intake and diet quality.

Based on data from a representative sample of the French adult population, the present study examined if there was an association between drinking water intake and diet quality assessed by several dietary indices. We hypothesised that the largest drinking water consumers had a better diet quality. We also estimated the adherence of men and women to the AI proposed by the EFSA and analysed the contributions of the different TWI sources.

2. Materials and Methods

2.1. Study Population

The second Individual and National Food Consumption Survey (INCA2) was carried out by ANSES (the French Agency for Food, Environmental, and Occupational Health) between December 2005 and May 2007 among representative samples of French adults and children to collect information on habitual food and beverage consumption. The samples were obtained using a multi-stage cluster sampling technique, established by the National Institute for Statistics and Economic Studies (INSEE). The sampling frame was approved by the French National Commission for Computed Data and Individual Freedom (Commission Nationale de l'Informatique et des Libertés, CNIL). The present analyses used data from the adult sample of the INCA2 ($n = 1918$) including men ($n = 776$) and women ($n = 1142$) aged 18–79 years old. INCA2 remains the most recent version of a population-based survey available in France providing dietary intake information. A detailed survey methodology is available elsewhere [13,24].

2.2. Demographic, Socio-Economic and Behavioural Variables

Individual socio-economic variables were collected using a self-reported questionnaire and an interview. The following information was available: sex, age, socio-occupational status, family status, education level, income per consumption unit, food insecurity, perception of household financial situation, educational level, residency, season of protocol completion, physical activity, and smoking status. A detailed description of these variables is available elsewhere [25].

Socio-occupational status was classified into four categories: 'low', 'intermediate', 'high', and 'economically inactive'. 'High' was assigned to executive, top-management, and professional classes; 'intermediate' to middle professions (office employees, technicians, and similar); and 'low' to manual workers and unemployed people. The fourth class, labelled as 'economically inactive', included retired people, students, and housewives/househusbands.

Family status was divided into 'couples with children', 'couples without children', 'single parent households', and 'single without children'.

Education level was divided into 'high', 'intermediate', and 'low'. 'High' was assigned to university education; 'intermediate' to high school; and 'low' to mid-secondary or below [26].

Income per consumption unit (ICU) was calculated as the self-reported household total net income divided by the number of consumption units in the household. The number of consumption units was calculated using the Organization for Economic Co-operation and Development (OECD) modified equivalent scale (one consumption unit for the householder, 0.5 for other household members aged 14 or over and 0.3 to each child aged less than 14 years old) [27]. For the analysis, the ICU was transformed into quintiles according to sex.

Food insecurity was classified into 'yes' or 'no' based on the perception of the actual situation in the household about having enough food or not, and the reason for a lack of food [25]. Individuals having reported 'getting enough, but not always the kinds of food they want to eat', or 'sometimes' or 'often not getting enough to eat' because of 'lack of money' were classified as living in a household experiencing food insecurity.

The perception of household financial situation ('living comfortably', 'getting by', 'finding it difficult', 'impossible without debt') was assessed [28] and further aggregated into two classes: 'high' and 'low'.

Residency was recorded based on eight different regions of France: Northwest; East; Ile de France; West; Centre; Centre-East; Southwest; and Southeast.

Level of physical activity was based on the International Physical Activity Questionnaire (IPAQ) score [29], which assesses physical activity, including exercise, leisure time, domestic and gardening activities, work-related and transport-related activity.

2.3. Dietary Assessment

Diet was assessed using a seven-day open-ended food record. Each day of the food record was divided into three main meals (breakfast, lunch, and dinner) and three between-meals snacks. The individuals were asked to describe, as precisely as possible, all food and beverage intakes for seven consecutive days: food name, origin (home-made or industrial product), and features (low fat, low sugar, fortified, dietetic, as well as fresh, canned, or frozen). Portion sizes were expressed by weight or household measures (spoon) or estimated using a photographic booklet (SU.VI.MAX) [30]. Average daily nutritional intakes (excluding all alcoholic beverages) were evaluated matching food intakes with the 2013 French food composition database of the CIQUAL led by ANSES [31]. Daily TWI, expressed in grams per day, was estimated by assessing the amount of the nutrient "water", from fluids and from food moisture. Energy and quantity of alcoholic beverages were estimated separately.

2.4. Foods and Fluids Categorization

All the foods and fluids declared as consumed in INCA2 were categorised into nine food groups and 27 food subgroups (Supplementary Materials Table S1). In our study, the food group "drinking water" contained tap water, and non-carbonated and carbonated non-caloric bottled water. The food group "beverages" included fruit juices, hot drinks, sugar-sweetened beverages, and diet sweet beverages. "Fluids" referred to the food groups "drinking water", "beverages", and the "milk" subgroup.

2.5. Nutritional Quality of Diet

Solid energy density (SED), mean adequacy ratio (MAR), mean excess ratio (MER), probability of adequate intakes (PANDiet) scores, and food variety were used as indicators of nutritional quality for each individual diet. The MAR, the PANDiet, and the MER are reliable indicators of the nutritional quality of diets at the population or individual level [32–34]. SED (kcal/100 g) was defined as the ratio of the total energy consumed from solid foods and the total weight consumed from solid foods [35,36]. A low SED diet has been associated with a good overall nutritional quality [35].

The MAR (% of adequacy) was used as an indicator of good nutritional quality and was calculated for each individual diet as the mean percentage of sex- and age-specific French Recommended Dietary Allowances (RDA) [32] for 23 key nutrients [37]. The MER (% of excess) was calculated as the mean daily percentage of the French maximum recommended values for saturated fatty acids (22.2 g), free sugars (50 g), and sodium (3153 mg), as proposed by Vieux [34]. The MAR and MER values range between 0% and 100%.

The PANDiet score was composed of adequacy probabilities for 24 nutrients grouped into two sub-scores: the adequacy sub-score (AS) and moderation sub-score (MS) [32,38]. The AS assessed the probability of adequacy for items for which the usual intake should be above a reference value, whereas the MS evaluated the probability of adequacy for several items—recently adapted and including free sugar—for which the usual intake should not exceed a reference value [38]. PANDiet scores range between 0 and 100; where 100 represents 100% of the usual intake adequacy for the 24 nutrients.

Food variety was estimated as the number of different foods and fluids (except alcohol) declared as consumed by each individual during the seven-day food record.

2.6. Diet Cost

Diet cost was calculated by multiplying the quantity of each food in the diet by its mean national price. A detailed methodology has been previously described [39]. Diet cost was expressed either per day or per 2000 kcal (i.e., energy cost). Mean national prices, expressed in euros per 100 g of edible food, were previously obtained from the 2006 Kantar-World Panel database, which gives the annual food expenditures of a representative sample of 12,000 French households [40].

2.7. Statistical Analysis

All analyses accounted for the complex INCA2 sampling frame design [24]. Data were weighted for unequal sampling probabilities and for differential non-responses by region, agglomeration size, age, sex, occupation of the household head, size of the household and season [13,24]. All analyses were conducted separately by sex due to the sex-specific EFSA AI of TWI (>2.5 L for men and >2 L for women). Small, medium, and large consumers were identified based on the tertiles of drinking water intake (including non-consumers). Socio-demographic characteristics were described and statistically compared between tertiles of drinking water intake using the chi-squared test (for qualitative variables) and general linear models (GLM, for continuous variables). Water intakes from fluids and food moisture, expressed in g/day and in percentage of TWI, were evaluated and represented graphically. The prevalence of adherence to the AI of TWI was assessed by tertile of drinking water intake and by sex using binomial logistic regression. The distance between TWI and the AI (i.e., TWI shortfall) for individuals considered in inadequacy was assessed. Distribution of TWI and the average TWI shortfall were graphically represented by tertile of water consumption by sex, and compared two by two using GLM, with Bonferroni correction.

Food intakes, food variety, SED, MAR (%), MER (%), PANDiet, diet cost (€/day), energy cost (€/2000 kcal), and macro- and micronutrient intakes (those used in the MAR or PANDiet) were statistically compared using GLM according to tertiles of drinking water intake in observed diets. Linear trends in diet quality and food intakes were also evaluated by tertile and by sex.

A *p*-value of 5% was used as the threshold of significance. Values are survey-weighted means and adjusted for total energy intake. When specified, adjustments were made for the level of education, socio-occupational status, season, level of physical activity, smoking status, region of residence, and quintile of ICU. Based upon the weighting factors, all results are representative of the French population. Analyses were conducted using SAS version 9.4 (SAS Institute, Cary, NC, USA).

3. Results

3.1. Drinking Water Intake

Figure 1 shows the cumulative distribution of drinking water intake (g/day) by tertile and by sex. The mean intake of drinking water in the male and female sample was 768 g/day and 808 g/day, respectively. Small consumers were identified as men and women having a consumption of drinking water ≤474 g/day (including 18.3% of non-consumers) and ≤500 g/day (including 8.0% of non-consumers), respectively. Large consumers were defined as individuals consuming drinking water in an amount superior to 879 g/day among men and to 934 g/day among women.

Demographic, socio-economic, and behavioural variables by tertile of drinking water intake and by sex are presented in Table 1. Among both men and women, tertiles of drinking water intake were significantly associated with socio-occupational status and season. For men only, consumers at the highest level of drinking water intake had a significantly higher education level, higher physical activity level, higher income per consumption unit, and were more likely to be non-smokers.

3.2. Water Intakes from Fluids and Food Moisture

Figure 2 shows the average TWI (g/day, Figure 2a,b) and the average contribution of water intake from fluids and food moisture (%, Figure 2c,d) by tertile of drinking water intake for men and women.

TWI from food moisture significantly increased from the lowest to the highest tertile (799–859 g/day among men and 701–765 g/day among women) (Figure 2a,b), while food moisture contribution to TWI decreased, both among men (from 47% to 31%, *p* for trend = 0.008) and women (from 43% to 28%, *p* for trend = 0.002) (Figure 2c,d).

Both the TWI from fluids (g/day) and fluids' contribution to TWI (%) increased significantly from the first to the third tertile (*p* for trend < 0.0001), both among men (from 53% to 69%, i.e., 893–1897 g/day) and women (from 57% to 72%, i.e., 931–1938 g/day) (Figure 2a–d).

The contribution to TWI of all sources of drinking water (tap water, still water in a bottle, and carbonated water in a bottle) significantly increased from the lowest to the highest tertile, whereas the contribution of water from the other fluids (except fruit juices among women) significantly decreased (Figure 2c,d).

The main contributor of TWI among both men and women in the first tertile was hot drinks (with 22% for men and 25% for women) followed by tap water (with 7% for men and 10% for women), whereas in the third tertile, the main contributors were tap water (with 23% for both men and women) and still water in a bottle (with 23% for men and 28% for women). In the second tertile, contributions to TWI from hot drinks and still water in a bottle were equivalent (around 16% for men and 18%–19% for women).

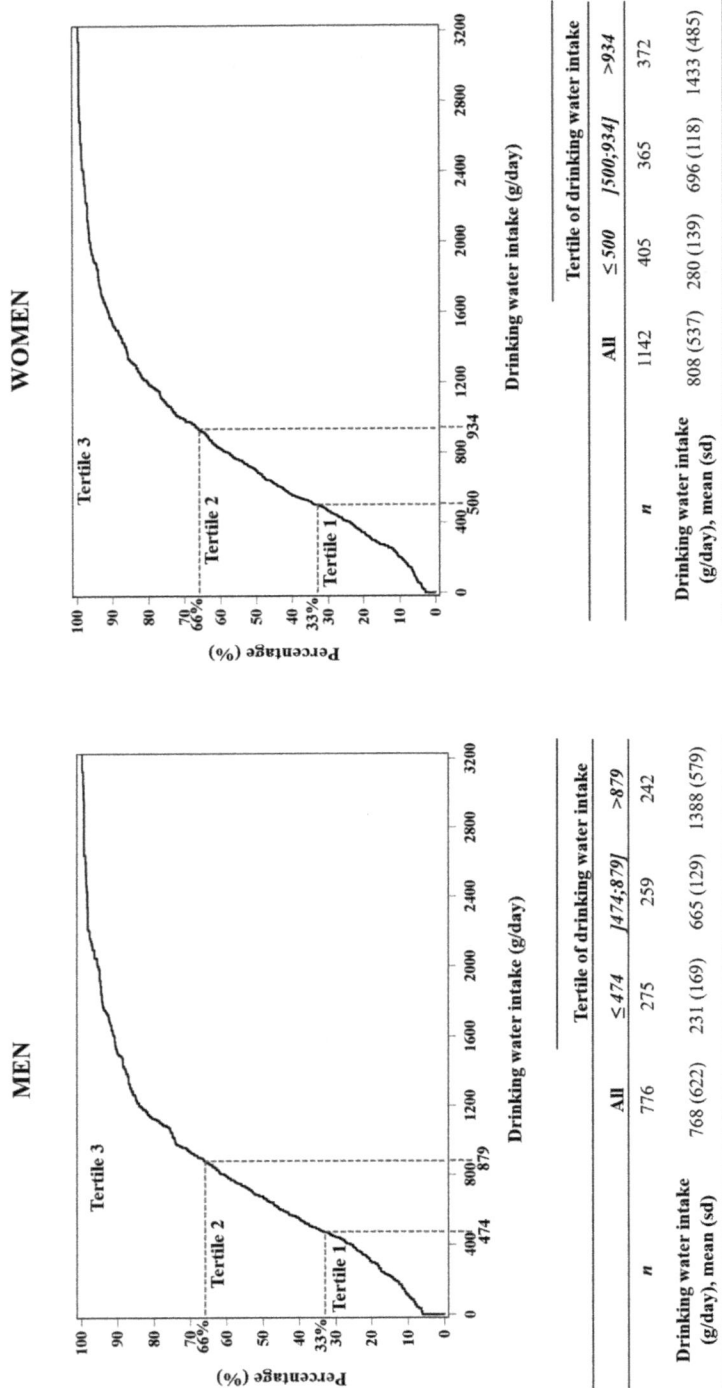

Figure 1. Cumulative distribution* (%) of drinking water intake and average of drinking water intake (g/day) by tertile, among men (n = 776) (a) and among women (n = 1142) (b). * The survey-weight coefficients were applied to the distribution.

MEN

	Tertile of drinking water intake		
	All	≤474	]474;879]	>879
n	776	275	259	242
Drinking water intake (g/day), mean (sd)	768 (622)	231 (169)	665 (129)	1388 (579)

(a)

WOMEN

	Tertile of drinking water intake		
	All	≤500	]500;934]	>934
n	1142	405	365	372
Drinking water intake (g/day), mean (sd)	808 (537)	280 (139)	696 (118)	1433 (485)

(b)

Table 1. Demographic, socio-economic, and behavioural variables by tertile of drinking water intake (g/day) and by sex [1].

	Men					Women				
		Tertile of Drinking Water Intake					Tertile of Drinking Water Intake			
	All	≤474 mL/Day	474–879 mL/Day	>879 mL/Day	p	All	≤500 mL/Day	500–932 mL/Day	>934 mL/Day	p
n	776	275	259	242		1142	1142	405	365	
	Mean ± SD					Mean ± SD				
Age (years)	49.0 ± 17.8	50.5 ± 16.9	48.7 ± 19.1	47.9 ± 17.2	0.333	45.2 ± 15.0	45.4 ± 15.1	45.1 ± 15.4	45.0 ± 14.6	0.977
	(%)					(%)				
Socio-occupational status					0.001					0.009
Low	20.4	19.1	18.1	23.9		10.1	6.9	10.1	13.4	
Intermediate	26.2	25.2	21.2	32.0		40.4	41.7	38.4	41.0	
High	10.7	8.6	11.1	12.2		7.3	5.7	5.5	10.6	
Economically inactive	42.7	47.1	49.6	31.9		42.2	45.7	46.1	34.9	
Familial status					0.182					0.204
Couple with children	26.5	25.7	22.7	30.8		33.0	33.3	31.5	34.2	
Couple without child	47.9	52.2	47.2	44.4		34.4	29.6	35.8	37.8	
Single parent household	6.3	4.9	8.8	5.2		7.0	9.1	5.9	6.0	
Single without children	19.3	17.2	21.3	19.5		25.4	27.9	26.4	22.1	
No answer	0.0	0.0	0.0	0.0		0.1	0.0	0.4	0.0	
Quintile of ICU [†]					0.009					0.154
1	20.2	25.2	18.2	17.3		20.6	23.5	20.9	17.5	
2	19.3	21.3	22.3	14.3		19.9	19.1	19.2	21.2	
3	23.1	14.9	27.3	26.9		19.6	21.5	18.9	18.6	
4	19.6	19.2	17.8	21.8		23.2	20.7	24.9	24.0	
5	17.8	19.4	14.3	19.8		16.7	15.1	16.1	18.7	
Food insecurity					0.339					0.303
Yes	9.9	9.3	11.9	8.3		11.9	14.0	10.2	11.5	
No	85.9	84.2	83.7	89.6		83.2	81.7	86.0	81.9	
No answer	4.3	6.4	4.3	2.1		4.9	4.4	3.8	6.6	
Perception of household financial situation					0.242					0.174
High	6.4	8.7	5.3	5.3		94.7	92.8	94.8	96.6	
Low	93.0	90.5	93.9	94.6		5.0	7.0	4.7	3.4	
No answer	0.5	0.7	0.8	0.1		0.3	0.2	0.6	0.0	
Level of education					0.010					0.599
Low	15.4	21.0	17.0	8.4		20.1	22.1	20.2	18.1	
Intermediate	55.5	53.4	53.8	59.2		48.6	49.1	49.5	47.2	
High	29.0	25.7	29	32.2		31.2	28.8	30.0	34.7	
No answer	0.1	0.0	0.2	0.2		0.1	0.0	0.3	0.0	
Region of residence					0.128					0.008
Northwest	13.8	12.8	13.3	15.2		15	11.2	19	15	
East	8.9	10.0	11.2	5.6		9.7	8.5	8.7	11.8	
Ile De France	17.7	19.7	14.7	18.8		17.3	22.5	15.0	14.3	

Table 1. Cont.

	Men					Women				
		Tertile of Drinking Water Intake					Tertile of Drinking Water Intake			
	All	≤474 mL/Day	474–879 mL/Day	>879 mL/Day	p	All	≤500 mL/Day	500–932 mL/Day	>934 mL/Day	p
n	776	275	259	242			1142	405	365	
		Mean ± SD						Mean ± SD		
West	14.1	15.2	13.8	13.3		14.4	12.5	18.1	12.6	
Centre	10.4	10.4	13.6	7.4		9.6	10.3	9.5	9.1	
Centre-east	11.6	10.1	7.9	16.5		12.6	14.8	12.2	10.8	
South-west	11.2	10.4	12.8	10.3		10.0	9.2	6.2	14.4	
South-east	12.4	11.5	12.6	13.0		11.5	11.1	11.4	12.0	
Season of protocol completion					0.004					<0.001
Winter	23.8	27.4	25.0	19.0		26.9	33.1	25.3	22.5	
Spring	26.4	22.4	25.4	31.4		23.5	23.6	22.1	24.7	
Summer	24.0	21.2	20.3	30.3		26.9	16.8	28.9	35.0	
Autumn	25.9	29.0	29.3	19.4		22.6	26.5	23.7	17.8	
Level of physical activity (IPAQ score)					0.017					0.808
Low	20.7	24.6	20.6	17.0		24.0	23.3	24.3	24.5	
Middle	29.6	31.8	33.9	23.2		32.4	34.2	33.4	29.7	
High	48.6	43.3	45.3	56.9		42.4	41.6	41.1	44.5	
No answer	1.1	0.2	0.2	2.8		1.1	0.9	1.2	1.2	
Smoker					0.004					0.164
Smoker	28.1	36.5	22.3	25.7		23.3	26.9	19.9	23.0	
Not smoker	71.9	63.5	77.7	74.3		76.7	73.1	80.1	77.0	

Abbreviations: ICU, income per consumption unit; IPAQ, International Physical Activity Questionnaire. [1] Values are survey-weighted means with standard deviations; [†] quintiles of ICU were ≤700:]700;976];]976;1367];]1367;1867]; >1867 and ≤580;]580;915];]915;1306];]1306;1867]; among men and women, respectively.

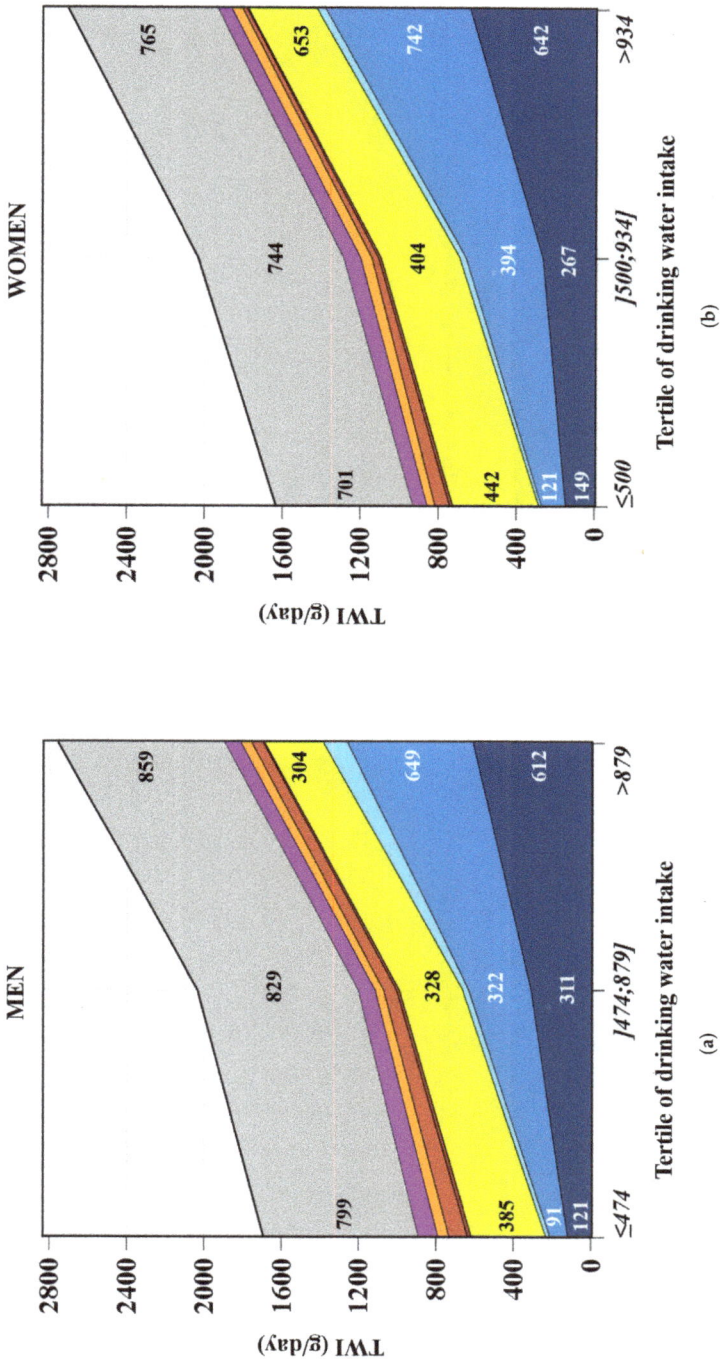

Figure 2. *Cont.*

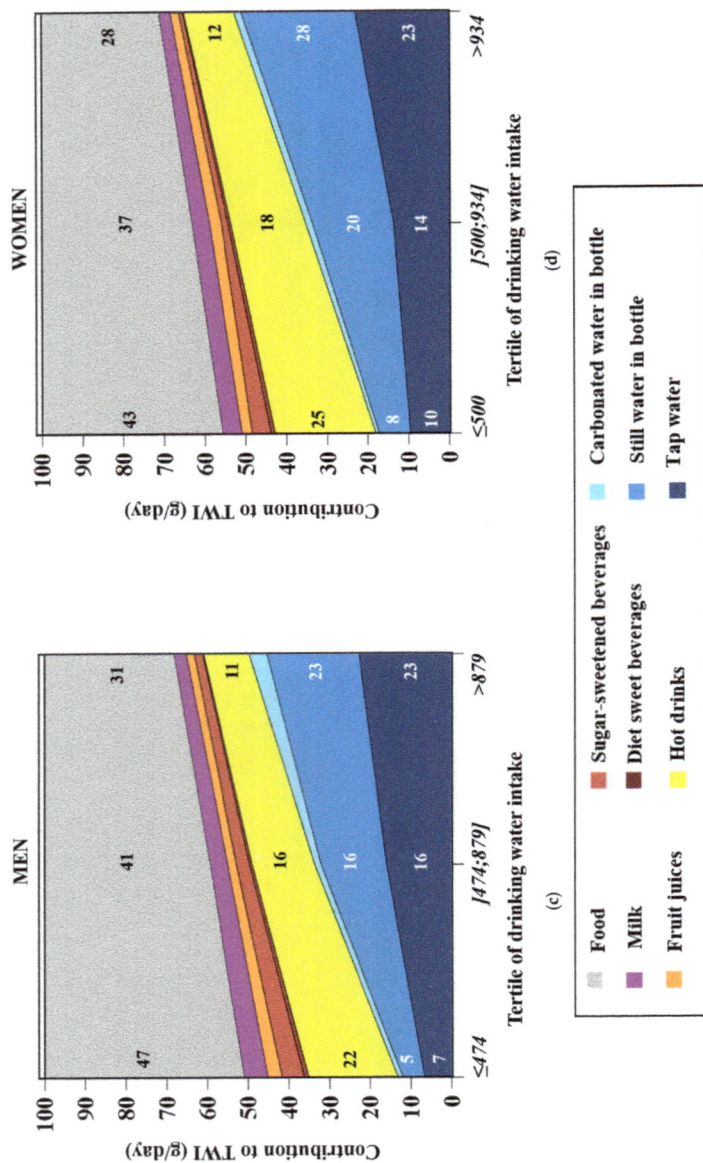

Figure 2. Total water intake (g/day) [1] by tertile of drinking water among men (n = 776) (**a**) and women (n = 1142) (**b**) (means are adjusted for energy) and the contribution (%) of fluids and food moisture to the total water intake [2,3] by tertile of drinking water among men (n = 776) (**c**) and women (n = 1142) (**d**). [1] Among men and women, p for trend was significant for: sugar-sweetened beverages, hot drinks, carbonated water in a bottle, still water in a bottle, and tap water; [2] Among men, p for trend was significant for: milk, fruit juices, sugar-sweetened beverages, diet sweet beverages, hot drinks, carbonated water in a bottle, still water in a bottle, and tap water; [3] Among women, p for trend was significant for: milk, sugar-sweetened beverages, diet sweet beverages, hot drinks, carbonated water in a bottle, still water in a bottle, and tap water.

3.3. TWI and Adherence to EFSA AI

Total water intakes by tertile of drinking water intake and by sex are presented in Table 2. The daily mean TWI was 2160.8 g/day (2.16 L) for men and 2122.3 g/day (2.12 L) for women (Table 2).

Figure 3 shows the proportion of individuals (non-)adhering to the AI of TWI by tertile by drinking water intake and by sex. Seventy-two percent of men and 46% of women had a TWI below the EFSA AI (Figure 3a,c). Among both men and women, the proportion of non-adherence to AI decreased from the lowest to the highest tertile of drinking water intake (from 95% to 34%, respectively, for men, and from 81% to 9%, respectively, for women) (Figure 3a,c).

Individuals in the first and second tertile were less likely to fulfil the EFSA AI than those in the third tertile among men ($p < 0.0001$, OR = 38.8, and OR = 13.3, respectively) and women ($p < 0.0001$, OR = 49.4, and OR = 11.0 respectively) after full adjustment. No significant interaction between season and the probability of inadequacy was found (data not shown).

The average shortfall of TWI among individuals in inadequacy significantly decreased from the lowest to the highest tertile of water consumption (917 g/day to 317 g/day for men; 603 g/day to 143 g/day for women) (p for trend < 0.05) (Figure 3b,d).

Among male and female individuals adhering to the AI, total TWI increased significantly from the first to the third tertile but was not different between the first and second tertile (2726 vs. 2691, $p = 0.836$ and 2412 vs. 2375, $p = 0.627$ among men and women, respectively, after adjustment) (Figure 3b,d).

3.4. Drinking Water Intake and Nutritional Quality of Diet

Table 2 describes the nutrient intakes and diet quality indicators of observed diets by tertile of drinking water intake and by sex. Among men and women, energy intake was significantly different between tertiles and increased (from 2290 to 2518 kcal/day, p for trend = 0.008 for men, and from 1779–1901 kcal/day, p for trend = 0.004 for women) with full adjustment. The total weight consumed also increased, steered by the strong increase of the weight of fluids from the first to the third tertile and a slight increase of the weight of solid foods (Table 2).

For men and women, the PANDiet score and adequacy subscore, MAR (%/day), food variety, daily cost, and energy cost significantly increased with adjustment for energy intake only, from the lowest to the highest tertile (all p for trend < 0.05). For men only, MER (%/day) was close to a significant decrease (adjusted $p = 0.065$) and, for women only, SED decreased significantly from the first to the third tertile (p for trend < 0.0001) (Table 2). After full adjustments, diet cost and energy cost remained significant for men and women (p for trend < 0.0001), as well as PANDiet, MAR, food variety, and SED for women only (p for trend < 0.0001). Women with the largest consumption of drinking water intake had higher diet quality and less energy dense diets.

For both men and women, there were no differences in macronutrient intakes, with all adjustments, except an increase of fibre from the lowest to the highest tertile (p for trend = 0.015 among men, and p for trend < 0.001 among women) and a decrease of free sugar (% energy) only for women (p for trend = 0.028). Only among women, intakes of sodium increased (p for trend < 0.001) (Table 2). Both among men and women, the level of consumption of drinking water was not strongly related to macronutrient intake.

Vitamin and mineral intakes by tertile of drinking water and by sex are presented in Supplementary Materials Table S2. After all adjustments, significant differences were found between tertiles of drinking water. Among men, magnesium, calcium, and vitamin A intake significantly increased from the lowest to the highest tertile. Among women, linolenic fatty acid, magnesium, calcium, copper, iron, iodin, zinc, vitamin B6, folic acid, and vitamin C intake increased from the first to the third tertile.

3.5. Food Intake Compared to Levels of Drinking Water Intake

The food group intakes by tertile of drinking water intake and by sex are presented in Table 3.

Table 2. Observed nutrient intakes and diet quality indicators by tertile of drinking water intake (g/day) and by sex (means are adjusted for energy)[1].

			Men				
			Tertile of Drinking Water Intake				
Variables	All	≤474 mL/Day	474–879 mL/Day	>879 mL/Day	p[†]	p[‡]	p for Trend[§]
	Mean ± SD	Mean ± SD	Mean ± SD	Mean ± SD			
Energy (kcal/day)	2403.8 ± 592.0	2289.7 ± 529.3	2400.1 ± 551.3	2518.0 ± 671.2	<0.001	0.003	0.001
Total water (TWI[2], g/day)	2160.8 ± 28.8	1691.6 ± 25.2	2034.1 ± 19.9	2756.7 ± 41.2	<0.001	<0.001	<0.001
Water from foods (g/day)	829.1 ± 16.9	798.9 ± 15.7	829.2 ± 18.0	859.3 ± 17.2	0.041	0.032	0.009
Water from fluids (g/day)	1331.7 ± 27.3	892.7 ± 24.1	1204.9 ± 17.9	1897.3 ± 40.0	<0.001	<0.001	<0.001
Total weight (g/day)	2668.3 ± 29.1	2199.9 ± 25.3	2540.4 ± 20.4	3264.7 ± 41.7	<0.001	<.0001	<0.001
Weight of solid foods (g/day)	1304.6 ± 18.1	1270.4 ± 17.4	1306.0 ± 18.8	1337.3 ± 18.3	0.036	0.022	0.006
Weight of fluids (g/day)	1363.8 ± 28.3	929.5 ± 25.6	1234.3 ± 18.6	1927.5 ± 40.6	<0.001	<0.001	<0.001
Food variety	56.1 ± 1.1	53.2 ± 1.0	57.6 ± 1.2	57.5 ± 1.1	0.003	0.121	
Energy from alcohol	180.4 ± 194.4	216.2 ± 211.9	154 ± 171.4	171.5 ± 191.1	0.008	0.007	0.030
Alcoholic drinks	255.4 ± 21.2	294.7 ± 20.9	222.8 ± 22.4	248.7 ± 20.4	0.053	0.077	
SED (kcal/100 g)	179.9 ± 2.1	183.0 ± 2.2	180.0 ± 2.3	176.8 ± 2.0	0.119	0.084	
PANDiet	62.5 ± 0.5	61.4 ± 0.4	62.6 ± 0.5	63.7 ± 0.5	0.001	0.084	
Adequacy subscore	69.6 ± 0.7	68.1 ± 0.7	69.7 ± 0.7	71.0 ± 0.6	0.005	0.274	
Moderate subscore	55.5 ± 0.7	54.7 ± 0.7	55.4 ± 0.7	56.3 ± 0.7	0.235	0.299	
MAR (% adequacy)	83.3 ± 0.4	82.3 ± 0.5	83.4 ± 0.4	84.2 ± 0.4	0.006	0.093	
MER (% excess)	44.4 ± 1.2	47.2 ± 1.2	43.9 ± 1.2	42.1 ± 1.2	0.004	0.065	
Cost (€/day)	7.3 ± 0.1	7.0 ± 0.1	7.3 ± 0.1	7.7 ± 0.1	<0.001	<0.001	<0.001
Cost (€/2000 kcal)	6.2 ± 0.2	5.8 ± 0.2	6.1 ± 0.2	6.5 ± 0.2	<0.001	0.084	
Proteins (% energy)	16.9 ± 2.9	17.0 ± 3.3	17.0 ± 2.8	16.6 ± 2.7	0.326	0.369	
Carbohydrates (% energy)	43.0 ± 6.9	43.0 ± 7.2	42.6 ± 6.6	43.4 ± 7.0	0.459	0.751	
Total fat (% energy)	37.9 ± 6.2	37.8 ± 6.0	38.2 ± 5.9	37.7 ± 6.7	0.681	0.885	
Saturated fat (% energy)	14.6 ± 3.3	14.9 ± 3.1	14.7 ± 3.2	14.3 ± 3.6	0.141	0.306	
Free sugar (% energy)	9.0 ± 5.6	9.4 ± 5.9	8.7 ± 5.3	8.9 ± 5.5	0.372	0.243	
Fiber (g)[†]	20.6 ± 0.3	20.1 ± 0.3	20.5 ± 0.3	21.1 ± 0.4	0.099	0.038	0.015
Saturated fat (g/day)	39.3 ± 0.6	39.9 ± 0.5	39.4 ± 0.5	38.5 ± 0.7	0.229	0.421	
Free sugar (g/day)	56.0 ± 2.2	59.7 ± 2.3	54.6 ± 2.3	53.7 ± 2.1	0.119	0.105	
Sodium (mg/day)	3664.1 ± 49.9	3652.5 ± 45.4	3684.0 ± 58.4	3655.8 ± 45.7	0.895	0.769	

Nutrients **2016**, _8_, 689

Table 2. *Cont.*

Variables	All Mean ± SD	Tertile of Drinking Water Intake ≤500 mL/Day Mean ± SD	500–934 mL/Day Mean ± SD	>934 mL/Day Mean ± SD	p[†]	p[‡]	p for Trend[§]
Energy (kcal/day)	1866.1 ± 427.1	1779.4 ± 421.9	1910.9 ± 407.7	1908.6 ± 440.5	0.001	0.003	0.004
Total water (TWI[2], g/day)	2122.3 ± 34.2	1631.4 ± 33.5	2033.0 ± 34.8	2702.6 ± 34.4	<0.001	<0.001	<0.001
Water from foods (g/day)	736.3 ± 13.7	700.9 ± 14.9	743.5 ± 13.0	764.5 ± 13.1	0.004	0.006	0.002
Water from fluids (g/day)	1386.1 ± 30.2	930.6 ± 25.2	1289.5 ± 35.5	1938.1 ± 29.9	<0.001	<0.001	<0.001
Total weight (g/day)	2512.2 ± 34.7	2021.0 ± 33.8	2422.3 ± 35.6	3093.4 ± 34.8	<0.001	<0.001	<0.001
Weight of solid foods (g/day)	1100.2 ± 14.6	1063.0 ± 15.8	1105.9 ± 14.0	1131.7 ± 14.0	0.004	0.005	0.001
Weight of fluids (g/day)	1412.1 ± 30.7	958.0 ± 25.9	1316.4 ± 36.3	1961.8 ± 29.9	<0.001	<0.001	<0.001
Food variety	59.8 ± 0.8	55.5 ± 0.6	62.9 ± 1.0	61.1 ± 0.8	<0.001	<0.001	<0.001
Energy from alcohol	49.5 ± 70.5	45.1 ± 65.4	53.4 ± 67.1	50.2 ± 78.5	0.397	0.257	0.438
Alcoholic drinks	63.2 ± 6.0	57.9 ± 5.7	66.2 ± 5.8	65.4 ± 6.5	0.547	0.438	
SED (kcal/100 g)	165.5 ± 2.0	171.7 ± 2.5	164.3 ± 1.9	160.5 ± 1.7	0.001	0.001	<0.001
PANDiet	62.3 ± 0.5	60.6 ± 0.5	62.6 ± 0.4	63.6 ± 0.5	<0.001	<0.001	<0.001
Adequacy subscore	64.3 ± 0.6	60.7 ± 0.6	65.8 ± 0.5	66.5 ± 0.6	<0.001	<0.001	<0.001
Moderate subscore	60.2 ± 0.7	60.5 ± 0.6	59.3 ± 0.7	60.7 ± 0.7	0.295	0.188	
MAR (% adequacy)	79.1 ± 0.4	76.4 ± 0.5	79.9 ± 0.4	80.8 ± 0.4	<0.001	<0.001	<0.001
MER (% excess)	21.7 ± 0.9	23.3 ± 1.1	21.7 ± 1.0	20.2 ± 0.7	0.089	0.199	
Cost (€/day)	6.2 ± 0.2	5.8 ± 0.2	6.3 ± 0.2	6.5 ± 0.2	<0.001	<0.001	<0.001
Cost (€/2000 kcal)	6.8 ± 0.1	6.3 ± 0.1	6.9 ± 0.1	7.2 ± 0.1	<0.001	<0.001	<0.001
Proteins (% energy)	16.2 ± 2.7	16.2 ± 2.8	16.1 ± 2.7	16.3 ± 2.7	0.608	0.810	
Carbohydrates (% energy)	42.5 ± 5.7	42.8 ± 6.1	42.3 ± 5.9	42.4 ± 5.2	0.507	0.427	
Total fat (% energy)	38.8 ± 5.3	38.6 ± 5.3	39.2 ± 5.5	38.8 ± 5.1	0.552	0.388	
Saturated fat (% energy)	14.6 ± 2.8	14.6 ± 2.9	14.8 ± 2.7	14.6 ± 2.9	0.592	0.508	
Free sugar (% energy)	9.9 ± 4.8	10.2 ± 5.7	10.2 ± 4.4	9.4 ± 4.0	0.066	0.028	0.028
Fibre (g)[†]	16.9 ± 0.3	16.3 ± 0.2	16.7 ± 0.3	17.5 ± 0.2	0.003	<0.001	<0.001
Saturated fat (g/day)	30.4 ± 0.4	30.3 ± 0.3	30.6 ± 0.4	30.3 ± 0.4	0.769	0.662	
Free sugar (g/day)	47.4 ± 1.5	49.8 ± 1.7	48.1 ± 1.5	44.2 ± 1.2	0.015	0.006	0.003
Sodium (mg/day)	2687.1 ± 40.6	2577.2 ± 30.8	2712.3 ± 54.8	2771.9 ± 36.4	<0.001	<0.001	<0.001

Abbreviations: TWI, total water intake; SED, solid energy density; PANDiet, probability of adequate intakes; MAR, mean adequacy ratio; MER, mean excess ratio. [1] Values are survey-weighted means with standard deviations; [2] TWI, total water intake; [†] adjustment for energy intake (except for energy and variables expressed in %energy); [‡] adjustment for energy intake (except for energy and variables expressed in %energy), level of education, socio-occupational group, season, level of physical activity, smoker status, region, and quintile of income per consumption unit (ICU); [§] calculated only for significant differences.

241

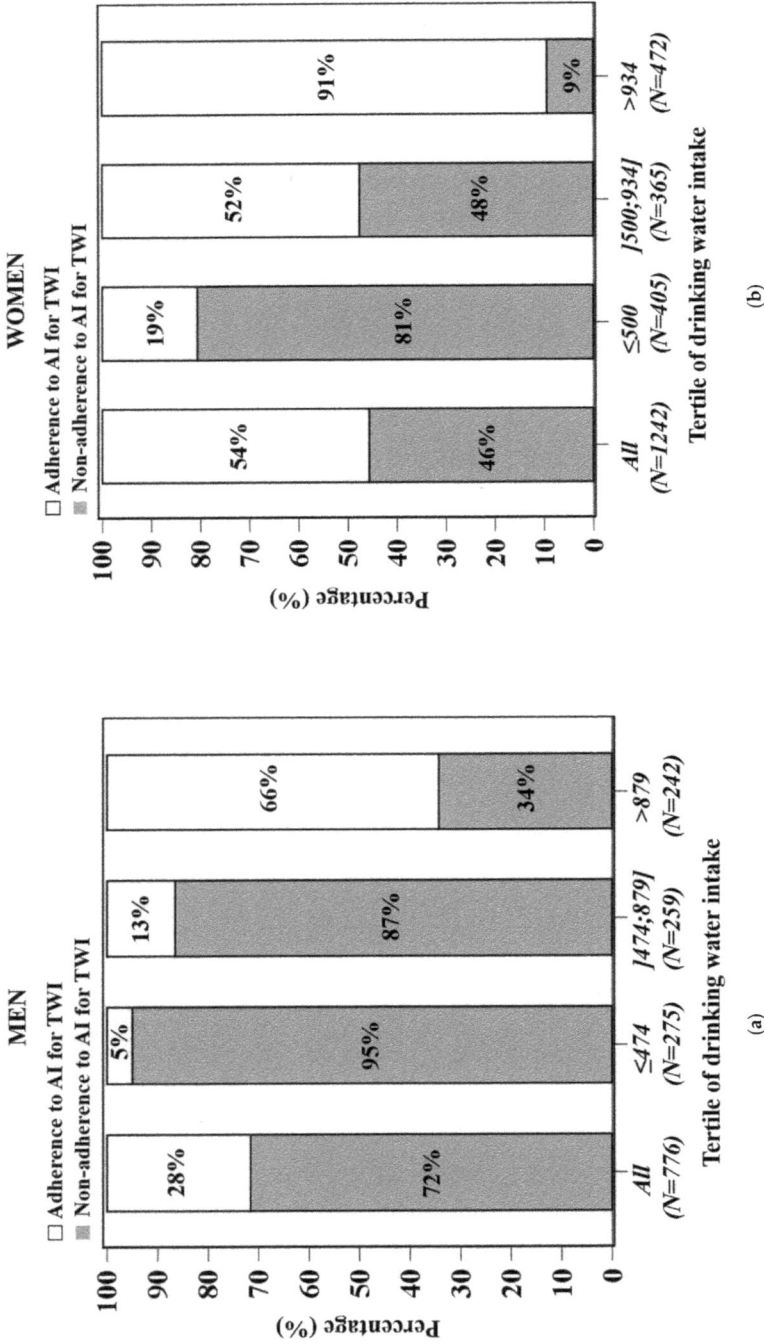

Figure 3. *Cont.*

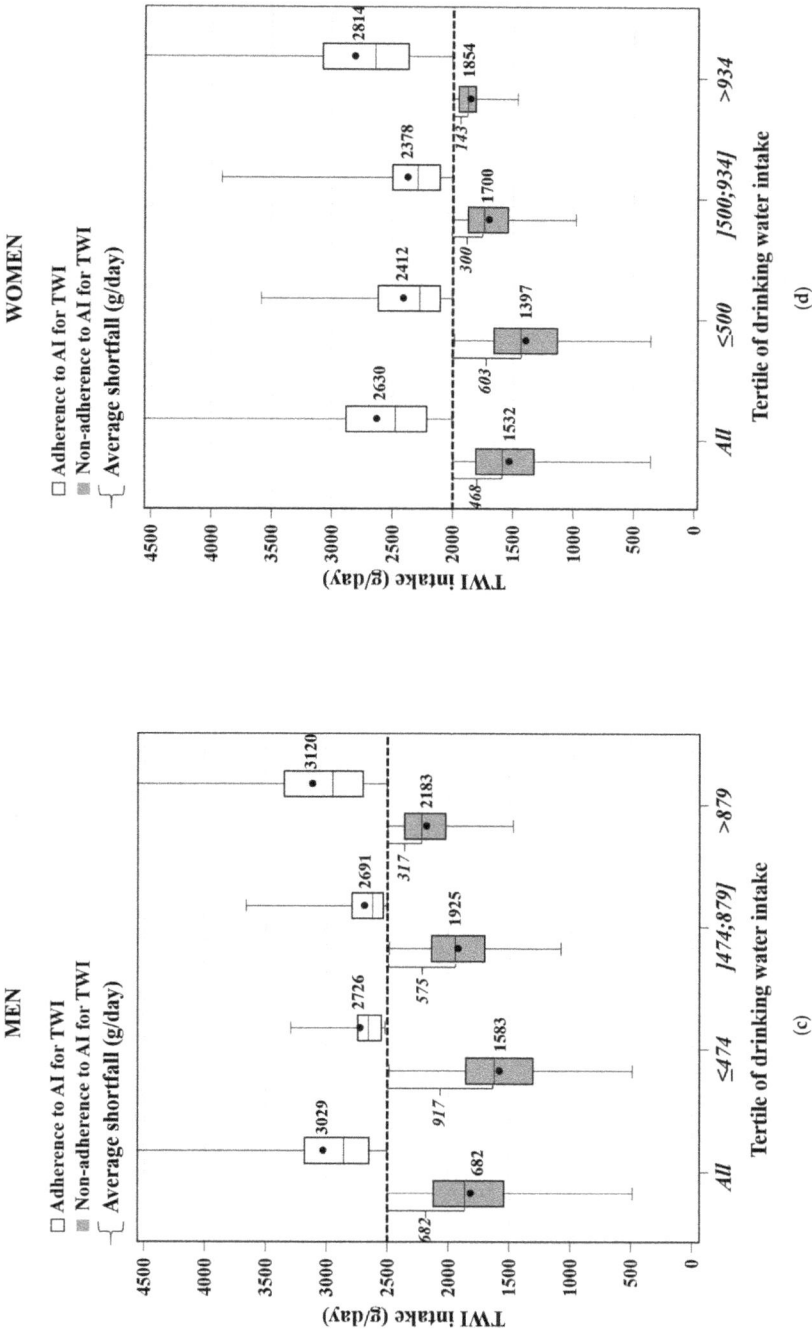

Figure 3. Adherence to adequate intake (AI) of total water intake (TWI) (%) by tertile of drinking water among men (*n* = 776) (**a**) and women (*n* = 1142) (**b**); survey-weighted daily average TWI in subjects meeting or failing to meet EFSA AI by tertile of drinking water among men (*n* = 776) (**c**) and women (*n* = 1142) (**d**).

Table 3. Food intakes by food groups and subgroups by tertile of drinking water (g/day) and by sex (means are adjusted for energy) [1].

Food Groups and Subgroups (g/Day)	Men						
		Tertile of Drinking Water Intake					
	All	≤474 mL/Day	474–879 mL/Day	>879 mL/Day	p[†]	p[‡]	p for Trend[§]
	Mean ± SD	Mean ± SD	Mean ± SD	Mean ± SD			
Fruits and vegetables	368.1 ± 19.1	336.6 ± 16.3	370.4 ± 21.3	397.4 ± 19.7	0.069	0.076	
Vegetables, soup and crudités	210.0 ± 11.6	201.2 ± 12.1	215.1 ± 11.8	213.6 ± 10.8	0.602	0.449	0.015
Fresh and processed fruits	155.9 ± 11.1	132.4 ± 7.6	153.3 ± 12.3	181.9 ± 13.4	0.008 *	0.048 *	
Nuts	2.3 ± 0.4	3.0 ± 0.5	2.0 ± 0.4	1.9 ± 0.3	0.139	0.209	
Starches	306.3 ± 7.5	303.1 ± 8.1	304.6 ± 6.2	311.3 ± 8.0	0.742	0.355	
Refined starches	212.0 ± 6.3	206.0 ± 7.5	210.7 ± 5.9	219.4 ± 5.4	0.316	0.093	
Unrefined starches	89.8 ± 4.0	91.3 ± 3.7	89.6 ± 3.4	88.5 ± 4.9	0.907	0.869	
Cereals for breakfast	4.5 ± 1.3	5.8 ± 1.8	4.4 ± 1.1	3.4 ± 1.0	0.504	0.200	
Meats/fishes/eggs	190.9 ± 4.7	181.1 ± 4.6	194.5 ± 4.4	197.3 ± 5.1	0.026 *	0.034 *	0.027
Eggs	16.2 ± 1.2	15.2 ± 1.1	17.1 ± 1.3	16.2 ± 1.3	0.530	0.503	
Fishes	30.2 ± 2.1	27.6 ± 2.1	31.9 ± 2.1	31.2 ± 2.1	0.271	0.514	
Meat	144.6 ± 4.6	138.3 ± 4.6	145.5 ± 4.1	149.9 ± 5.2	0.270	0.253	
Mixed dishes and sandwiches	153.6 ± 7.6	175.1 ± 7.3	148.3 ± 8.6	137.4 ± 6.9	<0.001 *	0.001 *	0.001
Ready-made dishes and stocks	90.9 ± 5.6	101.4 ± 5.1	90.6 ± 5.5	80.7 ± 6.2	0.018 *	0.063	
Sandwiches and savoury puff pastries	62.7 ± 5.3	73.7 ± 6.1	57.6 ± 5.0	56.7 ± 4.8	0.018 *	0.002 *	0.001
Dairy products	214.1 ± 14.3	219.3 ± 20.9	211.1 ± 11.9	211.7 ± 10.0	0.924	0.603	
Milk	101.9 ± 13.1	114.7 ± 20.2	98.0 ± 10.5	93.1 ± 8.5	0.563	0.247	
Fresh dairy products	70.9 ± 5.8	61.4 ± 5.1	71.2 ± 5.1	80.1 ± 7.4	0.075	0.167	
Cheese	41.2 ± 2.8	43.2 ± 2.8	42.0 ± 2.7	38.5 ± 2.8	0.332	0.502	
Sweet products	123.6 ± 4.7	126.4 ± 4.6	125.9 ± 4.9	118.5 ± 4.6	0.367	0.601	
Dairy dessert	18.6 ± 2.2	20.6 ± 2.2	17.5 ± 2.2	17.8 ± 2.2	0.550	0.532	
Cakes, tarts, sweet pastries	67.5 ± 3.8	67.8 ± 4.2	70.0 ± 4.1	64.6 ± 3.1	0.585	0.564	
Biscuits and sweets	37.5 ± 2.4	38.0 ± 2.1	38.4 ± 3.1	36.0 ± 2.0	0.791	0.774	
Drinking water	761.5 ± 18.5	232.4 ± 11.1	664.8 ± 8.5	1387.3 ± 35.8	<0.001 *	<0.001 *	<0.001
Tap water	348.2 ± 24.2	120.9 ± 11.3	311.2 ± 22.2	612.6 ± 38.9	<0.001 *	<0.001 *	<0.001
Still water in a bottle	354.1 ± 28.1	90.7 ± 10.9	322.3 ± 24.1	649.2 ± 49.3	<0.001 *	<0.001 *	<0.001
Carbonated water in a bottle	59.2 ± 14.0	20.8 ± 4.7	31.3 ± 5.5	125.5 ± 31.8	0.005 *	0.025 *	0.007
Beverages	500.3 ± 21.1	582.4 ± 21.9	471.5 ± 21.3	447.0 ± 20.2	<0.001 *	<0.001 *	<0.001
Hot drinks (Tea. Coffee)	343.6 ± 18.5	389.8 ± 20.4	332.4 ± 17.4	308.7 ± 17.7	0.011 *	0.010 *	0.003
Diet sweet beverages	14.4 ± 4.8	20.3 ± 5.8	14.8 ± 5.7	8.1 ± 3.0	0.086	0.351	
Sugar-sweetened beverages	82.2 ± 12.4	106.8 ± 14.7	74.0 ± 10.9	65.9 ± 11.5	0.035 *	0.055	
Fruit juices	60.1 ± 6.7	65.6 ± 8.4	50.3 ± 4.9	64.4 ± 6.9	0.092	0.064	
Fat products	47.0 ± 1.9	42.5 ± 1.5	47.8 ± 2.1	50.6 ± 2.0	0.003 *	0.003 *	0.001
Animal fat	14.7 ± 0.9	14.7 ± 0.8	14.6 ± 1.2	14.7 ± 0.8	0.993	0.844	
Vegetable fat	23.2 ± 1.4	19.7 ± 1.3	23.6 ± 1.6	26.3 ± 1.2	0.001 *	0.001 *	<0.001
Spices and sauces	9.1 ± 0.9	8.2 ± 0.7	9.6 ± 0.7	9.6 ± 1.3	0.183	0.286	

Table 3. *Cont.*

	Women									
			Tertile of Drinking Water Intake							
	All		≤500 mL/Day		500–934 mL/Day		>934 mL/Day				
Food Groups and Subgroups (g/Day)	Mean	SD	Mean	SD	Mean	SD	Mean	SD	$p^\dagger$	$p^\ddagger$	p for Trend§
Fruits and vegetables	374.7	13.4	345.8	16.9	378.7	12.5	399.5	10.7	0.047	0.008	0.003
Vegetables, soup and crudités	213.7	8.6	203.0	10.3	216.4	7.9	221.6	7.7	0.333	0.105	
Fresh and processed fruits	159.3	8.3	141.2	8.5	160.5	7.5	176.0	8.8	0.025	0.037	0.011
Nuts	1.8	0.3	1.6	0.2	1.8	0.3	1.9	0.3	0.777	0.712	
Starches	202.4	4.8	207.7	5.4	192.8	4.1	206.7	5.1	0.019	0.005	0.551
Refined starches	126.8	3.5	130.4	3.2	120.7	3.4	129.1	3.9	0.084	0.084	
Unrefined starches	70.3	3.5	73.5	3.7	66.6	2.8	70.9	3.9	0.342	0.223	
Cereals for breakfast	5.4	1.0	3.8	0.8	5.5	1.0	6.7	1.1	0.056	0.299	
Meats/fishes/eggs	138.1	3.0	134.7	2.7	137.8	3.3	141.8	3.0	0.165	0.579	
Eggs	14.4	1.3	15.0	1.6	12.9	1.0	15.4	1.4	0.285	0.194	
Fishes	29.8	1.6	27.9	1.4	31.3	1.9	30.3	1.5	0.229	0.345	
Meat	93.9	2.7	91.9	2.5	93.7	2.9	96.2	2.6	0.495	0.793	
Mixed dishes and sandwiches	106.5	4.5	107.7	5.8	113.1	4.0	98.8	3.8	0.035	0.003	0.214
Ready-made dishes and stocks	64.8	3.3	61.7	2.9	70.8	3.7	61.8	3.2	0.122	0.043	
Sandwiches and savoury puff pastries	41.7	2.9	46.0	4.2	42.3	2.4	36.9	2.1	0.159	0.008	0.023
Dairy products	199.4	9.6	185.5	8.8	213.1	11.2	199.5	8.7	0.182	0.353	
Milk	86.3	7.6	82.0	6.3	97.3	8.3	79.5	8.2	0.217	0.240	
Fresh dairy products	86.6	4.6	78.5	4.1	89.2	5.0	92.0	4.6	0.080	0.603	
Cheese	26.5	1.4	25.0	1.3	26.7	1.3	27.9	1.6	0.309	0.114	
Sweet products	111.9	4.2	114.9	3.5	116.1	5.7	104.7	3.5	0.047	0.004	0.002
Dairy dessert	18.1	2.3	16.9	1.4	19.7	3.2	17.8	2.4	0.734	0.711	
Cakes, tarts, sweet pastries	61.1	3.4	62.8	3.6	65.2	3.9	55.2	2.6	0.057	0.013	
Biscuits and sweets	32.7	1.8	35.2	2.0	31.2	1.6	31.7	1.9	0.238	0.419	
Drinking water	802.5	14.9	284.0	8.3	693.2	8.1	1430.3	28.2	<0.001	<0.001	<0.001
Tap water	352.8	23.6	148.8	8.3	266.7	18.0	642.9	44.6	<0.001	<0.001	<0.001
Still water in a bottle	419.2	21.6	121.2	8.5	394.1	20.1	742.4	36.3	<0.001	<0.001	<0.001
Carbonated water in a bottle	30.5	5.2	14.0	3.6	32.3	5.2	45.1	6.7	<0.001	<0.001	<0.001
Beverages	523.3	29.5	592.0	27.5	526.0	35.7	451.9	25.4	<0.001	<0.001	<0.001
Hot drinks (Tea, Coffee)	404.1	27.8	447.0	23.8	408.4	34.6	356.8	25.1	0.011	0.018	0.005
Diet sweet beverages	12.2	3.5	16.2	4.9	13.7	3.9	6.8	1.6	0.016	0.014	0.100
Sugar-sweetened beverages	48.4	10.4	82.9	17.6	37.5	9.5	24.8	4.2	0.006	0.007	0.002
Fruit juices	58.6	6.4	45.9	8.7	66.3	5.2	63.5	5.2	0.069	0.049	0.150
Fat products	45.1	1.2	43.0	0.9	45.1	1.1	47.1	1.4	0.033	0.029	0.008
Animal fat	13.3	0.8	13.5	0.7	12.9	0.7	13.6	0.8	0.786	0.489	
Vegetable fat	23.4	0.9	22.2	0.8	23.6	0.8	24.5	1.1	0.117	0.189	
Spices and sauces	8.3	0.7	7.3	0.6	8.6	0.5	9.0	0.9	0.198	0.300	

[1] Values are survey-weighted means with standard deviations; † adjustment for energy intake; ‡ adjustment for energy intake, level of education, socio-occupational group, season, level of physical activity, smoker status, region, and quintile of income per consumption unit (ICU); § calculated only for significant differences.

For both men and women, and with full adjustment, consumption of fluids was characterised by a significant increase from the lowest to the highest tertile of all types of drinking water (drinking water, tap water, still water in a bottle) (p for trend < 0.0001) and a decrease in other beverages (p for trend < 0.0001). In particular, the consumption of hot drinks significantly decreased (p for trend = 0.003 among men and p for trend = 0.005 among women) (Table 3).

For both sexes, the fruits and vegetables food group was characterised by an increase from the lowest to the highest tertile, being significant only among women (p for trend = 0.003 after full adjustment). This result was steered by the fresh and processed fruits subgroup (p for trend < 0.05 for men and p for trend = 0.011 for women). For men and women, after full adjustment, the consumption of fat products significantly increased from the first to the third tertile (p for trend = 0.001 for men and p for trend = 0.08 for women), steered among men by a significant increase in the vegetable fat subgroup (p for trend = 0.001). Among men, after full adjustment, a significant increase from the lowest to the highest tertile was found for consumption of the meat/fishes/eggs group (p for trend = 0.027) and a significant decrease was found for the mixed dishes and sandwiches group (p for trend = 0.001). Among women, sweet products consumption decreased from the first to the third tertile (p for trend = 0.002) and the consumption of starches and mixed dishes was significantly different between tertiles but with no linear trend (Table 3).

4. Discussion

This study was the first representative study of French adults investigating the associations by sex between drinking water patterns and diet quality in light of socio-economic determinants and adherence to EFSA AI for TWI. Our findings confirmed our hypothesis that an elevated drinking water intake was positively associated with diet quality, as large drinking water consumers were more likely to adhere to the EFSA AI, had diets of higher nutritional quality and, mostly among women, seemed to make healthier food choices (e.g., more fruits and vegetables and fewer sweets). Seventy-two percent of men and 46% of women in the French adult population were below the EFSA AI for TWI. In our sample, large drinking water consumers were more likely to have a high socio-occupational status and, among men only, to have a higher education level, a higher physical activity level, a higher income per consumption unit, and were more likely to be non-smokers.

It stems from our results that a higher drinking water intake was associated with higher nutritional quality of the diet, assessed by several dietary indices. In our study, the MAR and the PANDiet were positively associated with drinking water while differing in their methods, as the MAR is a simple mean percentage of sex- and age-specific French RDA [37], whereas the PANDiet is a score that takes into account different parameters, including the number of days of dietary data, the mean nutrient intake and its day-to-day variability, the nutrient reference value, and inter-individual variability [38]. Using different indices is useful to show that our observations are consistent and do not depend on a certain methodology of assessing diet quality. All relationships between tertiles of drinking water and dietary indices, SED, and energy cost, even though not all were significant, were congruent in the same direction. Full adjustment revealed that the association between drinking water intake and diet quality was particularly noticeable for women, for whom drinking water increased, as did the indicators of nutritional quality (i.e., higher MAR and PANDiet scores, and lower SED values). Results are consistent with Kim et al., who found a positive association, among both Korean men and women, between drinking water intake and the MAR [41]. When not using dietary indices, other relationships between drinking water intake and nutrients have been found in the literature that we could consider as good indicators of nutritional quality. In the US, Yang and Chun found a positive association between TWI, drinking water, and moisture in foods with dietary and serum minerals, vitamins, and carotenoids [22]. Those nutrients positively associated with TWI can be compared to identical components of the MAR, and are in line with our results. In a recent national study of US adults, an increase in the proportion of daily drinking water in TWI was found to be associated with a decreased daily intake of total energy, energy from sugar-sweetened beverages, discretionary foods, and total fat, saturated fat, sugar, sodium, and cholesterol [21]. Most of those nutrients, the intake of which is negatively associated with drinking water, are similar to the components of the MER, and are also slightly decreased in our results among men. Higher intakes of sodium found in women could possibly explain why the MER did not significantly decrease. In previous studies, a positive association was found between drinking water and sodium intakes [4,41], similar to our results among women, although the cause-consequence relationship is unknown.

In terms of fluid patterns, our results indicate that large drinking water consumers seemed to favour a higher intake of only water and not necessarily all other fluids. A similar observation was made by Illescas-Zarate et al. in her study among Mexican adults, in which a negative association was found between drinking water intake and sugar-sweetened beverages [42].

In terms of food choices, large drinking water consumers seemed to favour diets rich in moisture-abundant foods, especially fresh fruits. This finding is in line with the literature reporting the opposite observation, i.e., low levels of fruit and vegetable intake among low drinking water consumers [23,41]. Similarly, a negative association between drinking water intake and beverage moisture, but a positive association with food moisture, was found among US adults [20,22]. Kant et al. suggested some substitution effect of drinking water intake on other fluid consumption and possibly higher fruit and vegetable intake [20]. According to Hedrick et al., consumption of water, unsweetened tea/coffee, low-fat milk, artificially sweetened beverages, and fruit/vegetable juice is closely aligned with a "prudent" dietary pattern (usually including vegetables, fruits, legumes, whole grains, fish, and poultry); conversely, the consumption of high-fat milk, alcohol, and sugar-sweetened beverages is strongly associated with a "Western" dietary pattern (usually including red meat, processed meat, refined grains, sweets and dessert, French fries, and high-fat dairy products) [43]. This last point is particularly illustrated in our results with the decrease of mixed dishes and sandwiches among men and of sweet products among women from the first to third tertile of drinking water intake. Large drinking water consumers tended to consume more moisture-abundant foods, also rich in nutrients and vitamins, implying that people fulfilling their water intake requirements have higher quality diets and make food choices more likely to fulfil their nutritional requirements.

Identifying characteristics of large drinking water consumers can be useful to identify individuals more likely to have healthier dietary behaviours. In the literature, associations have been found between drinking water intake and some socioeconomic determinants, such as sex [42,44], age [22,23,41,45], education level [22,23], income [23,45], level of physical activity [22,23,41], and smoking status [11,23, 41]. The novelty of our study is that drinking water patterns were explored in light of several factors combined (socio-demographics, lifestyle determinants, and overall dietary intake). Moreover, a major strength of our study is the investigation of socioeconomic determinants of drinking water intake by sex in order to identify gender specificities, which has only been done before, to our knowledge, by Kim et al. [41]. In our study, both among men and women, drinking water intake was positively associated with socioeconomic position. However, female drinking water intake appears to be less influenced by socioeconomic factors, considering the numerous additional associations for men, notably with education, physical activity, income, and smoking status. Thus, among men, drinking water intake may be considered as a reliable indicator of socioeconomic differences. This male specificity has not been noticed by Kim et al. among Korean adults [41]. Among men, the association between drinking water intake and diet quality was explained by their socio-economic status, as men in higher socio-economic strata had a higher nutritional quality and higher drinking water intake. However, among women, the association between drinking water intake and a healthy dietary pattern was independent of the social level. Gender contrasts in food choices are influenced by views on food and health, the ethical dimensions of food production and food selection, nutritional attitudes and choices, dietary change, food work, and body image [46]. One hypothesis could be that, regarding beverages, women appear to be more 'health-conscious' [47] than males, who consume more alcohol [14,48,49] and sweet beverages regularly [14,49]. More research is needed to fully apprehend divergent associations found in the literature and to verify if women and men follow a distinct drinking water pattern elsewhere than in France.

In the current study, daily means of TWI were consistent with results from previous European studies [11,14,50]. However, a remarkable observation was made in that the sex difference in TWI was less pronounced in France than in some other countries: estimated TWI was slightly lower for men and slightly higher for women than those of Irish [11], British [14], and German [50] adults (2.16 L vs. 2.52 L, 2.53 L, and 2.48 L for men, and 2.12 L vs. 2.09 L, 2.03 L, and 2.05 L for women, respectively). This is, on one hand, in contrast to a tendency reported in the literature with men systematically having a higher TWI than women [4,11,14,20,22,45,50] while, on the other hand, fluid surveys in 13 countries showed few significant differences in fluid intake between both sexes. The latter suggests that if there is a gender difference in TWI, the difference could be due to a difference in water from food moisture, a result that was also observed in our study, but needs to be confirmed further.

Several strengths and limitations of this study should be acknowledged. The INCA2 data were collected in 2006–2007 and the observations may already be obsolete. However, INCA2 is still the most recent version of a population-based survey available in France and remains the standard source of reliable information about dietary intakes. Furthermore, between the first version of the national survey (INCA1) and the second (INCA2), the food group 'waters' increased from six items to 50 items, increasing the robustness of data from this food group, which is of particular importance for the present study [51]. A potential additional limitation could come from numerous low drinking water consumers interviewed during the winter. However, no interaction effect was found between the season and drinking consumption patterns on the level of adequacy (data not shown). Another limitation, inherent to any dietary survey, is the fact that the nutritional intake data is self-reported. Especially collecting data to evaluate TWI is not without limitations: accurate recording of drinking water and other beverages, as well as estimating water from food moisture, might be prone to bias [52]. A final point of discussion is the exclusion of alcohol. Since several publications report a major contribution of alcoholic beverages to water intake [11,14,22,41,45], excluding these beverages could lead to an overestimation of the proportion of French adults below the EFSA AI of TWI. However, this could also be interpreted as a limitation in our case, since having an adequate intake of TWI should be achieved mainly with drinking water.

5. Conclusions

This is the first description of total water intakes among small, medium, and large drinking water consumers considering socio-demographic determinants and diet quality among men and women in France. It shows that large drinking water consumers have healthier fluid intake and nutritional patterns, independent of the social level among women. In the future, more research should be performed to demonstrate the role of a high water intake, as part of a high quality diet, in the prevention of chronic disease. In the meantime, these results could already imply that the guidelines for disease prevention should not only mention a high quality diet, but also a high intake of water. Nevertheless, inadequacy of TWI remains prevalent at all levels of drinking water intake for both sexes. Advice regarding the importance of drinking water intake is still necessary to help individuals to reach adequate water intake.

Supplementary Materials: The following are available online at http://www.mdpi.com/2072-6643/8/11/689/s1, Table S1: Nine food groups and 27 food subgroups, Table S2: Vitamin and mineral intakes by sex and tertile.

Acknowledgments: R.G., J.S. and M.M. have received research grants from Danone Research. R.G. was financially supported by MS-Nutrition and ANRT (Agence Nationale de la Recherche et de la Technology).

Author Contributions: R.G., J.S., M.M., I.G. and A.L. were involved in developing the analysis plan, data interpretation and manuscript redaction. Data analysis was performed by R.G., J.S. and M.M.

Conflicts of Interest: A.L. and I.G. are full-time employees of Danone Research. The other authors declare no conflict of interest.

References

1. Popkin, B.M.; D'Anci, K.E.; Rosenberg, I.H. Water, hydration, and health. *Nutr. Rev.* **2010**, *68*, 439–458. [CrossRef] [PubMed]
2. Pross, N.; Demazières, A.; Girard, N.; Barnouin, R.; Santoro, F.; Chevillotte, E.; Klein, A.; Le Bellego, L. Influence of progressive fluid restriction on mood and physiological markers of dehydration in women. *Br. J. Nutr.* **2013**, *109*, 313–321. [CrossRef] [PubMed]
3. EFSA Panel on Dietetic Products Nutrition and Allergies (NDA). Scientific Opinion on the substantiation of health claims related to water and maintenance of normal physical and cognitive functions (ID 1102, 1209, 1294, 1331), maintenance of normal thermoregulation (ID 1208) and "basic requirement of all living things. *EFSA J.* **2011**, *9*, 2075.
4. Sontrop, J.M.; Dixon, S.N.; Garg, A.X.; Buendia-Jimenez, I.; Dohein, O.; Huang, S.-H.S.; Clark, W.F. Association between water intake, chronic kidney disease, and cardiovascular disease: A cross-sectional analysis of NHANES data. *Am. J. Nephrol.* **2013**, *37*, 434–442. [CrossRef] [PubMed]
5. Muckelbauer, R.; Sarganas, G.; Grüneis, A.; Müller-Nordhorn, J. Association between water consumption and body weight outcomes: A systematic review. *Am. J. Clin. Nutr.* **2013**, *98*, 282–299. [CrossRef] [PubMed]
6. Roussel, R.; Fezeu, L.; Bouby, N.; Balkau, B.; Lantieri, O.; Alhenc-Gelas, F.; Marre, M.; Bankir, L. Low water intake and risk for new-onset hyperglycemia. *Diabetes Care* **2011**, *34*, 2551–2554. [CrossRef] [PubMed]
7. Clark, W.F.; Sontrop, J.M.; Macnab, J.J.; Suri, R.S.; Moist, L.; Salvadori, M.; Garg, A.X. Urine volume and change in estimated GFR in a community-based cohort study. *Clin. J. Am. Soc. Nephrol.* **2011**, *6*, 2634–2641. [CrossRef] [PubMed]
8. Strippoli, G.F.; Craig, J.C.; Rochtchina, E.; Flood, V.M.; Wang, J.J.; Mitchell, P. Fluid and nutrient intake and risk of chronic kidney disease. *Nephrology* **2011**, *16*, 326–334. [CrossRef] [PubMed]
9. EFSA Panel on Dietetic Products Nutrition and Allergies (NDA). Scientific Opinion on Dietary Reference Values for water/European Food Safety Authority. *EFSA J.* **2010**, *8*, 48.
10. Institute of Medicine. *Dietary Reference Intakes for Water, Potassium, Sodium, Chloride, and Sulfate*; National Academies Press: Washington, DC, USA, 2005.
11. O'Connor, L.; Walton, J.; Flynn, A. Water intakes and dietary sources of a nationally representative sample of Irish adults. *J. Hum. Nutr. Diet.* **2014**, *27*, 550–556. [CrossRef] [PubMed]
12. Nissensohn, M.; Sánchez-Villegas, A.; Ortega, R.; Aranceta-Bartrina, J.; Gil, Á.; González-Gross, M.; Varela-Moreiras, G.; Serra-Majem, L. Beverage Consumption Habits and Association with Total Water and Energy Intakes in the Spanish Population: Findings of the ANIBES Study. *Nutrients* **2016**, *8*, 232. [CrossRef] [PubMed]
13. Cartier, T.; Dubuisson, C.; Panetier, P.; Volatier, J.-L. Human water consumption in France: Results from the INCA2 diet study. *Environ. Risques Santé* **2012**, *11*, 479–491.
14. Gibson, S.; Shirreffs, S.M. Beverage consumption habits "24/7" among British adults: Association with total water intake and energy intake. *Nutr. J.* **2013**, *12*, 9. [CrossRef] [PubMed]
15. Bellisle, F.; Thornton, S.N.; Hébel, P.; Denizeau, M.; Tahiri, M. A study of fluid intake from beverages in a sample of healthy French children, adolescents and adults. *Eur. J. Clin. Nutr.* **2010**, *64*, 350–355. [CrossRef] [PubMed]
16. Guelinckx, I.; Ferreira-Pêgo, C.; Moreno, L.A.; Kavouras, S.A.; Gandy, J.; Martinez, H.; Bardosono, S.; Abdollahi, M.; Nasseri, E.; Jarosz, A.; Ma, G.; et al. Intake of water and different beverages in adults across 13 Countries. *Eur. J. Nutr.* **2015**, *54*, 45–55. [CrossRef] [PubMed]
17. Vieux, F.; Maillot, M.; Constant, F.; Drewnowski, A. Water and beverage consumption among children aged 4–13 years in France: Analyses of INCA 2 (Étude Individuelle Nationale des Consommations Alimentaires 2006–2007) data. *Public Health Nutr.* **2016**, *19*, 2305–2314. [CrossRef] [PubMed]
18. Popkin, B.M.; Armstrong, L.E.; Bray, G.M.; Caballero, B.; Frei, B.; Willett, W.C. A new proposed guidance system for beverage consumption in the United States. *Am. J. Clin. Nutr.* **2006**, *83*, 529–542. [PubMed]
19. Duffey, K.J.; Popkin, B.M. Adults with healthier dietary patterns have healthier beverage patterns. *J. Nutr.* **2006**, *136*, 2901–2907. [PubMed]
20. Kant, A.K.; Graubard, B.I.; Atchison, E.A. Intakes of plain water, moisture in foods and beverages, and total water in the adult US population—Nutritional, meal pattern, and body weight correlates: National Health and Nutrition Examination Surveys 1999–2006. *Am. J. Clin. Nutr.* **2009**, *90*, 655–663. [CrossRef] [PubMed]

21. An, R.; McCaffrey, J. Plain water consumption in relation to energy intake and diet quality among US adults, 2005–2012. *J. Hum. Nutr. Diet.* **2016**, *29*, 624–632. [CrossRef] [PubMed]

22. Yang, M.; Chun, O.K. Consumptions of plain water, moisture in foods and beverages, and total water in relation to dietary micronutrient intakes and serum nutrient profiles among US adults. *Public Health Nutr.* **2015**, *18*, 1180–1186. [CrossRef] [PubMed]

23. Goodman, A.B.; Blanck, H.M.; Sherry, B.; Park, S.; Nebeling, L.; Yaroch, A.L. Behaviors and attitudes associated with low drinking water intake among US adults, Food Attitudes and Behaviors Survey, 2007. *Prev. Chronic Dis.* **2013**, *10*, E51. [CrossRef] [PubMed]

24. Dubuisson, C.; Lioret, S.; Touvier, M.; Dufour, A.; Calamassi-Tran, G.; Volatier, J.-L.; Lafay, L. Trends in food and nutritional intakes of French adults from 1999 to 2007: Results from the INCA surveys. *Br. J. Nutr.* **2010**, *103*, 1035–1048. [CrossRef] [PubMed]

25. Bocquier, A.; Vieux, F.; Lioret, S.; Dubuisson, C.; Caillavet, F.; Darmon, N. Socio-economic characteristics, living conditions and diet quality are associated with food insecurity in France. *Public Health Nutr.* **2015**, *18*, 2952–2961. [CrossRef] [PubMed]

26. Lioret, S.; Touvier, M.; Lafay, L.; Volatier, J.-L.; Maire, B. Are eating occasions and their energy content related to child overweight and socioeconomic status? *Obesity (Silver Spring).* **2008**, *16*, 2518–2523. [CrossRef] [PubMed]

27. National Institute of Statistics and Economic Studies (INSEE). Definitions and Methods. Definitions. Consumption Unit. Available online: http://www.insee.fr/en/methodes/default.asp?page=definitions/unite-consommation.htm (accessed on 15 June 2016).

28. Kendrick, T.; King, F.; Albertella, L.; Smith, P.W. GP treatment decisions for patients with depression: An observational study. *Br. J. Gen. Pract.* **2005**, *55*, 280–286. [PubMed]

29. International Physical Activity Questionnaire (IPAQ). Guidelines for Data Processing and Analysis of the International Physical Activity Questionnaire (IPAQ)—Short and Long Forms. Available online: https://www.researchgate.net/file.PostFileLoader.html?id=56f92d66615e27d49a658031&assetKey=AS%3A344600888791041%401459170662924 (accessed on 17 April 2016).

30. Le Moullec, N.; Deheeger, M.; Preziosi, P.; Montero, P.; Valeix, P.; Rolland-Cachera, M.; Potier de Courcy, G.; Christides, J.; Galan, P.; Hercberg, S. Validation du manuel-photos utilisé pour l'enquête alimentaire de l'étude SUVIMAX. *Cah. Nutr. Diet* **1996**, *31*, 158–164.

31. Agence Nationale de Sécurité Sanitaire de L'alimentation, de L'environnement et du Travail (ANSES). French Food Composition Table Ciqual 2013. Available online: https://pro.anses.fr/TableCIQUAL/index.htm (accessed on 23 March 2016).

32. Verger, E.O.; Mariotti, F.; Holmes, B.A.; Paineau, D.; Huneau, J.-F. Evaluation of a diet quality index based on the probability of adequate nutrient intake (PANDiet) using national French and US dietary surveys. *PLoS ONE* **2012**, *7*, e42155. [CrossRef] [PubMed]

33. Guthrie, H.A.; Scheer, J.C. Validity of a dietary score for assessing nutrient adequacy. *J. Am. Diet Assoc.* **1981**, *78*, 240–245. [PubMed]

34. Vieux, F.; Soler, L.-G.; Touazi, D.; Darmon, N. High nutritional quality is not associated with low greenhouse gas emissions in self-selected diets of French adults. *Am. J. Clin. Nutr.* **2013**, *97*, 569–583. [CrossRef] [PubMed]

35. Ledikwe, J.H.; Blanck, H.M.; Khan, L.K.; Serdula, M.K.; Seymour, J.D.; Tohill, B.C.; Rolls, B.J. Low-energy-density diets are associated with high diet quality in adults in the United States. *J. Am. Diet. Assoc.* **2006**, *106*, 1172–1180. [CrossRef] [PubMed]

36. Stubbs, J.; Ferres, S.; Horgan, G. Energy density of foods: Effects on energy intake. *Crit. Rev. Food Sci. Nutr.* **2000**, *40*, 481–515. [CrossRef] [PubMed]

37. Darmon, N.; Caillavet, F.; Joly, C.; Maillot, M.; Drewnowski, A. Low-cost foods: How do they compare with their brand name equivalents? A French study. *Public Health Nutr.* **2009**, *12*, 808–815. [CrossRef] [PubMed]

38. Verger, E.O.; Holmes, B.A.; Huneau, J.F.; Mariotti, F. Simple changes within dietary subgroups can rapidly improve the nutrient adequacy of the diet of French adults. *J. Nutr.* **2014**, *144*, 929–936. [CrossRef] [PubMed]

39. Masset, G.; Vieux, F.; Verger, E.O.; Soler, L.G.; Touazi, D.; Darmon, N. Reducing energy intake and energy density for a sustainable diet: A study based on self-selected diets in French adults. *Am. J. Clin. Nutr.* **2014**, *99*, 1460–1469. [CrossRef] [PubMed]

40. Kantar Worldpanel. French Household Consumer Panel—Kantar Worldpanel. Available online: http://www.kantarworldpanel.com/global/Sectors (accessed on 5 May 2013).

41. Kim, J.; Yang, Y.J. Plain water intake of Korean adults according to life style, anthropometric and dietary characteristic: The Korea National Health and Nutrition Examination Surveys 2008–2010. *Nutr. Res. Pract.* **2014**, *8*, 580–588. [CrossRef] [PubMed]

42. Illescas-Zarate, D.; Espinosa-Montero, J.; Flores, M.; Barquera, S. Plain water consumption is associated with lower intake of caloric beverage: Cross-sectional study in Mexican adults with low socioeconomic status. *BMC Public Health* **2015**, *15*, 405. [CrossRef] [PubMed]

43. Hedrick, V.E.; Davy, B.M.; Duffey, K.J. Is Beverage Consumption Related to Specific Dietary Pattern Intakes? *Curr. Nutr. Rep.* **2014**, *4*, 72–81. [CrossRef]

44. Özen, A.E.; Bibiloni, M.D.M.; Pons, A.; Tur, J.A. Fluid intake from beverages across age groups: A systematic review. *J. Hum. Nutr. Diet.* **2015**, *28*, 417–442. [CrossRef] [PubMed]

45. Drewnowski, A.; Rehm, C.D.; Constant, F. Water and beverage consumption among adults in the United States: Cross-sectional study using data from NHANES 2005–2010. *BMC Public Health* **2013**, *13*, 1068. [CrossRef] [PubMed]

46. Beardsworth, A.; Bryman, A.; Keil, T.; Goode, J.; Haslam, C.; Lancashire, E. Women, men and food: The significance of gender for nutritional attitudes and choices. *Brit. Food J.* **2002**, *104*, 470–491. [CrossRef]

47. Hattersley, L.; Irwin, M.; King, L.; Allman-Farinelli, M. Determinants and patterns of soft drink consumption in young adults: A qualitative analysis. *Public Health Nutr.* **2009**, *12*, 1816–1822. [CrossRef] [PubMed]

48. Martinez, H. Fluid intake in Mexican adults; a cross-sectional study. *Nutr. Hosp.* **2014**, *29*, 1179–1187. [PubMed]

49. Ferreira-Pêgo, C.; Babio, N.; Fenández-Alvira, J.M.; Iglesia, I.; Moreno, L.A.; Salas-Salvadó, J. Fluid intake from beverages in Spanish adults; cross-sectional study. *Nutr. Hosp.* **2014**, *29*, 1171–1178. [PubMed]

50. Manz, F.; Johner, S. A.; Wentz, A.; Boeing, H.; Remer, T. Water balance throughout the adult life span in a German population. *Br. J. Nutr.* **2012**, *107*, 1673–1681. [CrossRef] [PubMed]

51. Agence française de sécurité sanitaire des aliments (AFSSA). *Étude Individuelle Nationale des Consommations Alimentaires 2 (INCA 2) 2006–2007*; AFSSA: Paris, France, 2009.

52. Gandy, J. Water intake: Validity of population assessment and recommendations. *Eur. J. Nutr.* **2015**, *54*, 11–16. [CrossRef] [PubMed]

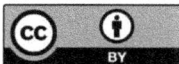

nutrients MDPI

Article

Substitution Models of Water for Other Beverages, and the Incidence of Obesity and Weight Gain in the SUN Cohort

Ujué Fresán [1], Alfredo Gea [1,2,3], Maira Bes-Rastrollo [1,2,3], Miguel Ruiz-Canela [1,2,3] and Miguel A. Martínez-Gonzalez [1,2,3,*]

[1] Department of Preventive Medicine and Public Health, University of Navarra, Medical School, Irunlarrea 1, 31008 Pamplona, Spain; ufresan@unav.es (U.F.); ageas@unav.es (A.G.); mbes@unav.es (M.B.-R.); mcanela@unav.es (M.R.-C.)
[2] Navarra Institute for Health Research (IdisNa), 31008 Pamplona, Spain
[3] CIBER Physiopathology of Obesity and Nutrition (CIBERobn), Carlos III Institute of Health, 28029 Madrid, Spain
*   Correspondence: mamartinez@unav.es; Tel.: +34-636-355-333

Received: 30 July 2016; Accepted: 26 October 2016; Published: 31 October 2016

Abstract: Obesity is a major epidemic for developed countries in the 21st century. The main cause of obesity is energy imbalance, of which contributing factors include a sedentary lifestyle, epigenetic factors and excessive caloric intake through food and beverages. A high consumption of caloric beverages, such as alcoholic or sweetened drinks, may particularly contribute to weight gain, and lower satiety has been associated with the intake of liquid instead of solid calories. Our objective was to evaluate the association between the substitution of a serving per day of water for another beverage (or group of them) and the incidence of obesity and weight change in a Mediterranean cohort, using mathematical models. We followed 15,765 adults without obesity at baseline. The intake of 17 beverage items was assessed at baseline through a validated food-frequency questionnaire. The outcomes were average change in body weight in a four-year period and new-onset obesity and their association with the substitution of one serving per day of water for one of the other beverages. During the follow-up, 873 incident cases of obesity were identified. In substitution models, the consumption of water instead of beer or sugar-sweetened soda beverages was associated with a lower obesity incidence (the Odds Ratio (OR) 0.80 (95% confidence interval (CI) 0.68 to 0.94) and OR 0.85 (95% CI 0.75 to 0.97); respectively) and, in the case of beer, it was also associated with a higher average weight loss (weight change difference = −328 g; (95% CI −566 to −89)). Thus, this study found that replacing one sugar-sweetened soda beverage or beer with one serving of water per day at baseline was related to a lower incidence of obesity and to a higher weight loss over a four-year period time in the case of beer, based on mathematical models.

Keywords: Mediterranean cohort; water; soft drinks; beer; obesity; body weight

1. Introduction

Obesity is a major epidemic in the 21st century for developed countries. In fact, 20%–30% of the Western adult population is obese [1], and the United States or some European countries have unacceptably high mean values of body mass index (BMI) [2]. In the last decade, its prevalence has risen seriously [3], and, although it is predicted to plateau by 2033, if the actual trend continues, around 30% of USA population would be overweight and obese [4]. These huge figures require new preventive measures and policy actions [4,5], as obesity is a risk factor for many chronic diseases such as cardiovascular disease, diabetes, some types of cancer and all-cause mortality [6]. Obesity is a multifactorial disorder [7,8]. Although sedentary lifestyle and epigenetics contribute to obesity, excessive caloric intake is a key determinant that needs to be addressed [9].

Beverages are major components of the daily diet. As for food, there are guidelines for beverage consumption in order to contribute to healthy diet [10,11]. Beverages can account for a substantial share of daily calories, even having low nutritional value, as it is the case of regular soft drinks and alcoholic beverages [12,13]. Solid and liquid preloads have been described as incomplete energy compensations [14], but beverages have a weaker satiety capacity than solids. Thus, a subsequent decompensated adjustment of calories intake takes place, causing an increase in total energy intake. Some beverages, like sugar-sweetened soda, are associated with weight gain and obesity [15,16]. Assessing alcoholic drinks, the relationship with these outcomes seems to depend on the type of alcohol analyzed because wine, beer and spirits may have different effects [17]. Water consumption has various health benefits, and a promising target for health promotion for obesity prevention could be to increase water intake at the expense of decreasing the consumption of other beverages [18,19].

Our objective was to evaluate the effect of substituting a serving per day of water for one of another beverage, or group of beverages according to the Spanish Society of Community Nutrition (Sociedad Española de Nutrición Comunitaria; SENC) recommendations, on obesity incidence and weight change in a Mediterranean cohort, using mathematical models.

2. Materials and Methods

2.1. Study Population

The Spanish project Seguimiento Universidad de Navarra (University of Navarra Follow-Up) (SUN) is a multipurpose, dynamic and prospective cohort, designed to establish relationships between diet and chronic conditions, such as obesity. All the participants are university graduates. Recruitment started in December 1999, and is permanently open. When participants are invited to enter the study, they receive, with the baseline questionnaire, a letter explaining the methodology, aims, data management and all information about the SUN cohort, including how to withdraw from the study. Informed consent was implied by the voluntary completion of the baseline questionnaire. Every two years, information from participants is collected by mailed or e-mailed questionnaires. When participants do not return a questionnaire, we send them a short exit questionnaire. The Research Ethics Committee of the University of Navarra approved the study. Further details of the study design and methods have been published elsewhere [20].

Up to March 2013, 21,686 participants were recruited. Among them, we excluded 2046 participants with total energy intake beyond predefined limits (<800 Kcal/day and <500 Kcal/day or >4000 Kcal/day and >3500 Kcal/day in men and women, respectively [21])—260 women who were pregnant at baseline or declared it in the second questionnaire, 1096 participants with a prevalent chronic disease such as cancer, diabetes and cardiovascular disease, and 513 participants with missing values in variables of interest in the analyses. Furthermore, 1706 people failed to answer the follow-up questionnaires (retention in the cohort: 90.7%), leaving a total of 16,065 participants. Finally, as this study was investigating the effect of beverage substitution on the incidence of obesity over time, we furthermore excluded people with prevalent obesity at baseline (n = 300). Therefore, the final number of participants for this analysis was 15,765.

2.2. Beverage Exposure Assessment

A semi-quantitative food frequency questionnaire (FFQ) was included in the baseline questionnaire. It was previously validated in Spain and recently re-evaluated [22,23]. The FFQ contained 17 beverage items (whole milk, reduced-fat milk, skim milk, milk shake, red wine, other kind of wine, beer, spirits, sugar-sweetened soda beverages (SSSBs), diet soda beverages, regular coffee, decaffeinated coffee, fresh orange juice, fresh non-orange fruit juice, bottled juice (any kind of fruit), tap water and bottled water). For each of them, frequencies of consumption were measured in nine categories, ranking from never/almost never to >6 servings/day. Serving size differed between beverages: coffee = 50 mL, wine = 100 mL, beer = 330 mL, spirits = 50 mL and, for the remaining beverages, a serving was equivalent to 200 mL.

All beverages reported were grouped according to SENC recommendations [11] and other publications [24] into six groups: two items on water (tap and bottled water), three items on low/non-caloric beverages (LNCBs) (non-sugared coffee (decaffeinated and regular) and diet soda beverages), nine items on milk, juice and sugared coffee (whole, reduced-fat and skim milk, milk shake, fresh orange and non-orange fruit juice, and any kind of fruit bottled juice, and sugared coffee (decaffeinated and regular), two items on occasional consumption (SSSBs and spirits), two items on wine (red and other kind of wine) and one item on beer (beer). The SENC has put together beverages into groups according to the evidence of quantity of energy and nutrients, benefits and harmful effects, and hydration capacity of each beverage. Liquids consumed as part of a food item are not taken into account. Our questionnaire did not distinguish between coffee with or without sugar. To make this distinction, we assumed that if the sugar intake was equal to or bigger than servings of coffee (both the decaffeinated and the regular one), coffee was drunk with sugar. Conversely, if sugar consumption was smaller than servings of coffee, coffee was assumed to be taken without sugar.

2.3. Outcome Assessment

Weight information was self-reported at baseline and in the follow-up questionnaires every two years. BMI was calculated as weight in kilograms divided by the square of height in meters. The validity of these measures has been assessed in a subsample of this cohort [25]. The mean relative error in self-reported weight was 1.45%, and the correlation coefficient between measured and self-reported weight was 0.99 (95% confidence intervals (95% CI) 0.98 to 0.99). For BMI, the mean relative error was 2.64% with a correlation coefficient of 0.94 (95% CI 0.91 to 0.97) [25]. The outcomes were incidence of obesity and weight change. A participant was classified as an incident case of obesity if his/her BMI was lower than 30 kg/m^2 at baseline and equal to or higher than 30 during the follow-up. Average change in body weight was assessed between baseline and the four-year follow-up questionnaire, subtracting the first from the second.

2.4. Assessment of Other Variables

The baseline questionnaire also inquired about socio-demographic factors, medical history, and health-related habits. To quantify physical activity during free time, we assessed time spent in 17 activities at baseline, in order to compute an activity metabolic equivalent index (MET). Each activity was assigned a multiple of resting metabolic rate (MET score) [26] and time spent in each activity was multiplied by its specific MET score. Self-reported weekly MET-h correlated with energy expenditure objectively measured in a subsample of the cohort (Spearman r = 0.51; 95% CI 0.232 to 0.707) [27]. Adherence to Mediterranean diet was evaluated using the nine-item Mediterranean diet score developed by Trichopoulou and colleagues [28]. When the beverage that we were analyzing was included in this score, we recalculated it after excluding the item that we were studying, to avoid overlapping with the main exposure.

2.5. Statistical Analyses

We evaluated the association between substituting one serving per day of water for each beverage or beverage group (increasing one serving of water and decreasing one serving of the beverage/group in question) and incident obesity using mathematical models [29]. These replacements referred only to reported consumption at baseline; changes in beverage intake over time were not assessed. We fitted generalized estimating equations (GEE) models to evaluate the association of the described substitutions with obesity incidence. We assumed a binomial distribution, a logit link function, and an exchangeable correlation matrix. All completed observations from each participant were included, from the baseline to either the questionnaire in which the participant was classified as an incident case of obesity or the last follow-up questionnaire. Data received from participants after their classification as an incident case of obesity were excluded. As mentioned before, exposure was assumed constant for this model. If women reported a pregnancy during follow-up were censored at the questionnaire previous to their pregnancy. The Odds Ratio (OR) and 95% CI were estimated as the difference between β coefficients of exchanged beverages and then exponentiated [29]. Linear regression models were used to assess the association between the beverage replacements and four-year weight change. We estimated the adjusted absolute mean weight change (and 95% CI) of the beverage substitutions as the difference between β of exchanged beverages [29]. We fitted a crude univariate model, an age- and sex-adjusted model, and a multiple-adjusted model adjusted for the following potential confounders: sex, age, age squared, baseline BMI (kg/m^2), physical activity (MET-h/week), smoking habit (never smoker, current smoker, former smoker), personal and family history of obesity, following a special diet, adherence to the Mediterranean dietary pattern, snacking between meals, weight change during the five years prior to baseline, and total energy intake from other sources than the exchanged beverages. When the analyses were carried out for group of beverages, we additionally adjusted for servings per day of other groups. Interactions were assessed using the Wald test for the two product terms between each beverage involved in the substitution and the characteristic evaluated.

In order to calculate the contribution of each beverage (or group of them) to the between-person variability in fluid intake, we conducted nested regression analyses after a stepwise selection algorithm. The contribution of each beverage is shown in the cumulative R^2 change. Furthermore, we estimated their contribution related to total fluid intake as the mL consumed from each beverage divided by total fluid intake (%).

To ensure that the method of dealing with missing values did not influence the results, we performed a sensitivity analysis using multiple imputation technique to impute missing values in weight during follow-up. We imputed weight change over four years according to sex, age, BMI, physical activity, smoking status, if a special diet was followed, adherence to Mediterranean diet and snacking between meals, generating 20 complete datasets. Furthermore, we refitted the models in different sensitivity analyses to assess the robustness of our results: excluding participants who answered less than 10% of beverage items; excluding participants with weight change in previous five years due to pregnancy; excluding participants with personal history of obesity; excluding participants with family history of obesity; excluding participants with baseline BMI $\geq$ 27.5 kg/m^2; excluding participants with a total energy intake under or over limits of daily calorie requirements, which is the basal metabolic rate (BMR) value multiplied by a factor depending on the activity level. We excluded people under BMR*1.2 and/or over BMR*1.9. BMR was estimated with the Mifflin–St Jeor equation [30]. Analyses were repeated after stratifying by sex, age (under or over the median) or physical activity (under or over the median of MET-h/week). Finally, we refitted the analysis using Cox regression. Hazard ratios (HRs) and 95% CI were estimated as the difference between β coefficients of exchanged group of beverage and then exponentiated [29]. All *p*-values presented are two-tailed; $p < 0.05$ was considered statistically significant. Analyses were performed using STATA/SE V.12.1 (StataCorp, College Station, TX, USA).

3. Results

Our analysis included a total of 16,065 participants (6455 men and 9610 women). The principal baseline characteristics of participants across quintiles of water consumption are presented in Table 1. The median water intake was five servings per day, and the interquartile range was 2.5–7; these are equivalent to 1000 mL, 500–1400 mL, respectively. The mean age of the sample was 37.9 years (standard deviation (SD): 11.7) and the mean BMI was 23.49 kg/m^2 (SD: 3.5). Participants in the fifth quintile of water consumption compared to those in the first quintile were more likely to be women, younger and with a personal and/or family history of obesity; more participants in the top quintile of water intake had lost weight in the previous five years and their total energy intake was higher; on average, they consumed snacks between main meals more frequently, they were more likely to have followed a special diet and had better adherence to Mediterranean diet; they had higher fibre intake and their intake of almost every nutrient analyzed was higher, except for alcohol, which was slightly smaller;

they were more active, spent less time having a sleeping siesta and were less prone to be a former smokers than those in the first quintile. According to other beverage consumption, they drank more servings of beverages included in LNCBs, spirits, and milk, juice and sugared coffee groups, and less SSSBs and wine, although the differences were small.

Table 1. Distribution of baseline characteristics of participants across quintiles of water consumption [1].

	Quintiles of Water Consumption					
	Q1	Q2	Q3	Q4	Q5	*p*-Value *
N	5227	1457	3250	4000	2131	
Water intake [1] (mL)	357 (0, 500)	529 (513, 700)	1000 (1000, 1000)	1400 (1013, 1400)	1500 (1413, 2800)	<0.001
Sex (men %)	44.4	44.0	39.0	37.2	34.6	<0.001
Age (years)	40.8 (12.0)	38.3 (11.4)	38.2 (11.8)	35.8 (11.1)	34.1 (10.3)	<0.001
Baseline body mass index (kg/m^2)	23.7 (3.42)	23.4 (3.33)	23.4 (3.50)	23.4 (3.49)	23.3 (3.53)	0.052
Current smoker (%)	21.8	20.9	20.4	21.8	22.9	<0.001
Former smoker (%)	31.1	26.1	29.4	26.6	25.2	<0.001
Personal history of obesity (%)	7.21	6.18	7.51	7.23	8.40	0.149
Family history of obesity (%)	21.6	22.9	23.0	24.3	23.0	0.047
Weight loss in the previous 5 years (%)	20.4	20.5	22.6	26.2	28.3	<0.001
Weight gain in the previous 5 years (%)	52.2	54.4	50.2	48.9	48.4	<0.001
Physical activity (MET-h/week)	19.1 (21.2)	20.6 (20.9)	21.1 (19.9)	23.8 (24.1)	25.8 (27.0)	<0.001
Total energy intake (kcal/day)	2233 (620)	2397 (602)	2369 (600)	2394 (596)	2430 (620)	0.047
Snacking between meals (%)	31.6	34.0	33.1	32.7	35.5	0.023
Following special diet (%)	6.62	5.97	7.23	8.18	10.09	<0.001
Adherence to Mediterranean diet (0–9)	3.98 (1.74)	4.10 (1.79)	4.14 (1.77)	4.30 (1.76)	4.40 (1.78)	0.690
Fat intake (g/day)	90.9 (30.7)	98.8 (30.9)	97.6 (30.4)	98.0 (30.5)	99.5 (31.5)	0.397
Saturated fatty acids intake (g/day)	31.5 (12.3)	33.9 (12.0)	33.1 (11.7)	33.0 (12.1)	33.6 (12.4)	0.025
Monounsaturated fatty acids intake (g/day)	38.7 (14.2)	42.3 (14.4)	42.0 (14.3)	42.2 (14.3)	42.8 (14.8)	0.383
Polyunsaturated fatty acids intake (g/day)	13.1 (5.72)	14.3 (5.94)	13.9 (5.91)	13.9 (5.80)	14.0 (5.69)	0.115
Carbohydrates intake (g/day)	244 (83.9)	262 (81.8)	259 (82.5)	263 (83.7)	265 (85.3)	0.362
Protein intake (g/day)	101 (28.0)	106 (26.4)	105 (26.5)	107 (27.3)	110 (28.9)	<0.001
Alcohol intake (g/day)	4.84 (9.03)	4.99 (7.59)	4.59 (7.80)	4.43 (7.62)	4.64 (6.94)	0.0734
Dietary fibre intake (g/day)	26.4 (12.2)	27.1 (11.2)	27.9 (11.8)	28.9 (12.5)	29.3 (12.4)	<0.001
Sleeping hours (h/day)	7.24 (0.91)	7.32 (0.78)	7.31 (0.80)	7.32 (0.84)	7.31 (0.82)	<0.001
Sleeping siesta (h/day)	0.34 (0.86)	0.29 (0.76)	0.28 (0.73)	0.30 (0.74)	0.27 (0.71)	<0.001
Groups of beverages (servings/week)						
1. Water [#]	11.0 (6.69)	20.2 (2.72)	35.0 (0.00)	43.9 (6.03)	58.3 (13.86)	<0.001
2. Low/non-caloric beverages	7.01 (10.3)	7.49 (10.0)	7.21 (9.9)	7.39 (10.2)	7.77 (10.3)	0.105
Diet soda beverages [#]	0.81 (3.22)	0.78 (2.79)	0.70 (2.58)	0.85 (2.70)	1.11 (3.54)	<0.001
Coffee without sugar [†]	6.20 (9.52)	6.71 (9.47)	6.52 (9.34)	6.54 (9.63)	6.66 (9.50)	0.474

Table 1. *Cont.*

	Q1	Q2	Q3	Q4	Q5	*p*-Value *
	Quintiles of Water Consumption					
3. Milk, juice and sugared coffee	15.8 (11.4)	16.8 (10.9)	16.8 (10.6)	16.7 (11.4)	16.8 (11.7)	<0.001
Dairyproducts #	9.33 (8.09)	9.79 (7.63)	9.58 (7.14)	9.72 (7.67)	9.71 (7.77)	<0.001
Juices #	2.91 (4.29)	3.24 (4.13)	3.01 (3.86)	3.34 (4.83)	3.33 (4.60)	<0.001
Coffee with sugar †	3.57 (6.37)	3.79 (6.44)	4.17 (6.66)	3.62 (6.42)	3.81 (7.06)	<0.001
4. Occasional consumption	2.04 (3.85)	2.09 (3.09)	1.83 (3.00)	1.83 (2.78)	2.02 (3.25)	<0.001
SSSBs #	1.55 (3.41)	1.55 (2.65)	1.30 (2.29)	1.26 (2.11)	1.42 (2.87)	<0.001
Spirits †	0.49 (1.35)	0.54 (1.21)	0.53 (1.34)	0.57 (1.46)	0.60 (1.17)	<0.001
5.Wine ‡	3.64 (6.45)	3.30 (5.75)	2.74 (5.31)	2.30 (5.01)	2.11 (4.55)	<0.001
6. Beer •	1.34 (2.92)	1.37 (2.50)	1.25 (2.42)	1.14 (2.02)	1.23 (2.41)	<0.001

Mean and standard deviation (SD), or %. The SUN project 1999–2015. [1] Median and minimum and maximum; * Categorical variables were analyzed using X^2 test and expressed as percentages. Continuous variables were analyzed using analysis of variance (ANOVA) test and expressed as means and SD otherwise indicated; # A serving of water, diet soda beverages, dairy products (whole, reduced-fat and skim milk, and milk shake), juices (fresh orange and non-orange fruit juice, and any kind of fruit bottled juice) and sugar-sweetened soda beverages (SSSBs) is defined as 200 mL; † A serving of any kind of coffee and spirits is defined as 50 mL; ‡ A serving of wine is defined as 100 mL. • A serving of beer is defined as 330 mL.

There were 873 incident cases of obesity during the follow-up. The incidence of obesity was estimated according to the substitution of one of the beverages gathered in the questionnaire by one glass of water per day, in crude and multivariable-adjusted models (Table 2). The substitution of beer with water was associated with a lower incidence of obesity (OR 0.81 (95% CI 0.69 to 0.94)). The association was also significant in the case of SSSBs (OR 0.85 (95% CI 0.75 to 0.97)).

Table 2. The Odds Ratio (OR) (95% confidence interval (CI)) for incident obesity associated with the substitution of one serving/day of water for several beverages (increasing 1 serving/day of water and decreasing 1 serving/day of the beverage in question) at baseline, using mathematical models.

Substitution	Crude Model	Age- & Sex-Adjusted Model	Multiple-Adjusted Model [1]
Water for beer	0.63 (0.55 to 0.71)	0.78 (0.67 to 0.91)	0.81 (0.69 to 0.94)
Water for SSSBs [2]	0.80 (0.71 to 0.90)	0.82 (0.73 to 0.91)	0.85 (0.75 to 0.97)
Water for bottled juice	0.96 (0.78 to 1.19)	0.94 (0.79 to 1.13)	0.86 (0.73 to 1.02)
Water for diet soda beverages	0.77 (0.71 to 0.85)	0.75 (0.69 to 0.82)	0.91 (0.80 to 1.04)
Water for red wine	0.78 (0.72 to 0.84)	0.95 (0.87 to 1.04)	0.92 (0.84 to 1.00)
Water for other wines (non-red)	0.75 (0.64 to 0.87)	0.91 (0.76 to 1.10)	0.93 (0.76 to 1.13)
Water for skim milk	0.93 (0.86 to 1.00)	0.92 (0.86 to 0.99)	0.94 (0.87 to 1.03)
Water for whole milk	1.07 (0.97 to 1.18)	1.12 (1.00 to 1.24)	0.96 (0.87 to 1.06)
Water for regular coffee	0.89 (0.85 to 0.94)	0.94 (0.89 to 0.99)	0.97 (0.91 to 1.02)
Water for spirits	0.69 (0.55 to 0.85)	0.84 (0.67 to 1.04)	1.02 (0.77 to 1.34)
Water for decaffeinated coffee	0.87 (0.79 to 0.97)	0.93 (0.84 to 1.03)	1.05 (0.94 to 1.18)
Water for reduced-fat milk	1.10 (1.01 to 1.21)	1.08 (0.99 to 1.19)	1.06 (0.96 to 1.16)
Water for fresh non-orange fruit juice	1.09 (0.75 to 1.58)	1.13 (0.80 to 1.59)	1.06 (0.73 to 1.52)
Water for fresh orange juice	1.10 (0.93 to 1.31)	1.14 (0.97 to 1.33)	1.06 (0.90 to 1.24)
Water for milk shake	1.94 (0.89 to 4.25)	1.56 (0.83 to 2.97)	1.32 (0.79 to 2.22)

873 incident cases of obesity. [1] Additionally adjusted for baseline body mass index, physical activity, smoking habit, personal history of obesity, family history of obesity, following a special diet, adherence to the Mediterranean dietary pattern, snacking between meals, weight change in the past five years, and total energy intake from other sources than the exchanged beverages; [2] SSSBs: sugar-sweetened soda beverages.

Figure 1a shows the assessment of the incidence of obesity depending on the substitution of water for beverage groups made according to SENC recommendations. In the multiple-adjusted model, we observed an 11% lower incidence of obesity for the group of occasional consumption (SSSBs and spirits) (OR 0.89 (95% CI 0.80 to 0.99)), 8% lower for the group of wine (OR 0.92 (95% CI 0.86 to 0.99)) and 19% lower for beer (OR 0.81 (95% CI 0.69 to 0.94)).

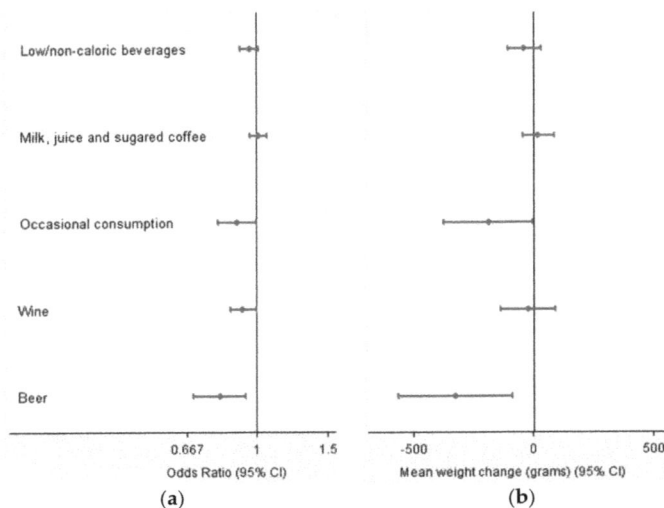

Figure 1. Substitution for group of beverages of one serving/day of water at baseline, using mathematical models. Low/non-caloric beverages contains: non-sugared coffee (decaffeinated and regular) and diet soda beverages; Milk, juice and sugared coffee contains whole, reduced-fat and skim milk, milk shake, fresh orange and non-orange fruit juice, and any kind of fruit bottled juice, and sugared coffee (decaffeinated and regular); Occasional consumption contains sugar-sweetened soda beverages and spirits; (**a**) the Odds Ratio (OR) (95% confidence interval (CI)) for incident obesity; and (**b**) four-year mean absolute weight change (g) (95% CI). Multiple-adjusted model.

When we estimated the odds ratio additionally adjusted for the consumption of other beverage groups, the statistical significance was maintained for the beer group (OR 0.84 (95% CI 0.71 to 0.98)) but it was no longer significant for the group of SSSBs and spirits (OR 0.92 (95% CI 0.82 to 1.03)) or wine (OR 0.94 (95% CI 0.87 to 1.02)). We did not observe any significant association with obesity for people in the fifth quintile of water consumption versus those in the first quintile (OR 1.03 (95% CI 0.82 to 1.30)).

SENC recommends the use of water or, if not, low/non-caloric beverages instead of caloric options. For that reason, we performed the same analysis but replacing by LNCBs. When low/non-caloric options were assumed to be used to replace a serving of beer, this change was associated with a lower incidence of obesity (OR 0.84 (95% CI 0.71 to 1.00) $p = 0.05$), but this was not observed for the substitution of LNCBs neither for SSSBs and spirits (OR 0.94 (95% CI 0.83 to 1.06)) nor for wine (OR 0.96 (95% CI 0.88 to 1.05)).

Table 3 shows the absolute four-year mean weight change (g) associated with substituting each beverage by a serving/day of water. The replacement of water for beer assumed a reduction of 328 g (95% CI −566 to −89). Refitting the models after using multiple imputations to impute missing values of weight change over four years, we obtained similar results, with the only statistically significant substitution being water for beer (−319 (−555 to −83)).

Table 3. Mean four-year absolute weight change (95% CI) associated with the substitution of one serving/day of water for several beverages (increasing 1 serving/day of water and decreasing 1 serving/day of the beverage in question) at baseline, using mathematical models.

Substitution	Crude Model	Age- & Sex-Adjusted Model	Multiple-Adjusted Model [1]
Water for milk shake	−554 (−1205 to 98)	−482 (−1134 to 171)	−399 (−1049 to 250)
Water for fresh non-orange fruit juice	−303 (−724 to 118)	−336 (−757 to 85)	−342 (−760 to 76)
Water for beer	−226 (−458 to 6)	−272 (−511 to −34)	−328 (−566 to −89)
Water for spirits	−265 (−695 to 166)	−274 (−713 to 165)	−226 (−667 to 216)
Water for SSSBs [2]	−291 (−508 to −75)	−215 (−435 to 5)	−205 (−425 to 16)
Water for bottled juice	−203 (−469 to 63)	−172 (−437 to 94)	−137 (−400 to 127)
Water for diet soda beverages	−152 (−367 to 62)	−122 (−336 to 93)	−86 (−300 to 129)
Water for other wines (non-red)	86 (−270 to 441)	−24 (−382 to 335)	−41 (−397 to 315)
Water for red wine	60 (−75 to 195)	−24 (−167 to 119)	−38 (−181 to 104)
Water for regular coffee	−49 (−126 to 28)	−56 (−135 to 22)	−21 (−101 to 58)
Water for decaffeinated coffee	48 (−104 to 199)	−14 (−168 to 139)	5 (−148 to 157)
Water for reduced-fat milk	31 (−76 to 138)	31 (−76 to 138)	6 (−100 to 113)
Water for fresh orange juice	81 (−115 to 276)	43 (−153 to 239)	7 (−189 to 202)
Water for skim milk	52 (−57 to 160)	23 (−86 to 133)	28 (−82 to 137)
Water for whole milk	4 (−107 to 115)	20 (−92 to 132)	61 (−55 to 177)

[1] Additionally adjusted for baseline body mass index, physical activity, smoking habit, personal history of obesity, family history of obesity, following a special diet, adherence to the Mediterranean dietary pattern, snacking between meals, weight change in the past five years, and total energy intake from other sources than the exchanged beverages; [2] SSSBs: sugar-sweetened soda beverages.

When performing the study for beverage groups, we observed the already described change in weight for reducing beer at the expense of increasing water. In the case of beverages recommended as occasional consumption (SSSBs and spirits), this substitution is also statistically significant, decreasing 187 g (95% CI −374 to 0; $p = 0.05$) (Figure 1b). When we additionally adjusted for the consumption of other beverage groups, the significance was maintained for beer (−308 (95% CI −550 to −65)), but not for SSSBs and spirits (−164 (95% CI −352 to 24)). We did not observe any relationship when analyzing the body weight change of participants in the fifth versus the lowest quintile of water consumption (−187 (95% CI −477 to 103)). Substitution of LNCBs for beer was associated with a reduction of 291 g in body weight in a four-year period (95% CI −535 to −47), but this association was not observed for the group of SSSBs and spirits (49 (95% CI −25 to 123)).

After analyzing the contribution of each beverage to the total intake of fluids, we concluded that water was the main source of fluid consumption among all beverage items (56.28%) and also the main source of variability ($R^2 = 0.715$) in our population (Table 4).

Table 4. Sources of variability (cumulative R^2) and main sources (%) in total liquid intake.

Beverage	Cumulative R^2	% of Total Liquid Intake
Water	0.715	56.28
Reduced-fat milk	0.740	6.90
Whole milk	0.765	6.78
Regular coffee	0.786	4.56
Skim milk	0.847	5.77
Bottled juice	0.861	1.71
Fresh orange juice	0.891	3.93
Diet soda beverage	0.914	1.57
SSSBs [1]	0.933	3.07
Beer	0.978	4.26
Decaffeinated coffee	0.981	0.96
Red wine	0.992	2.10
Milk shake	0.994	0.54
Fresh non-orange fruit juice	0.998	0.84
Another type of wine (non-red)	0.999	0.43
Spirits	1.000	0.30

[1] SSSBs: sugar-sweetened soda beverages.

We performed several sensitivity analyses in order to discard potential biases due to our assumptions and to test the robustness of our results (Table 5). When we refitted the analysis using Cox regression instead of GEE, we did not detect significant differences between the two models, but significance for wine group replacement was lost (HR: 0.96 (95% CI 0.89 to 1.04)). Results of the sensitivity analyses did not substantially change in any of these scenarios, except for the analysis of the incidence of obesity after stratifying the population according to sex and leisure-time physical activity (dichotomous: under or equal and over the median, 16.10 MET-h/week). We observed that the substitution of one serving of water for one of the group of SSSBs and spirits was significantly associated with a lower incidence of obesity in women (OR: 0.78 (95% CI 0.63 to 0.96)) but not in men (OR: 0.96 (95% CI 0.84 to 1.10)). However, the interaction was not statistically significant ($p = 0.65$). Furthermore, this replacement was associated with a lower incidence of obesity in those who were less active (OR: 0.83 (95% CI 0.73 to 0.95)) but not among participants who practiced more physical activity (OR: 1.02 (95% CI (0.82 to 1.26)). Again, the interaction was not statistically significant ($p = 0.16$). Stratifying by sex, there was a difference as well for the substitution for wine group (OR: 1.23 (95% CI 0.95 to 1.59) for women, and OR: 0.92 (95% CI 0.85 to 1.00) for men), but the interaction was not significant ($p = 0.11$).

4. Discussion

The results from the present study indicate that replacing a serving of water for beer or sugar-sweetened soda beverages at baseline (using mathematical models) was associated with a lower incidence of obesity, and, in the case of beer, this potential intervention would reduce average weight in a four-year period. Furthermore, water was the main source of fluid consumption among all beverage items as well as the main source of variability in our population.

It is assumed that excessive alcohol consumption increases the risk of obesity because it is a source of energy per se and because energy from alcohol is not substitutive for the calories coming from food; instead, they are extra added calories [24]. Our results showed that the replacement of water for each group that contains alcoholic beverages (occasional consumption (SSSBs and spirits), wine and beer groups) was associated with a lower incidence of obesity. However, when we analyzed them separately, we only observed a statistically significant association for beer, but not for any kind of wine or spirits. Once again, the only one with a significant association with weight change was beer. In the literature, the evidence about the relationship between alcohol intake and body weight is contradictory [17]. In several investigations, a positive correlation has been described, while, in others, alcohol consumption was not related to body weight or to reducing the risk of weight gain and obesity. It seems that the positive association is more evident in heavy drinkers [31,32], whereas moderate consumption does not have an association [33], or it is negative [34]. Apart from the quantity of alcohol intake, it has been shown that not all types of alcoholic beverages have the same effect on body weight [35].

The positive correlation between beer consumption and weight gain and the risk of being overweight or obesity has been already published by our group for people whose BMI at baseline was lower than 25 kg/m^2 [24]. However, in that study, the effect of beer was not analyzed alone, but with spirits. This time, we analyzed them separately due to their different effects on health. The SENC recommends alcohol-free beer intake due to its hydration capacity and because it is a source of vitamin B, fibre, minerals and antioxidants. Furthermore, it has been suggested that a moderate consumption of regular beer could be accepted in a healthy diet because moderate drinking may have some health benefits. For instance, a crossover study showed that moderate consumption of beer facilitates the recovery of the hormonal and immunological metabolism in active individuals after physical exercise [36].

Table 5. Sensitivity analyses. OR (95% CI) for incident obesity associated with the substitution of beverages by one serving/day of water.

	Cases	Low/Non-Caloric Beverages [1]	Milk, Juice and Sugared Coffee [2]	Occasional Consumption [3]	Wine	Beer
Overall	873	0.96 (0.91 to 1.01)	1.01 (0.96 to 1.06)	0.89 (0.80 to 0.99)	0.92 (0.86 to 0.99)	0.81 (0.69 to 0.94)
Excluding participants who answered ≤10% beverage items	862	0.95 (0.91 to 1.00)	1.00 (0.95 to 1.05)	0.89 (0.80 to 1.00)	0.92 (0.85 to 0.99)	0.80 (0.69 to 0.94)
Excluding participants with weight change in the previous 5 years due to pregnancy	854	0.96 (0.91 to 1.02)	1.01 (0.96 to 1.06)	0.90 (0.80 to 1.01)	0.92 (0.86 to 1.00)	0.80 (0.68 to 0.95)
Excluding participants with personal history of obesity	623	0.93 (0.87 to 0.98)	1.03 (0.97 to 1.09)	0.91 (0.81 to 1.02)	0.92 (0.84 to 1.01)	0.76 (0.64 to 0.89)
Excluding participants with family history of obesity	587	0.96 (0.90 to 1.01)	1.03 (0.97 to 1.10)	0.96 (0.84 to 1.09)	0.93 (0.85 to 1.01)	0.81 (0.67 to 0.97)
Excluding participants with BMI ≥ 27.5	369	0.94 (0.87 to 1.01)	1.04 (0.96 to 1.12)	0.89 (0.77 to 1.03)	0.90 (0.80 to 1.02)	0.77 (0.61 to 0.96)
Energy limits: under or over limits of daily calories needs, according to BMR [‡]	441	0.98 (0.91 to 1.05)	0.92 (0.86 to 0.98)	0.79 (0.69 to 0.90)	0.87 (0.78 to 0.97)	0.81 (0.67 to 0.98)
Assessing only women	358	0.97 (0.89 to 1.05)	1.01 (0.93 to 1.09)	0.78 (0.63 to 0.96) [†]	1.23 (0.95 to 1.59) [¥]	0.71 (0.42 to 1.20)
Assessing only men	515	0.96 (0.90 to 1.03)	1.00 (0.94 to 1.07)	0.96 (0.84 to 1.10) [†]	0.92 (0.85 to 1.00) [¥]	0.79 (0.68 to 0.91)
Assessing only people under 35 years old	281	0.92 (0.85 to 1.00)	1.06 (0.98 to 1.16)	0.90 (0.75 to 1.08)	0.83 (0.67 to 1.01)	0.72 (0.56 to 0.94)
Assessing only people 35 year olds or older	592	0.98 (0.92 to 1.05)	0.99 (0.93 to 1.05)	0.90 (0.78 to 1.03)	0.92 (0.85 to 1.01)	0.84 (0.70 to 1.02)
Assessing only less active people (under the median)	500	0.95 (0.89 to 1.01)	1.03 (0.97 to 1.10)	0.83 (0.73 to 0.95) *	0.93 (0.84 to 1.04)	0.82 (0.67 to 1.02)
Assessing only more active people (in and over the median)	373	0.97 (0.90 to 1.06)	0.98 (0.91 to 1.05)	1.02 (0.82 to 1.26) *	0.89 (0.80 to 0.99)	0.79 (0.63 to 0.99)

Adjusted for sex, age, age squared, baseline body mass index (BMI), physical activity, smoking habit, personal history of obesity, following a special diet, adherence to the Mediterranean dietary pattern, snacking between meals, weight change in the past 5 years, and total energy intake from other sources than the exchanged beverages. [1] Non-sugared decaffeinated/regular coffee and diet soda beverages; [2] Any king of juice and dairy product, and sugared decaffeinated/regular coffee; [3] Sugar-sweetened soda beverages and spirits; [†] *p* for interaction = 0.6527; [¥] *p* for interaction = 0.1145; [‡] *p* for interaction = 0.198; * The daily calorie needs is the basal metabolic rate multiplied by a factor with a value between 1.2 and 1.9, depending on the activity level. The basal metabolic rate (BMR) is estimated with the Mifflin–St Jeor equation.

Nothing is stated in the SENC recommendations about spirits. We decided to classify it in the occasional consumption group with SSSBs, allowing a maximum of one serving per week. We did not observe any correlation between the substitution for a serving of spirit with a serving of water neither in incidence of obesity nor in weight change. This finding may explain that the previously reported effect on weight gain and the risk of obesity by the group composed of beer and spirits could be attributable only to beer [24], and in the present study, to the effect of SSSBs, as was shown by analyzing sugared sodas separately. In fact, increasing beer consumption was associated with waist circumference in the prospective Copenhagen City Heart Study, and although they reported an association between moderate-to-large spirits consumption and high waist circumference in both sexes, they concluded that their result was non-conclusive because of the large CI [35]. In another Danish prospective cohort, consumption of spirits was statistically associated with higher waist circumference in women after five years of follow-up, but the absolute change did not have relevance from a practical point of view due to its small magnitude [37].

The SENC suggests that beer and wine consumption should both be moderate. However, deriving from our previous investigations where we did not observe a correlation between wine intake and changes on body weight or the risk of obesity [24], we decided to analyze it separately from beer. In fact, moderate consumption of wine, especially red wine, has been negatively or not associated with body weight. This lack of association (or its protector effect at lower levels of consumption [37]) has been explained not only because wine drinkers usually follow a healthier diet [38] (all of our analyses were adjusted for multiple covariates, including diet quality, decreasing the potential residual confounding) but also because of the inherent properties of wine due to its components [39,40]. Indeed, a clinical trial carried out in 14 healthy young men showed that the addition of two servings of wine per day over six weeks did not affect anthropometric parameters [41]. When we analyzed the replacement of water for red or other types of wine separately, one of them predicted the outcomes, although the substitution for red wine was close to the statistical significance for obesity incidence (OR 0.92 (95% CI 0.84 to 1.00); $p = 0.062$). Furthermore, for the replacement of a serving from the group of both types of wine, we found an association for obesity incidence, but not for weight change in a four-year period. In the Danish study previously described, they found a U-shape relationship between wine consumption and waist circumference [37], so maybe our results are due to the moderate-high consumption of wine in our sample. If the association between wine consumption and weight gain follows a U-shape, a substitution in lower levels would result in a different effect than a substitution for higher levels of consumption.

Many studies have examined the association between intake of SSSBs and later weight change, and most of them suggested that their consumption increases the risk of obesity [42]. We have previously demonstrated that, among people with a previous history of weight gain, those in the fifth quintile of SSSB consumption (more than three servings per week) increased by 60% the odds of weight gain during a 28.5 month follow-up when compared to those with the lowest quintile (never/almost never intake) [43]. Previous studies have analyzed the effect of the real substitution of water for a caloric soft drink, or the other way around. Short-term clinical trials have investigated the consequences of the replacement of SSSBs for water before or during meals [43]. They concluded that this change supposed an increase of 7.8% in total energy intake. With data from a 12-month "A TO Z" intervention, consisting of increasing water intake in substitution for SSSBs, this replacement was associated with lower energy intake in premenopausal overweight women [44], and a significant reduction of weight and fat [45]. However, it should be noted that this study was designed as a weight loss intervention; therefore, it was expected that energy intake and body weight would decrease. Our analyses did not show a correlation between water substitution for SSSBs and weight change in a four-year period, independently of total energy intake, but in the case of the group in which SSSBs were gathered, the association was just statistically significant (-187 g (95% CI -374 to 0; p for trend = 0.05)). Our results suggested that this replacement could be associated with a lower incidence of obesity. Olsen and Heitmann [42] informed readers that the most consistent studies that analyzed the association between calorically sugared beverages and body weight/obesity are those whose follow-up period is five years or more. This may be a potential reason why we could not appreciate in full the effect of the replacement for SSSBs on average body weight given that the follow-up analyzed was shorter than that recommended by these authors. In fact, when we studied the incidence of obesity over a longer period, the replacement of water for SSSB was correlated with the reduction in that risk. It was proposed that the mechanism by which the increase of this type of beverages in decrement of water affects body weight is the subsequent increase of energy intake. However, some studies that affirm a positive correlation between SSSBs and obesity do not present any differences in their results when data are adjusted for energy intake [42]. Thus, there must be more biological mechanisms that relate them, along with the increment of energy intake. Other studies proposed that the intake of SSSBs may fail to trigger physiological satiety mechanisms or that the consumption of this type of beverages may cause a lower thermogenesis, resulting in an increase of energy intake [42]. Furthermore, although the available data about the relationship between increasing water consumption and body weight is not very conclusive, it has been suggested that drinking water could control body weight by inducing thermogenesis [46]. This effect of water, combined with the decrease of SSSB intake, could give an explanation of the effect on the body via a thermogenesis pathway. We did not find any correlation between increasing water consumption at baseline either with less weight gain nor incidence of obesity. In fact, all of the studies which correlate water and body weight, although interesting, are based on short-term studies, thus they may not be applicable to long-term effects [43,45].

The SENC suggests always drinking water, or, if not, low/non-caloric beverages to control body weight. When we analyzed the effect of substituting one serving of low/non-caloric beverages for one serving of beer, we could observe a correlation with a decrease in body weight and in obesity incidence. However, in replacement of one serving of LNCBs for one of the group in which SSSBs are gathered, we have not seen any association nor with reduction of weight neither in the risk of obesity. It was also not observed for obesity incidence when the replacement was made for a wine group. Available evidence is not very clear about the topic of diet soda beverages and weight loss [19,47]. Studies about the effects of diet drink consumption could be affected by an unmeasured confounding factor (for example, people who prefer dieting instead of regular soft drinks may be healthier or perform other strategies that could influence in body weight). It is possible that the correlation between diet soda beverage intake and weight loss are only evident in overweight and obese people, as was reported in three American prospective cohorts [19], or even in clinical trials [48]. In randomized controlled trials in adults whose BMI exceeded the healthy value, the replacement of water or diet soft drinks for SSSBs achieved a 5% weight loss compared to the control group [49] and a reduction on total energy intake [50], as expected as part of a weight loss program. A longer follow-up trial with overweight and obese adolescents showed a reduction in BMI from replacing sugar-sweetened soda beverages with the diet version after one year, but not at the two-year follow-up [48]. This effect was also reported for healthy weight children in a double-blind, 18-month clinical trial, which showed that the intake of non-caloric soft drinks instead of the regular version was associated with lower weight gain, confirming that the replacements may have effects on body weight not only in overweight people but also in those with healthy weight at baseline [51]. On the other hand, water was not superior to non-nutritive sweetened beverages in a weight loss intervention trial [52]. Our cohort included people independently of their baseline BMI and the analysis was adjusted for total energy intake. More studies are needed before recommendations can be made to the general population regarding the consumption of diet soda drinks as a substitute of regular soft drinks instead of water.

We did not find any correlation between the replacement of water for any type of juice analyzed with weight change in a four-year period, nor with the incident of obesity. In a previous study, we found a 16% (OR 1.16 (95% CI 0.99 to 1.36)) increase in body weight when we compared people in the fifth quintile of sugared fruit juice consumption (six or more servings per week) with those in the first quintile (less than one serving per week) [53]. Three American cohorts concluded that the consumption of fruit juice increased weight, whereas its substitution by water caused a weight reduction [19]. However, these investigations did not take into account different types of juices. Only a few studies have analyzed the effect of fruit juice consumption on weight in adults, thus more are needed, in particular distinguishing between different types of juice [15].

Our analysis did not find any relationship between the substitution of water for any dairy product and weight gain or obesity. These findings are consistent with the results obtained from other cohorts [19,54,55] and a meta-analysis of randomized clinical trials [56], in which no correlation was found between dairy products consumption and weight change or obesity incidence.

The strengths of our study include its prospective design, which avoids the possibility of reverse causation bias potentially present in other types of studies, the previous validation of the questionnaires used, the use of a wide range score for beverage consumption, and a relatively large sample size. Additionally, we were able to control for multiple possible confounding variables and conducted various sensitivity analyses. The generalizability of the findings may be considered to be weak because the SUN cohort participants are all university graduates, and therefore the sample is not representative of the Spanish population. However, this enhanced the internal validity of our study because of the homogeneity of the population and the high education level and socioeconomic status, which reduces potential confounding.

Some potential limitations should be noted, as we used self-reported information. Although there is a tendency for participants to overestimate their height and underestimate their weight, self-reported weight and height was found to be valid in our cohort [25]. Beverage consumption was self-reported, and so it is susceptible to information bias. However, this method is arguably the best way to ascertain food habits in large cohorts that are followed over long periods [21]. Another limitation that should be taken into account is that the FFQ does not distinguish between coffee with or without sugar. We resolved this by considering that if the servings of sugar consumed per day are equal to or bigger than those of coffee (both the regular and decaffeinated kind), then that participant takes sugar-added coffee, and if the sugar servings are less than the coffee ones, then sugar-free coffee is taken. The item "bottle juice" does not specify between 100% fruit juice or juice from concentrates, or with or without added-sugar. Apart from that, our analysis was done using mathematical substitution models, thus real replacements may not show the same results. However, this technique has been widely used in nutritional epidemiology [29,57,58]. Furthermore, we have just measured baseline consumption, and not variations over time, thus changes in body weight could be a consequence of these disparities.

5. Conclusions

This study found that replacing one sugar-sweetened soda beverage (but not other sugared drinks, like fruit juices) or beer with one serving of water per day at baseline was related to a lower incidence of obesity and to a higher weight loss over a four-year period time in the case of beer, based on mathematical models. Nevertheless, longitudinal investigations based on real interventions are needed to confirm these potential effects. As obesity carries a high risk for the development of other diseases like diabetes or cardiovascular disease, the possible effects of the substitution for these beverages with water is an important target to consider in future public health research.

Acknowledgments: The authors would like to thank Natalie Parletta for her English review. The Seguimiento Universidad de Navarra (SUN) Project has received funding from the Spanish Ministry of Health (Grants PI14/01668, PI14/01764, PI14/01798), the Navarra Regional Government (122/2014), and the University of Navarra. We would also like to thank the participants of the SUN cohort for their continuous involvement in the project and all members of the SUN study for their support and collaboration.

Author Contributions: Conception and design: U.F., A.G. and M.B.-R., Acquisition, analysis and interpretation of data: U.F., A.G. and M.B.-R., Drafting of the manuscript: U.F., Critical revision of the manuscript for important intellectual content: A.G., M.-A.M.-G. and M.R.-C., Statistical analysis: U.F. and A.G., Obtaining funding: M.-A.M.-G. and M.B.-R., Supervision: A.G. and M.B.-R.

Conflicts of Interest: The authors declare no conflicts of interest.

References

1. Flegal, K.M.; Carroll, M.D.; Ogden, C.L.; Johnson, C.L. Prevalence and trends in obesity among us adults, 1999–2000. *JAMA* **2002**, *288*, 1723–1727. [CrossRef] [PubMed]
2. World Health Organization. *The Challenge of Obesity in the WHO European Region and the Strategies for Response*; World Health Organization: Geneva, Switzerland, 2007.
3. Stevens, G.A.; Singh, G.M.; Lu, Y.; Danaei, G.; Lin, J.K.; Finucane, M.M.; Bahalim, A.N.; McIntire, R.K.; Gutierrez, H.R.; Cowan, M.; et al. National, regional, and global trends in adult overweight and obesity prevalences. *Popul. Health Metr.* **2012**, *10*, 22. [CrossRef] [PubMed]
4. Thomas, D.M.; Weedermann, M.; Fuemmeler, B.F.; Martin, C.K.; Dhurandhar, N.V.; Bredlau, C.; Heymsfield, S.B.; Ravussin, E.; Bouchard, C. Dynamic model predicting overweight, obesity, and extreme obesity prevalence trends. *Obesity* **2014**, *22*, 590–597. [CrossRef] [PubMed]
5. Swinburn, B.A.; Sacks, G.; Hall, K.D.; McPherson, K.; Finegood, D.T.; Moodie, M.L.; Gortmaker, S.L. The global obesity pandemic: Shaped by global drivers and local environments. *Lancet* **2011**, *378*, 804–814. [CrossRef]
6. Guh, D.P.; Zhang, W.; Bansback, N.; Amarsi, Z.; Birmingham, C.L.; Anis, A.H. The incidence of co-morbidities related to obesity and overweight: A systematic review and meta-analysis. *BMC Public Health* **2009**, *9*, 88. [CrossRef] [PubMed]
7. Marti, A.; Moreno-Aliaga, M.J.; Hebebrand, J.; Martinez, J.A. Genes, lifestyles and obesity. *Int. J. Obes. Relat. Metab. Disord. J. Int. Assoc. Study Obes.* **2004**, *28* (Suppl. S3), S29–S36. [CrossRef] [PubMed]
8. Gesta, S.; Bluher, M.; Yamamoto, Y.; Norris, A.W.; Berndt, J.; Kralisch, S.; Boucher, J.; Lewis, C.; Kahn, C.R. Evidence for a role of developmental genes in the origin of obesity and body fat distribution. *Proc. Natl. Acad. Sci. USA* **2006**, *103*, 6676–6681. [CrossRef] [PubMed]
9. Hawkes, C.; Smith, T.G.; Jewell, J.; Wardle, J.; Hammond, R.A.; Friel, S.; Thow, A.M.; Kain, J. Smart food policies for obesity prevention. *Lancet* **2015**, *385*, 2410–2421. [CrossRef]
10. Popkin, B.M.; Armstrong, L.E.; Bray, G.M.; Caballero, B.; Frei, B.; Willett, W.C. A new proposed guidance system for beverage consumption in the united states. *Am. J. Clin. Nutr.* **2006**, *83*, 529–542. [PubMed]
11. Sociedad Española de Nutrición Comunitaria. Guía para una hidratación saludable. La Declaración de Zaragoza. SENC, 2008. *Rev. Esp. Nutr. Comunitaria* **2009**, *15*, 225–230.
12. Wolf, A.; Bray, G.A.; Popkin, B.M. A short history of beverages and how our body treats them. *Obes. Rev. Off. J. Int. Assoc. Study Obes.* **2008**, *9*, 151–164. [CrossRef] [PubMed]
13. Garriguet, D. Beverage Consumption of Canadian Adults. Available online: http://www.statcan.gc.ca/pub/82-003-x/2008004/article/6500240-eng.htm (accessed on 30 June 2016).
14. Almiron-Roig, E.; Palla, L.; Guest, K.; Ricchiuti, C.; Vint, N.; Jebb, S.A.; Drewnowski, A. Factors that determine energy compensation: A systematic review of preload studies. *Nutr. Rev.* **2013**, *71*, 458–473. [CrossRef] [PubMed]
15. Malik, V.S.; Schulze, M.B.; Hu, F.B. Intake of sugar-sweetened beverages and weight gain: A systematic review. *Am. J. Clin. Nutr.* **2006**, *84*, 274–288. [PubMed]
16. Vartanian, L.R.; Schwartz, M.B.; Brownell, K.D. Effects of soft drink consumption on nutrition and health: A systematic review and meta-analysis. *Am. J. Public Health* **2007**, *97*, 667–675. [CrossRef] [PubMed]
17. Sayon-Orea, C.; Martinez-Gonzalez, M.A.; Bes-Rastrollo, M. Alcohol consumption and body weight: A systematic review. *Nutr. Rev.* **2011**, *69*, 419–431. [CrossRef] [PubMed]
18. Muckelbauer, R.; Sarganas, G.; Gruneis, A.; Muller-Nordhorn, J. Association between water consumption and body weight outcomes: A systematic review. *Am. J. Clin. Nutr.* **2013**, *98*, 282–299. [CrossRef] [PubMed]
19. Pan, A.; Malik, V.S.; Hao, T.; Willett, W.C.; Mozaffarian, D.; Hu, F.B. Changes in water and beverage intake and long-term weight changes: Results from three prospective cohort studies. *Int. J. Obes.* **2013**, *37*, 1378–1385. [CrossRef] [PubMed]
20. Segui-Gomez, M.; de la Fuente, C.; Vazquez, Z.; de Irala, J.; Martinez-Gonzalez, M.A. Cohort profile: The 'Seguimiento Universidad de Navarra' (SUN) study. *Int. J. Epidemiol.* **2006**, *35*, 1417–1422. [CrossRef] [PubMed]
21. Willett, W. *Nutritional Epidemiology*, 3rd ed.; Oxford University Press: New York, NY, USA, 2013.
22. De la Fuente-Arrillaga, C.; Ruiz, Z.V.; Bes-Rastrollo, M.; Sampson, L.; Martinez-Gonzalez, M.A. Reproducibility of an ffq validated in spain. *Public Health Nutr.* **2010**, *13*, 1364–1372. [CrossRef] [PubMed]

23. Fernandez-Ballart, J.D.; Pinol, J.L.; Zazpe, I.; Corella, D.; Carrasco, P.; Toledo, E.; Perez-Bauer, M.; Martinez-Gonzalez, M.A.; Salas-Salvado, J.; Martin-Moreno, J.M. Relative validity of a semi-quantitative food-frequency questionnaire in an elderly Mediterranean population of Spain. *Br. J. Nutr.* **2010**, *103*, 1808–1816. [CrossRef] [PubMed]

24. Sayon-Orea, C.; Bes-Rastrollo, M.; Nunez-Cordoba, J.M.; Basterra-Gortari, F.J.; Beunza, J.J.; Martinez-Gonzalez, M.A. Type of alcoholic beverage and incidence of overweight/obesity in a Mediterranean cohort: The SUN project. *Nutrition* **2011**, *27*, 802–808. [CrossRef] [PubMed]

25. Bes-Rastrollo, M. Validation of self-reported weight and body mass index of the participants of a cohort of university graduates. *Rev. Esp. Obes.* **2005**, *3*, 352–358.

26. Ainsworth, B.E.; Haskell, W.L.; Herrmann, S.D.; Meckes, N.; Bassett, D.R., Jr.; Tudor-Locke, C.; Greer, J.L.; Vezina, J.; Whitt-Glover, M.C.; Leon, A.S. 2011 compendium of physical activities: A second update of codes and MET values. *Med. Sci. Sports Exerc.* **2011**, *43*, 1575–1581. [CrossRef] [PubMed]

27. Martinez-Gonzalez, M.A.; Lopez-Fontana, C.; Varo, J.J.; Sanchez-Villegas, A.; Martinez, J.A. Validation of the Spanish version of the physical activity questionnaire used in the Nurses' Health Study and the Health Professionals' follow-up Study. *Public Health Nutr.* **2005**, *8*, 920–927. [CrossRef] [PubMed]

28. Trichopoulou, A.; Costacou, T.; Bamia, C.; Trichopoulos, D. Adherence to a Mediterranean diet and survival in a Greek population. *N. Engl. J. Med.* **2003**, *348*, 2599–2608. [CrossRef] [PubMed]

29. Hu, F.B.; Stampfer, M.J.; Manson, J.E.; Rimm, E.; Colditz, G.A.; Rosner, B.A.; Hennekens, C.H.; Willett, W.C. Dietary fat intake and the risk of coronary heart disease in women. *N. Engl. J. Med.* **1997**, *337*, 1491–1499. [CrossRef] [PubMed]

30. Frankenfield, D.; Roth-Yousey, L.; Compher, C. Comparison of predictive equations for resting metabolic rate in healthy nonobese and obese adults: A systematic review. *J. Am. Diet. Assoc.* **2005**, *105*, 775–789. [CrossRef] [PubMed]

31. Wannamethee, S.G.; Field, A.E.; Colditz, G.A.; Rimm, E.B. Alcohol intake and 8-year weight gain in women: A prospective study. *Obes. Res.* **2004**, *12*, 1386–1396. [CrossRef] [PubMed]

32. Wannamethee, S.G.; Shaper, A.G. Alcohol, body weight, and weight gain in middle-aged men. *Am. J. Clin. Nutr.* **2003**, *77*, 1312–1317. [PubMed]

33. Alcacera, M.A.; Marques-Lopes, I.; Fajo-Pascual, M.; Puzo, J.; Blas Perez, J.; Bes-Rastrollo, M.; Martinez-Gonzalez, M.A. Lifestyle factors associated with BMI in a Spanish graduate population: The SUN Study. *Obes. Facts* **2008**, *1*, 80–87. [PubMed]

34. Wang, L.; Lee, I.M.; Manson, J.E.; Buring, J.E.; Sesso, H.D. Alcohol consumption, weight gain, and risk of becoming overweight in middle-aged and older women. *Arch. Intern. Med.* **2010**, *170*, 453–461. [CrossRef] [PubMed]

35. Vadstrup, E.S.; Petersen, L.; Sorensen, T.I.; Gronbaek, M. Waist circumference in relation to history of amount and type of alcohol: Results from the Copenhagen City Heart Study. *Int. J. Obes. Relat. Metab. Disord. J. Int. Assoc. Study Obes.* **2003**, *27*, 238–246. [CrossRef] [PubMed]

36. Jimenez-Pavon, D.; Cervantes-Borunda, M.S.; Diaz, L.E.; Marcos, A.; Castillo, M.J. Effects of a moderate intake of beer on markers of hydration after exercise in the heat: A crossover study. *J. Int. Soc. Sports Nutr.* **2015**, *12*, 26. [CrossRef] [PubMed]

37. Halkjaer, J.; Tjonneland, A.; Thomsen, B.L.; Overvad, K.; Sorensen, T.I. Intake of macronutrients as predictors of 5-y changes in waist circumference. *Am. J. Clin. Nutr.* **2006**, *84*, 789–797. [PubMed]

38. Sanchez-Villegas, A.; Toledo, E.; Bes-Rastrollo, M.; Martin-Moreno, J.M.; Tortosa, A.; Martinez-Gonzalez, M.A. Association between dietary and beverage consumption patterns in the SUN (Seguimiento Universidad de Navarra) cohort study. *Public Health Nutr.* **2009**, *12*, 351–358. [CrossRef] [PubMed]

39. Monteiro, R.; Soares, R.; Guerreiro, S.; Pestana, D.; Calhau, C.; Azevedo, I. Red wine increases adipose tissue aromatase expression and regulates body weight and adipocyte size. *Nutrition* **2009**, *25*, 699–705. [CrossRef] [PubMed]

40. Fischer-Posovszky, P.; Kukulus, V.; Tews, D.; Unterkircher, T.; Debatin, K.M.; Fulda, S.; Wabitsch, M. Resveratrol regulates human adipocyte number and function in a Sirt1-dependent manner. *Am. J. Clin. Nutr.* **2010**, *92*, 5–15. [CrossRef] [PubMed]

41. Cordain, L.; Bryan, E.D.; Melby, C.L.; Smith, M.J. Influence of moderate daily wine consumption on body weight regulation and metabolism in healthy free-living males. *J. Am. Coll. Nutr.* **1997**, *16*, 134–139. [CrossRef] [PubMed]

42. Olsen, N.J.; Heitmann, B.L. Intake of calorically sweetened beverages and obesity. *Obes. Rev. Off. J. Int. Assoc. Study Obes.* **2009**, *10*, 68–75. [CrossRef] [PubMed]
43. Daniels, M.C.; Popkin, B.M. Impact of water intake on energy intake and weight status: A systematic review. *Nutr. Rev.* **2010**, *68*, 505–521. [CrossRef] [PubMed]
44. Stookey, J.D.; Constant, F.; Gardner, C.D.; Popkin, B.M. Replacing sweetened caloric beverages with drinking water is associated with lower energy intake. *Obesity* **2007**, *15*, 3013–3022. [CrossRef] [PubMed]
45. Stookey, J.D.; Constant, F.; Popkin, B.M.; Gardner, C.D. Drinking water is associated with weight loss in overweight dieting women independent of diet and activity. *Obesity* **2008**, *16*, 2481–2488. [CrossRef] [PubMed]
46. Boschmann, M.; Steiniger, J.; Franke, G.; Birkenfeld, A.L.; Luft, F.C.; Jordan, J. Water drinking induces thermogenesis through osmosensitive mechanisms. *J. Clin. Endocrinol. Metab.* **2007**, *92*, 3334–3337. [CrossRef] [PubMed]
47. Pan, A.; Malik, V.S.; Schulze, M.B.; Manson, J.E.; Willett, W.C.; Hu, F.B. Plain-water intake and risk of type 2 diabetes in young and middle-aged women. *Am. J. Clin. Nutr.* **2012**, *95*, 1454–1460. [CrossRef] [PubMed]
48. Ebbeling, C.B.; Feldman, H.A.; Osganian, S.K.; Chomitz, V.R.; Ellenbogen, S.J.; Ludwig, D.S. Effects of decreasing sugar-sweetened beverage consumption on body weight in adolescents: A randomized, controlled pilot study. *Pediatrics* **2006**, *117*, 673–680. [CrossRef] [PubMed]
49. Tate, D.F.; Turner-McGrievy, G.; Lyons, E.; Stevens, J.; Erickson, K.; Polzien, K.; Diamond, M.; Wang, X.; Popkin, B. Replacing caloric beverages with water or diet beverages for weight loss in adults: Main results of the Choose Healthy Options Consciously Everyday (CHOICE) randomized clinical trial. *Am. J. Clin. Nutr.* **2012**, *95*, 555–563. [CrossRef] [PubMed]
50. Piernas, C.; Tate, D.F.; Wang, X.; Popkin, B.M. Does diet-beverage intake affect dietary consumption patterns? Results from the Choose Healthy Options Consciously Everyday (CHOICE) randomized clinical trial. *Am. J. Clin. Nutr.* **2013**, *97*, 604–611. [CrossRef] [PubMed]
51. de Ruyter, J.C.; Olthof, M.R.; Seidell, J.C.; Katan, M.B. A trial of sugar-free or sugar-sweetened beverages and body weight in children. *N. Engl. J. Med.* **2012**, *367*, 1397–1406. [CrossRef] [PubMed]
52. Peters, J.C.; Wyatt, H.R.; Foster, G.D.; Pan, Z.; Wojtanowski, A.C.; Vander Veur, S.S.; Herring, S.J.; Brill, C.; Hill, J.O. The effects of water and non-nutritive sweetened beverages on weight loss during a 12-week weight loss treatment program. *Obesity* **2014**, *22*, 1415–1421. [CrossRef] [PubMed]
53. Bes-Rastrollo, M.; Sanchez-Villegas, A.; Gomez-Gracia, E.; Martinez, J.A.; Pajares, R.M.; Martinez-Gonzalez, M.A. Predictors of weight gain in a Mediterranean cohort: The Seguimiento Universidad de Navarra Study 1. *Am. J. Clin. Nutr.* **2006**, *83*, 362–370. [PubMed]
54. Rajpathak, S.N.; Rimm, E.B.; Rosner, B.; Willett, W.C.; Hu, F.B. Calcium and dairy intakes in relation to long-term weight gain in US men. *Am. J. Clin. Nutr.* **2006**, *83*, 559–566. [PubMed]
55. Louie, J.C.; Flood, V.M.; Hector, D.J.; Rangan, A.M.; Gill, T.P. Dairy consumption and overweight and obesity: A systematic review of prospective cohort studies. *Obes. Rev. Off. J. Int. Assoc. Study Obes.* **2011**, *12*, e582–e592. [CrossRef] [PubMed]
56. Chen, M.; Pan, A.; Malik, V.S.; Hu, F.B. Effects of dairy intake on body weight and fat: A meta-analysis of randomized controlled trials. *Am. J. Clin. Nutr.* **2012**, *96*, 735–747. [CrossRef] [PubMed]
57. Bernstein, A.M.; de Koning, L.; Flint, A.J.; Rexrode, K.M.; Willett, W.C. Soda consumption and the risk of stroke in men and women. *Am. J. Clin. Nutr.* **2012**, *95*, 1190–1199. [CrossRef] [PubMed]
58. Guasch-Ferre, M.; Babio, N.; Martinez-Gonzalez, M.A.; Corella, D.; Ros, E.; Martin-Pelaez, S.; Estruch, R.; Aros, F.; Gomez-Gracia, E.; Fiol, M.; et al. Dietary fat intake and risk of cardiovascular disease and all-cause mortality in a population at high risk of cardiovascular disease. *Am. J. Clin. Nutr.* **2015**, *102*, 1563–1573. [CrossRef] [PubMed]

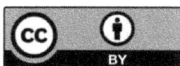

nutrients

Article

Fluid Intake of Pregnant and Breastfeeding Women in Indonesia: A Cross-Sectional Survey with a Seven-Day Fluid Specific Record

Saptawati Bardosono [1,*], Damar Prasmusinto [2], Diah R. Hadiati [3], Bangun T. Purwaka [4], Clementine Morin [5], Rizki Pohan [6], Diana Sunardi [1], Dian N. Chandra [1] and Isabelle Guelinckx [5]

[1] Department of Nutrition, Faculty of Medicine, Universitas Indonesia, Jakarta 10430, Indonesia; diana_sunardi@yahoo.com (D.S.); diannovitach@yahoo.com (D.N.C)

[2] Department of Obstetrics and Gynecology, Faculty of Medicine, University of Indonesia, Jakarta 10430, Indonesia; masdamar@yahoo.com

[3] Department of Obstetrics and Gynecology, Faculty of Medicine, Universitas Gadjah Mada, Yogyakarta 55281, Indonesia; rumekti@yahoo.com

[4] Department of Obstetrics and Gynecology, Faculty of Medicine, University of Airlangga, Surabaya 60112, Indonesia; b4ngun_tp@yahoo.com

[5] Hydration & Health Department, Danone Research, Palaiseau 91767, France; clementine.morin@danone.com (C.M.); isabelle.guelinckx@danone.com (I.G.)

[6] R&D AQUA Group, Jakarta 12950, Indonesia; Rizki.Pohan@danone.com

* Correspondence: tati.bardo@yahoo.com; Tel.: +62-817-149-629

Received: 29 July 2016; Accepted: 13 October 2016; Published: 22 November 2016

Abstract: During pregnancy and lactation, the adequate intake (AI) for total water intake is increased. This cross-sectional survey aimed to assess Total Fluid Intake (TFI; sum of drinking water and all other fluids) of 300 pregnant and 300 breastfeeding women in Indonesia. A seven-day fluid specific record was used to assess TFI. Mean TFI of pregnant and breastfeeding women were 2332 ± 746 mL/day and 2525 ± 843 mL/day, respectively. No significant difference in TFI between pregnancy trimesters was observed, while TFI of women breastfeeding for 12–24 months postpartum (2427 ± 955 mL/day) was lower than that of the two other groups (0–5 months: 2607 ± 754 mL/day; 6–11 months: 2538 ± 807 mL/day, respectively). Forty-two and 54% of the pregnant and breastfeeding subjects, respectively, did not reach the AI of water from fluids. These AI were actually known by only 14% and 23% of the pregnant and breastfeeding subjects. However, having the knowledge about the AI did not increase the odds of reaching the AI. Concluding that a high proportion of the pregnant and breastfeeding subjects did not reach the AI of water from fluid, it seems pertinent to further assess the fluid intake, as well as their hydration status, in other countries.

Keywords: fluid intake; pregnant; breastfeeding; hydration; Indonesia; seven-day fluid record

1. Introduction

During pregnancy, the water balance is altered due to an accretion in total body water. This total body water accretion measured by deuterium or antipyrine tracers is on average 7–8 L. For a gestational weight gain of about 12.5 kg, this total water gain is at term distributed in the fetus (2414 g), placenta (540 g), amniotic fluid (792 g), blood-free uterus (800 g), mammary gland (304 g), blood (1.267 g), and extracellular fluid (1.496 g) with no edema or leg edema [1]. Investigators found that the total body water accretion was positively correlated with birth weight [2,3] and the amount of amniotic fluid is a predictor of fetal well-being [4]. However, a direct association between total fluid intake, water intake or intake of any other fluid type and pregnancy outcome is rarely investigated. In an animal study vasopressin, a key player in water homeostasis was associated with a risk to develop preeclampsia;

however, this remains a preliminary finding [5]. Pregnant women with bacteriuria have an increased susceptibility to pyelonephritis [6]. Since an increased water intake seems to prevent recurrent urinary tract infections in non-pregnant women [7], it seems relevant to evaluate this, in the future, in pregnant women. The same applies for constipation, which is frequent during pregnancy (>30%) because of hormones and dietary factors [8]. A diet rich in fiber and an increased fluid intake is recommended; however, this is rather a practice-based than evidence-based recommendation [8]. While the physiological changes in body water content during pregnancy are known, the scientific literature on the consequences of inadequate hydration and the benefits of increased water intake remains scarce and superficial.

During lactation, the water balance is also altered. Through breast milk, composed of 87% water, breastfeeding women have an additional water loss of on average 700 mL/day at eight weeks postpartum [9,10]. To ensure the accretion in total body water during pregnancy and the compensation of the additional water loss via breast milk during lactation, the requirements for total water intake (TWI, water originates from fluids and food moisture) are increased during pregnancy and lactation [11].

The reference values of TWI for children, adolescents and adults are adequate intakes (AI) based on observed intakes. However, to the best of our knowledge, only one survey that aimed to assess total fluid intake (sum of drinking water and all other beverages) of pregnant and breastfeeding women was published. This survey was performed in Mexico and showed that a sample of 153 pregnant and 155 breastfeeding women drank on average 2.62 L/day and 2.75 L/day, respectively [12]. The Institute of Medicine (IOM) based the reference values of TWI for pregnant and breastfeeding women on the median TWI observed in National Health And Nutrition Examination Survey III (NHANES III). The AI was set at 3.0 L/day for pregnant women and 3.8 L/day for breastfeeding women, which is an increase of 0.3 L/day and 1.1 L/day, respectively, compared to non-pregnant/non-breastfeeding women [13]. In 2010, the European Food Safety Authorities (EFSA) had no European data available on observed water intakes of pregnant women. Since energy intake during pregnancy increases by 300 kcal/day, they recommend pregnant women to increase TWI by 300 mL/day compared to non-pregnant women. This resulted in an AI of TWI established at 2.3 L/day. For breastfeeding women, the EFSA established the AI of TWI also based on theoretical reasoning: In order to compensate for the water loss through breast milk, water requirement needs to increase by 700 mL/day compared to non-breastfeeding women [14]. In Indonesia, observed intakes of water among pregnant and breastfeeding women were also lacking. Like the EFSA, the Indonesian Ministry of Health consequently built recommendations based on the theoretical relationship between water intake and energy intake, meaning that for each kcal of energy intake, 1 to 1.5 mL of water needs to be consumed [15]. Pregnant women are therefore advised to add 300 mL/day of water to the AI of 2.3 L/day recommended to non-pregnant women. Breastfeeding women are recommended to increase TWI by 800 mL/day during the first six months postpartum and by 650 mL/day after six months postpartum.

To address the lack of available intake data, the primary aim of this cross-sectional survey was to assess the intake of drinking water and all other beverages of a sample of pregnant and breastfeeding women representative of three large cities in Indonesia. The secondary aim was to assess the knowledge about the requirement of fluid intake during pregnancy and lactation.

2. Materials and Methods

2.1. Survey Sampling and Protocol

This cross-sectional survey was conducted in Jakarta, Yogyakarta and Surabaya, representing Java Island in Indonesia. Data collection was performed from January to April 2014. All households with pregnant and breastfeeding women under the selected maternity clinic in each of the study areas were eligible for recruitment. A stratified sampling technique was applied: pregnant women were stratified into three strata, i.e., first, second and third trimester; the breastfeeding women into three strata, i.e., 0–5, 6–11 and 12–24 months post-partum. The study aimed to recruit 600 subjects in total, with 200 subjects per study location (i.e., 100 pregnant and 100 breastfeeding women).

All eligible subjects were given oral and written information about the study objectives and protocol. If willing to participate, a written informed consent was obtained. The study was approved on 23 December 2013 by the Ethics Committee of the Faculty of Medicine Universitas Indonesia (number 783/H2.F1/ETIK/2012).

Thereafter, eligible women were screened for the inclusion and exclusion criteria. Study inclusion criteria were: having signed the informed consent, being pregnant or (exclusively and non-exclusively) breastfeeding, having an age above 18 years, living in the study area for at last one year, having a middle-level of socio-economic status (level B and C based on household expenditure according to AC Nielsen criteria). There were 3 additional inclusion criteria for pregnant women: meeting the stratification of the pregnancy trimester, having a singleton pregnancy and having no pregnancy complication such as hyperemesis gravidarum, hypertension or (gestational) diabetes based on interview and physical examination. Breastfeeding women also had to be apparently healthy, i.e., no acute or chronic diseases based on interview and physical examination. The exclusion criteria were being illiterate and having difficulty with oral communication.

This screening visit was performed by trained physicians and nutritionists in the selected maternity clinic. During the same visit, the seven-day fluid diary was delivered and explained to the subjects during a face-to-face interview. Each day, the same nutritionist visited the subject at home to collect the fluid record of the previous day and to provide a new record for the next day. During the first visit, pregnant women reported their pre-pregnancy weight and height, and lactating women their current weight and height. On day 8, the nutritionist completed the questionnaire on fluid intake knowledge with the subjects. The aim of these daily home visits was to maintain a high participation rate and to avoid subjects copying the previous day's data into the next-day record. In total, 30 trained nutritionists were involved in the data collection. Each nutritionist was responsible for visiting a maximum of 10 subjects during the same period. This survey followed the same sampling method, protocol and fluid assessment as those taking part in the Liq.In[7] surveys [16,17].

2.2. Assessment of Fluid Intake with a Seven-Day Fluid Specific Record

The fluid record was structured to collect the following detailed information on each drinking act in open spaces on the record: the hour of consumption, the type of fluid, the brand of fluid, the volume of the recipient from which the volume was consumed and the volume actually consumed. To assist the subjects in estimating the consumed volumes, the records were supported by a photographic booklet of standard containers of fluids.

All fluids recorded were classified accordingly: water (bottled water and tap water. The latter one is because of safety reasons boiled before consumption), hot beverages (coffee and tea), milk and derivatives, soft drinks (carbonated and non-carbonated sweetened drinks, carbonated and non-carbonated non-calorically sweetened drinks, ice-based. coconut-based, chocolate-based, and energy drinks), juices (fruit and vegetable-based drinks) and other beverages (traditional drinks, cereal drinks, herbal drink, soy bean milk, and others). Total fluid intake (TFI) was defined as the sum of volumes of all these categories. Any addition (e.g., sugar) to a fluid was not taken into account during the fluid classification. The water content of food was not assessed, and consequently not taken into account.

An adequate fluid intake was defined as a TFI above or equal to 80% of AI or TWI since 70% to 80% of TWI is assumed to come from fluids and 20%–30% from food moisture [14]. Consequently the cut-offs used in this analysis to identify an adequate intake were 2080 mL/day for pregnant women, 2480 mL/day for breastfeeding women 0–6 months postpartum and 2360 mL/day for women 7–24 months postpartum [15].

2.3. Knowlegde on Fluid Intake Recommendation

The knowledge of the participants about the AI was assessed with 2 multiple-choice questions. The two questions were "In your opinion, how much water should a pregnant woman drink to have an adequate fluid intake?" and "In your opinion, how much water should a breastfeeding woman drink to have an adequate fluid intake?" The possible answers to the first question were the following:

○ Minimally 600 cc less than recommended for non-pregnant woman

○ Minimally 300 cc less than recommended for non-pregnant woman

○ As recommended for non-pregnant woman

○ Minimally 300 cc more than the non-pregnant recommendation

○ Minimally 600 cc more than the non-pregnant recommendation

○ Others: _____

The answers to the second question had a comparable format. Participants were requested to tick off only one answer.

2.4. Data Management and Analysis

Data were recorded daily using specific forms, and then checked, coded and entered into spread-sheets (SPSS version 21.0. SPSS Inc., Chicago, IL, USA). Subjects reporting a mean total daily fluid intake below 0.4 L/day or higher than 6 L/day, as well as subjects not completing all 7 days of the seven-day fluid record were excluded from the analysis. Data analysis was performed by using JMP (version 10, SAS Campus Drive, Cary, NC, USA). Continuous variables were presented as mean, standard deviation and percentiles and dichotomous variables as number and percentage. Statistical comparisons were performed by pregnancy trimesters, postpartum periods, and areas. The mean intakes are estimated values taking into account all consumers including non-consumers. A Wilcoxon paired test was used for multiple comparisons of continuous variable and chi-square for percentages. A p-value below 0.05 was considered significant.

3. Results

The analysis was done on five hundred and ninety-five women of which 296 were breastfeeding and 299 were pregnant. A flow chart of the survey is presented in Figure 1 and the demographics of the subjects in Table 1. Of the subjects who completed the survey, most (56%) graduated from senior high school and 72% were housewives. In the pregnant sample, subjects were mainly overweight and obese (51%) with the highest proportion (60%) in Jakarta. Among the breastfeeding women, there was more normal weight than overweight or obese subjects (54% and 38%, respectively). Of the pregnant and breastfeeding women, 4% and 8%, respectively, were underweight.

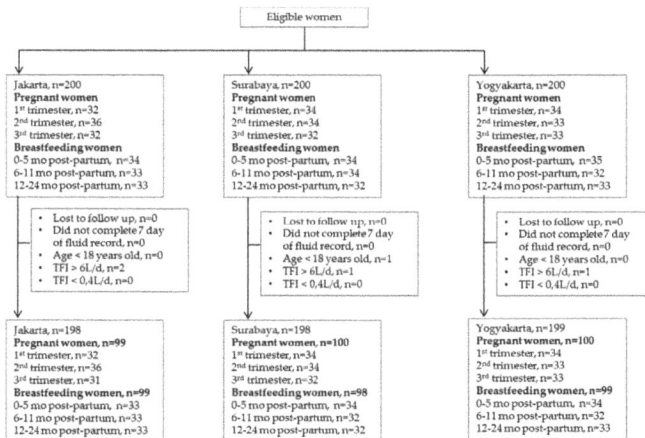

Figure 1. Flow chart of a cross-sectional survey recruiting pregnant and breastfeeding women in Indonesia.

Table 1. General characteristics of the pregnant and breastfeeding women categorized by study area.

Variables	Total	Jakarta	Surabaya	Yogyakarta
Age (years)				
Pregnant women	28.5 (4.3)	29.2 (4.4)	28.5 (4.1)	27.8 (4.3)
Breastfeeding women	28.6 (4.0)	28.9 (4.2)	28.5 (3.9)	28.5 (3.8)
Education Level				
None	4 (1)	0 (0)	1 (1)	3 (2)
Elementary school	41 (7)	20 (10)	14 (7)	7 (4)
Junior high school	109 (18)	38 (19)	33 (17)	38 (19)
Senior high school	335 (56)	117 (59)	103 (52)	115 (58)
Higher education	106 (18)	23 (12)	47 (24)	36 (18)
Working Status				
Any job	3 (1)	1 (1)	2 (1)	0 (0)
Housewife	428 (72)	159 (80)	133 (67)	136 (68)
College student	2 (0)	0 (0)	0 (0)	2 (1)
Labor	4 (1)	2 (1)	1 (1)	1 (1)
Service	5 (1)	2 (1)	1 (1)	2 (1)
Para/medical profession	20 (2)	0 (0)	10 (5)	0 (0)
Education	5 (1)	1 (1)	2 (1)	2 (1)
Finance/Business	29 (5)	6 (3)	7 (4)	16 (8)
Government employment	10 (2)	3 (2)	3 (2)	4 (2)
Private sector employment	98 (16)	24 (12)	39 (20)	35 (18)
Other	1 (0)	0 (0)	0 (0)	1 (1)
BMI Categories				
Pregnant women [1]				
Underweight	13 (4)	2 (2)	2 (2)	9 (9)
Normal weight	134 (45)	37 (37)	47 (47)	50 (50)
Overweight	110 (37)	37 (37)	41 (41)	32 (32)
Obese	42 (14)	23 (23)	10 (10)	9 (9)
Breastfeeding women				
Underweight	25 (8)	8 (8)	6 (6)	11 (11)
Normal weight	160 (54)	53 (54)	53 (54)	54 (55)
Overweight	76 (26)	29 (29)	25 (26)	22 (22)
Obese	35 (12)	9 (9)	14 (14)	12 (12)

Continuous data are presented as mean (SD) and dichotomous as *n* (%). [1] Body Mass Index (BMI) of pregnant women was calculated with pre-pregnancy weight.

3.1. Total Fluid Intake

Table 2 shows the mean and distribution in percentiles of TFI in both pregnant and breastfeeding women by study area, BMI classes, occupation and educational level. The mean TFI for pregnant and breastfeeding women was, respectively, 2332 ± 746 mL/day and 2525 ± 843 mL/day. In Jakarta, pregnant women had a higher TFI (2666 ± 681 mL/day) compared to those in Surabaya (2153 ± 732 mL/day; $p < 0.0001$) and Yogyakarta (2181 ± 717 mL/day; $p < 0.0001$). Among breastfeeding women, the same significant difference was observed between regions (Jakarta 2722 ± 897 mL/day; Surabaya 2 573 ± 899 mL/day; Yogyakarta 2280 ± 656 mL/day; $p = 0.0006$). No significant difference in TFI was found between pregnancy trimesters ($p = 0.50$), while the intake was different between the postpartum periods. Women breastfeeding for 12–24 months had a lower TFI (2427 ± 955 mL/day) than the two other groups of breastfeeding women (2607 ± 754 mL/day for 0–5 months postpartum; $p = 0.005$ and 2538 ± 807 mL/day for 6–11 months postpartum; $p = 0.035$). There was a significant difference in TFI between the BMI classess; however, this significant difference was only observed among pregnant women ($p = 0.0047$). There was no significant difference in TFI according to occupation or educational level among pregnant woman ($p = 0.0938$ and $p = 0.4707$, respectively). Similar observations were made among breasfeeding women (occupation $p = 0.5887$; educational level $p = 0.8650$).

Table 2. Total Fluid Intake (mL/day) of the pregnant and breastfeeding women categorized by study area, classes of body mass index, Occupation and Educational level.

Total Fluid Intake	n (%)	Mean (SD)	Percentiles						
			5	10	25	50	75	90	95
Pregnant Women									
Total	299 (100)	2332 (746)	1243	1436	1784	2229	2800	3307	3679
Jakarta	99 (33)	2666 (681)	1529	1784	2191	2721	3045	3643	3871
Surabaya	100 (33)	2153 (732)	1179	1343	1666	2000	2609	3298	3444
Yogyakarta	100 (33)	2181 (717)	1133	1441	1645	2039	2635	3129	3615
Underweight	13 (4)	1925 (535)	1129	1174	1607	1894	2195	2920	3119
Normal Weight	134 (45)	2210 (706)	1167	1416	1691	2129	2726	3142	3413
Overweight	110 (37)	2477 (771)	1315	1441	1876	2476	3053	3493	3857
Obesity	42 (14)	2469 (763)	1350	1606	1940	2356	2853	3567	4176
Housewife	186 (62)	2397 (779)	1183	1471	1795	2330	2900	3363	3861
Other occupation	113 (38)	2226 (678)	1272	1407	1726	2163	2693	3216	3473
Senior high school	163 (55)	2305 (751)	1226	1401	1750	2161	2833	3326	3580
Other educational level	136 (45)	2365 (740)	1313	1474	1837	2279	2791	3313	3850
Breastfeeding Women									
Total	296 (100)	2525 (843)	1491	1654	1971	2306	2901	3697	4357
Jakarta	99 (33)	2722 (897)	1463	1670	2024	2507	3240	3969	4581
Surabaya	100 (33)	2573 (899)	1599	1675	1952	2276	2979	3800	4404
Yogyakarta	99 (33)	2280 (656)	1476	1597	1907	2151	2476	3219	3519
Underweight	25 (8)	2430 (927)	1368	1460	1873	2266	2691	3559	5194
Normal Weight	160 (54)	2450 (778)	1582	1638	1910	2281	2777	3519	3942
Overweight	76 (26)	2655 (922)	1395	1647	2046	2438	3128	3840	4687
Obesity	35 (12)	2653 (871)	1718	1866	2000	2318	2957	4210	4643
Housewife	242 (82)	2530 (873)	1481	1638	1949	2285	2975	3764	4377
Other occupation	54 (18)	2500 (697)	1619	1724	2094	2410	2676	3324	3879
Senior high school	172 (58)	2522 (804)	1550	1661	1963	2306	2956	3709	4257
Other educational Level	124 (42)	2529 (897)	1433	1624	1979	2319	2825	3725	4396

3.2. Adherence to Indonesian Adequate Intake for Water from Fluids

Non-adherence to the AI was observed among 42% of the total sample of pregnant women. The lowest non-adherence to the AI was observed in Jakarta (18%) compared to 54% in Surabaya and 53% in Yogyakarta. No significant difference between stages of pregnancy was observed (1st trimester 46%; 2nd trimester 38%; 3rd trimester 42%; $p = 0.50$).

In the total sample of the breastfeeding women, 54% of women did not reach the AI for water from fluids. The highest non-adherence was observed in Yogyakarta (69%), then in Surabaya (56%) and the lowest proportion in Jakarta (37%). Non-adherence to the AI was the highest among women who were breastfeeding during 12–24 months (64%) compared to women breastfeeding during 0–5 months (50%) and those breastfeeding during 6–11 months (47%) ($p = 0.035$).

Table 3 shows the results of the assessment of the knowledge of the subjects on the AI of water from fluids. In the total sample, 14% and 23% of all subjects knew the AI for water from fluids of pregnant and beastfeeding women, respectively. Of the 47 pregnant women (16% of pregnant sample) who correctly identified the AI of water from fluids, 62% adhered to the AI and 38% did not. Of the 81 breastfeeding women (17% of breastfeeding sample) who knew the correct AI of water from fluids, 52% adhered to the AI of water from fluids for breastfeeding women and 48% did not. Having knowledge about the AI did not increase the odds of reaching the AI of water from fluids (pregnant women OR 1.18, 95% confidence interval 0.63–2.27; breastfeeding women OR 1.40, 95% confidence interval 0.84–2.34).

Table 3. Assessment of the knowledge of pregnant and breastfeeding women on the Indonesian Adequate intake for water from fluids.

		How Much Water Should a Pregnant Woman Drink Daily?	How Much Water Should a Breastfeeding Woman Drink Daily?
Total women	Incorrect answer	514 (86)	455 (77)
	Correct answer	81 (14)	140 (23)
Pregnant women	Incorrect answer	252 (84)	240 (80)
	Correct answer	47 (16)	59 (20)
Breastfeeding women	Incorrect answer	262 (88)	215 (73)
	Correct answer	34 (12)	81 (17)

Data expressed as *n* (%).

3.3. Consumption of Different Fluid Types

Table 4 shows the mean intake of the different fluid types by study area and Figure 2 the contribution of different fluid types to TFI. Among the different types of beverages, the highest intake in terms of volume and contribution to TFI was observed for water, especially boiled water for pregnant women in Jakarta and Yogyakarta (64% and 53% of drinking water, respectively) and bottled water for breastfeeding women in Jakarta and Surabaya (62% and 67% of drinking water, respectively). The second fluid type consumed the most were hot beverages with a daily intake ranging from 257 mL/day in Jakarta and 427 mL/day in Yogyakarta for breastfeeding women. For pregnant women, hot beverage intake was lower or similar to those of breastfeeding women, ranging from 181 mL/day in Surabaya and 293 mL/day in Jakarta. Soft drinks were the third most consumed beverages. Pregnant women had a significantly higher intake of soft drinks than brestfeeding women (115 ± 141 mL/day vs. 74 ± 116 mL/day, $p < 0.0001$). No significant differences was observed between study areas for pregnant women ($p = 0.99$), while for breastfeeding women, the intake of soft drinks ranged from 24 ± 61 mL/day in Jakarta to 123 ± 150 mL/day in Surabaya ($p < 0.0001$).

Table 4. Total daily consumption of different fluid types (mL/day) in the pregnant and breastfeeding women by study area.

	Pregnant Women (*n* = 299)				Breastfeeding Women (*n* = 296)			
	Total	Jakarta	Surabaya	Yogyakarta	Total	Jakarta	Surabaya	Yogyakarta
Water	1676 (737)	1806 (681)	1633 (755)	1590 (761)	1939 (885)	2199 (922)	2029 (904)	1591 (707)
Boiled water	877 (880)	1156 (912)	633 (780)	844 (872)	900 (1028)	845 (1173)	679 (961)	1173 (875)
Bottled water	799 (895)	650 (808)	1001 (1000)	746 (837)	1040 (1109)	1354 (1130)	1351 (1174)	418 (686)
Milk	191 (181)	282 (213)	139 (142)	152 (143)	97 (142)	116 (146)	75 (124)	99 (151)
Hot bev.	237 (199)	293 (195)	181 (186)	236 (202)	319 (275)	257 (204)	271 (243)	427 (329)
Coffee	12 (46)	12 (44)	12 (47)	13 (47)	28 (69)	30 (68)	16 (52)	39 (83)
Tea	224 (188)	281 (186)	169 (171)	223 (191)	290 (256)	227 (190)	256 (237)	388 (302)
Soft drinks	115 (141)	115 (139)	113 (147)	116 (138)	74 (116)	24 (61)	123 (150)	76 (96)
CSD	3 (13)	6 (19)	2 (9)	2 (9)	6 (22)	7 (29)	6 (18)	5 (17)
SSD	101 (126)	86 (96)	105 (143)	112 (133)	62 (104)	13 (38)	108 (135)	66 (94)
Functional & flavored drinks	11 (38)	23 (60)	6 (19)	2 (15)	6 (24)	4 (21)	9 (32)	5 (17)
Juices	63 (85)	80 (94)	43 (74)	68 (82)	47 (93)	64 (107)	37 (83)	41 (87)
Other bev.	51 (90)	90 (123)	43 (74)	20 (38)	48 (83)	62 (90)	37 (78)	46 (78)

Data expressed as mean (SD); Abbreviations: bev.: beverages; CSD: carbonated sweetened drinks; SSD: sugar sweetened drinks.

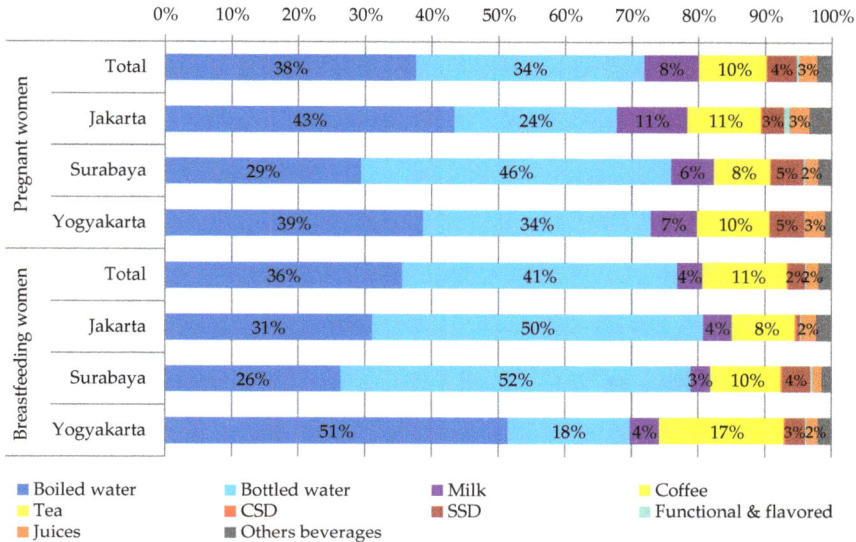

Figure 2. The contribution of different fluid types to total fluid intake of pregnant and breastfeeding women according to study area. Abbreviations: CSD: carbonated sweetened drinks; SSD: sugar sweetened drinks.

4. Discussion

To our knowledge, this is the first survey assessing the intake of water and all other beverages of a relatively large sample of Indonesian pregnant and breastfeeding women. The first finding of this survey was that the mean TFI of both the pregnant and breastfeeding women was 2.3 L/day and 2.5 L/day, respectively, which is different compared to published intake data among this target group. To the best of our knowledge, only two publications specifically focused on water or fluid intake among pregnant and breastfeeding women, and the mean TFI of a Mexican and Greek sample of pregnant woman was 2.6 L/day and 2.1 L/day, respectively [12,18]. The mean TFI of Mexican women breastfeeding during the first semester of lactation was 2.8 L/day [12]. Only hypotheses can be made to explain these intra-country differences. The methods used to assess the intake, climate and cultural factors could be possible explanations [19,20]. A second important observation is that compared to a Indonesian sample of non-pregnant and non-breastfeeding women previously investigated, the pregnant and breastfeeding women consumed on average only 0.26 L/day and 0.07 L/day more [16]. On one hand, this is similar to additional fluid intake (0.25 L/day) consumed by the pregnant Greek sample compared to the non-pregnant sample [18]. On the other hand, the additional TFI of the Mexican pregnant women (0.76 L/day) was much higher than that of non-pregnant Mexican women [12,16]. The Mexican women in the first semester of lactation increased their mean TFI with 0.96 L/day compared to the non-pregnant Mexican sample [12,16]. Even though the mean fluid increase of 0.26 L/day is relatively in line with the additional 300 mL/day of total water intake recommended by the Indonesian Ministry of Health, 42% of pregnant women in this sample still did not reach the AI of water from fluids. In the group of breastfeeding women, about half of the subjects (54%) did not adhere to the recommendation. Whether this increase was sufficient to cover the water requirements of the pregnant and breastfeeding women in this sample remains inconclusive due to lack of hydration biomarkers in the survey. A recent paper reported that urine color is also a valid marker of urine concentration among pregnancy and breastfeeding women, and consequently hydration status [21]. Using this hydration biomarker to have an indication of hydration status could be a suggestion for future large-scale surveys among this target.

The fluid type contributing the most to TFI among the pregnant and breastfeeding subjects was water (72%–77%). This was as expected since in a previous Indonesian adult sample drinking water contributed on average about 78% to TFI [17]. This is, however, an intake pattern specific to Indonesia. About 50% (1.44 L/day) of the water intake from fluids of the Greece pregnant women was drinking water and 33% (0.9 L/day) of the Mexican sample of pregnant women [12,18]. Among the Mexican sample of breastfeeding women, drinking water also contributed about 33% to TFI [12].

The observed difference in TFI between regions deserves a discussion. The pregnant and breastfeeding participants in Jakarta had a higher mean TFI and were consequently more likely to adhere to the AI than the participants in Surabaya and Yogyakarta. Since the socio-demographic characteristics of the participants were comparable at baseline, and since the climate, the method to assess fluid intake and period of data collection were comparable between regions, these factors could not explain the observed differences. In a national Total Diet Study, differences in nutrients and food intake were also observed, and differences in culture or habits was one of the suggested explanations [22]. The use of spices is, for example, different. Since capsaicin, a component of spicy food, can induce, via TRPV1, receptor thirst [23], this could be a potential explanation. That the regional differences were mainly related to a difference in water intake, and more specifically bottled or boiled water, could also suggest that water availability could be a factor influencing the intake of the participants. Intervention trials indeed showed that having water available stimulates consumption [24–26]. Besides water availability, education and having knowledge about the importance of water consumption was also identified as a key factor to effectively increase water intake [24–26]. In this survey, having the knowledge of the AI of water from fluids, however, did not increase the odds of adhering to the recommendations. This seems to be in line with previous evidence which indicated that one factor by itself (e.g., having the knowledge on AI) is not sufficient to induce a behavior, but a combination of multiple factors addressing the individual and their environment is required to maximize the chances for a behavior change [27]. A combination of factors could be providing nutritional education, ensuring access to water and providing them tools such as the urine color chart [21] to assess hydration status and/or measure fluid intake. Because many women are concerned about the health of their babies during pregnancy and are in frequent contact with their healthcare providers, pregnancy may be an especially powerful "teachable moment" for the promotion of healthy behaviors among women [28].

This survey does have limitations that we acknowledge. Data collection was performed in three cities, Jakarta. Surabaya and Yogyakarta, all three located on the Java Island. Since other nutritional surveys showed differences in nutritional intake between Indonesian provinces [22] and since ambient temperature and climate can be difference between the provinces, the findings of this study sample can therefore only be extrapolated to the pregnant and breastfeeding population of Java Island. Furthermore, this was a cross-sectional, and not a longitudinal survey in which subjects were followed from pre-pregnant status throughout pregnancy into the postpartum period. The comparison between pregnancy trimesters and between pregnant and breastfeeding should therefore be done with caution. The data collection was performed during one period of the year meaning that seasonality was not taken into account. However, since Java Island is situated around the equatorial line and the dry and rainy season do not differ in temperature, changes in fluid intake due to seasonality are expected to be limited. As mentioned previously, in the absence of hydration biomarkers, no conclusions can be drawn on the hydration status of the study sample.

Despite the limitations discussed above, this survey has several strengths and therefore contributed valuable information to the study of fluid consumption among specific target populations. Firstly, a large sample was recruited, with an equal distribution over pregnancy trimester and postpartum period. Moreover, the study was completed with a high compliance rate (i.e., >95%). Secondly, fluid intake was assessed used a seven-day fluid specific record, which is considered the reference method in nutritional assessment [29]. Moreover, this record was supported by a photographic booklet of standard containers, increasing the likelihood of having an accurate estimation of the consumption of the subjects. A potential risk of a dietary record is that the subject completes the record only the day after or even later, or that a subject copies the info recorded from one day to another day. Since the investigators visited the subject each day to check the completion, and recuperated the page of the fluid record, this risk was eliminated. In national surveys, a food frequency questionnaire, a 24 h dietary recall, or a mix of methods is more frequently used than a seven-day dietary record [30]. Since a 24 h recall tends to underestimate TFI [31], our results should be compared to other food surveys with caution.

5. Conclusions

To conclude, this survey indicated that a large proportion of this Indonesian pregnant and breastfeeding sample had an inadequate intake of water from fluids. Even though the evidence of potential positive health benefits of an increased water intake during pregnancy and lactation is currently limited, this finding suggests that the actions of midwives, general practitioners and other doctors to promote an increased water intake as part of a healthy lifestyle are pertinent.

Acknowledgments: The study was funded by a research grant from PT Tirta Investama (Danone AQUA, Jakarta 12950, Indonesia). The costs to publish in open access were covered by Danone Research.

Author Contributions: S.B., D.P., B.T.P., R.P. and D.R.H. conceived and designed the experiments; S.B., D.R.S. and D.N.C. performed the experiments; S.B. and C.M. analyzed the data; I.G. and C.M wrote the paper.

Conflicts of Interest: I.G. and C.M. are employees of Danone Research. R.P. is an employee of R&D AQUA Group. All other authors declare no conflict of interest.

References

1. Hytten, F.E.; Chamberlain, G. *Clinical Pysiology in Obstetrics*; Blackwell Scientific Publications: Oxford, UK, 1991.
2. Larciprete, G.; Valensise, H.; Vasapollo, B.; Altomare, F.; Sorge, R.; Casalino, B.; De Lorenzo, A.; Arduini, D. Body composition during normal pregnancy: Reference ranges. *Acta Diabetol.* **2003**, *40* (Suppl. S1), S225–S232. [CrossRef] [PubMed]
3. Butte, N.F.; Ellis, K.J.; Wong, W.W.; Hopkinson, J.M.; Smith, E.O. Composition of gestational weight gain impacts maternal fat retention and infant birth weight. *Am. J. Obstet. Gynecol.* **2003**, *189*, 1423–1432. [CrossRef]
4. Beall, M.H.; van den Wijngaard, J.P.; van Gemert, M.J.; Ross, M.G. Amniotic fluid water dynamics. *Placenta* **2007**, *28*, 816–823. [CrossRef] [PubMed]
5. Santillan, M.K.; Santillan, D.A.; Scroggins, S.M.; Min, J.Y.; Sandgren, J.A.; Pearson, N.A.; Leslie, K.K.; Hunter, S.K.; Zamba, G.K.; Gibson-Corley, K.N.; et al. Vasopressin in preeclampsia: A novel very early human pregnancy biomarker and clinically relevant mouse model. *Hypertension* **2014**, *64*, 852–859. [CrossRef] [PubMed]
6. Schnarr, J.; Smaill, F. Asymptomatic bacteriuria and symptomatic urinary tract infections in pregnancy. *Eur. J. Clin. Investig.* **2008**, *38* (Suppl. S2), 50–57. [CrossRef] [PubMed]
7. Eckford, S.D.; Keane, D.P.; Lamond, E.; Jackson, S.R.; Abrams, P. Hydration monitoring in the prevention of recurrent idiopathic urinary tract infections in pre-menopausal women. *Br. J. Urol.* **1995**, *76*, 90–93. [CrossRef] [PubMed]
8. Cullen, G.; O'Donoghue, D. Constipation and pregnancy. *Best Pract. Res. Clin. Gastroenterol.* **2007**, *21*, 807–818. [CrossRef] [PubMed]
9. Neville, M.C.; Keller, R.; Seacat, J.; Lutes, V.; Neifert, M.; Casey, C.; Allen, J.; Archer, P. Studies in human lactation: Milk volumes in lactating women during the onset of lactation and full lactation. *Am. J. Clin. Nutr.* **1988**, *48*, 1375–1386. [PubMed]
10. Bauer, J.; Gerss, J. Longitudinal analysis of macronutrients and minerals in human milk produced by mothers of preterm infants. *Clin. Nutr.* **2011**, *30*, 215–220. [CrossRef] [PubMed]
11. Institute of Medicine. *Nutrition during Lactation*; National Academies Press: Washington, DC, USA, 1991.
12. Martinez, H. Fluid consumption by Mexican women during pregnancy and first semester of lactation. *Biomed. Res. Int.* **2014**, *2014*, 603282. [CrossRef] [PubMed]

13. Institute of Medicine; Food and Nutrition Board. *Dietary Reference Intakes for Water, Potassium, Sodium, Chloride and Sulfate*; National Academies Press: Washington, DC, USA, 2004.

14. EFSA Panel on Dietetic Products Nutrition and Allergies (NDA). Scientific opinion on dietary reference values for water. *EFSA J.* **2010**, *8*, 1459.

15. Ministry of Health of the Republic of Indonesia. *Recommended Nutritional Intake for Indonesian Population*; Ministry of Health: Jakarta, Indonesia, 2013.

16. Ferreira-Pego, C.; Guelinckx, I.; Moreno, L.A.; Kavouras, S.A.; Gandy, J.; Martinez, H.; Bardosono, S.; Abdollahi, M.; Nasseri, E.; Jarosz, A.; et al. Total fluid intake and its determinants: Cross-sectional surveys among adults in 13 countries worldwide. *Eur. J. Nutr.* **2015**, *54* (Suppl. S2), 35–43. [CrossRef] [PubMed]

17. Guelinckx, I.; Ferreira-Pego, C.; Moreno, L.A.; Kavouras, S.A.; Gandy, J.; Martinez, H.; Bardosono, S.; Abdollahi, M.; Nasseri, E.; Jarosz, A.; et al. Intake of water and different beverages in adults across 13 countries. *Eur. J. Nutr.* **2015**, *54* (Suppl. S2), S45–S55. [CrossRef] [PubMed]

18. Malisova, O.; Protopappas, A.; Nyktari, A.; Bountziouka, V.; Antsaklis, A.; Zampelas, A.; Kapsokefalou, M. Estimations of water balance after validating and administering the water balance questionnaire in pregnant women. *Int. J. Food Sci. Nutr.* **2014**, *65*, 280–285. [CrossRef] [PubMed]

19. Malisova, O.; Bountziouka, V.; Panagiotakos, D.; Zampelas, A.; Kapsokefalou, M. Evaluation of seasonality on total water intake, water loss and water balance in the general population in Greece. *J. Hum. Nutr. Diet.* **2013**, *26* (Suppl. S1), 90–96. [CrossRef] [PubMed]

20. Gandy, J. Water intake: Validity of population assessment and recommendations. *Eur. J. Nutr.* **2015**, *54* (Suppl. S2), 11–16. [CrossRef] [PubMed]

21. McKenzie, A.L.; Munoz, C.X.; Ellis, L.A.; Perrier, E.T.; Guelinckx, I.; Klein, A.; Kavouras, S.A.; Armstrong, L.E. Urine color as an indicator of urine concentration in pregnant and lactating women. *Eur. J. Nutr.* **2015**. [CrossRef] [PubMed]

22. Health Research and Development; Ministry of Health Republic of Indonesia. *Total Diet Study: Food Consumption Survey of Indonesian Individual*; Ministry of Health: Jakarta, Indonesia, 2014.

23. Zheng, J. Molecular mechanism of TRP channels. *Compr. Physiol.* **2013**, *3*, 221–242. [PubMed]

24. Gomez, P.; Boesen-Mariani, S.; Lambert, J.L.; Monrozier, R. A water intervention program to improve fluid intakes among french women. *Nutr. Today* **2013**, *48*, S40–S42. [CrossRef]

25. Lahlou, S.; Boesen-Mariani, S.; Franks, B.; Guelinckx, I. Increasing water intake of children and parents in the family setting: A randomized controlled intervention using installation theory. *Ann. Nutr. Metab.* **2015**, *66*, 26–30. [CrossRef] [PubMed]

26. Storckdieck Gennant Bonsmann, S.; Mak, N.T.; Louro Caldeira, S.; Wollgast, J. *How to Promote Water Intake in Schools: A Toolkit*; Publications Office of the European Union: Luxembourg, 2016.

27. Huang, T.T.; Drewnowski, A.; Kumanyika, S.K.; Glass, T.A. A systems-oriented multilevel framework for addressing obesity in the 21st century. *Prev. Chronic Dis.* **2009**, *6*, A82. [PubMed]

28. Phelan, S. Pregnancy: A "teachable moment" for weight control and obesity prevention. *Am. J. Obstet. Gynecol.* **2010**, *202*, 135.e1–135.e8. [CrossRef] [PubMed]

29. Coulston, A.M.; Boushey, C.J. *Nutrition in the Prevention and Treatment of Disease*; Academic Press: Amsterdam, The Netherlands, 2008.

30. Gandy, J.; Martinez, H.; Guelinckx, I.; Moreno, L.A.; Bardosono, S.; Salas-Salvado, J.; Kavouras, S.A. Relevance of assessment methods for fluid intake. *Ann. Nutr. Metab.* **2016**, *68* (Suppl. S2), 1–5. [CrossRef] [PubMed]

31. Bardosono, S.; Monrozier, R.; Permadhi, I.; Manikam, N.R.; Pohan, R.; Guelinckx, I. Total fluid intake assessed with a seven-day fluid record versus a 24-h dietary recall: A crossover study in Indonesian adolescents and adults. *Eur. J. Nutr.* **2015**, *54* (Suppl. S2), 17–25. [CrossRef] [PubMed]

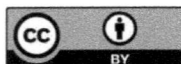

nutrients

MDPI

Article

Association between Plain Water and Sugar-Sweetened Beverages and Total Energy Intake among Mexican School-Age Children

Teresa Shamah-Levy, Claudia Gabriela García-Chávez and Sonia Rodríguez-Ramírez *

Centro de investigación en Nutrición y Salud, Instituto Nacional de Salud Pública, Avenida Universidad 655, Cuernavaca, Morelos 62100, Mexico; tshamah@insp.mx (T.S.-L.); gabriela.garcia@insp.mx (C.G.G.-C.)
* Correspondence: scrodrig@insp.mx; Tel.: +52-777-329-3000

Received: 29 July 2016; Accepted: 2 November 2016; Published: 18 December 2016

Abstract: Water consumption promotes a decrease in total diet energy intake, and one explanation for this fact is the replacement of sugar-sweetened beverages (SSBs) by plain water (PW). The objective of this study was to analyze the association between SSB and PW consumption as a part of the total energy intake. Dietary information was obtained by one 24 h recall of 2536 school-age children who participated in the National Nutrition Survey in Mexico. PW and SSB consumption was measured in mL and servings (240 mL), and consumption was stratified into two levels (<2 and ≥2 servings/day). Linear regression models were used to evaluate the association between PW and SSB consumption in relation to total energy intake. Models were adjusted for age, sex, the proportion of energy obtained from non-beverage food, area of residence, and socioeconomic status (based on information regarding housing conditions and ownership of home appliances). PW consumption at the national level was two servings/day, and was not associated with total energy intake. However, the combination of the high consumption of PW and the low consumption of SSB was associated with less total energy intake ($p < 0.05$). Promoting higher PW and lower SSB consumption provides a useful public health strategy for reducing total energy intake and preventing overconsumption among Mexican school-age children.

Keywords: plain water intake; energy intake; beverage consumption; children

1. Introduction

Water intake is necessary for life, and it should be the main beverage consumed by the population. Comprising 75% of body weight in infants to 55% in the elderly, it is essential for the maintenance of adequate hydration [1] and cellular homeostasis [2].

In addition to being the major component of the human body, water acts as a medium for numerous metabolic reactions, and assists in transporting nutrients, hormones, waste products and heat throughout the body. Hydration is thus fundamental for maintaining normal physical and cognitive performance [3].

Regarding diet, plain water (PW) consumption promotes a decrease in total energy intake [1,4,5]; it tends to replace caloric beverage intake, and creates a sensation of satiety, assuaging feelings of hunger and the desire to eat [5].

One recommendation for reducing the risk of major chronic disease through dietary changes is to replace sugar-sweetened beverages (SSBs) with PW and unsweetened beverages [6].

Some experimental trials have obtained a reduction in energy intake by replacing SSBs with PW [7]; however, various experimental studies of children have yielded less definitive results. One study showed that drinking PW instead of SSB before meals reduced the total energy intake in the short term, while another study found no such connection [4]. SSB consumption and its relationship to energy intake is well documented [8], but there have been no corresponding studies on the role of PW consumption [2,7].

It has been reported that in young to middle-aged adults without obesity, significant changes in energy intake do not correlate with the presence or absence of PW consumption [7]. On the other hand, some studies have shown that PW consumption is associated with healthier diets and reduced risk of chronic disease [9].

Recent studies have concluded that reducing SSB consumption can prevent weight gain in children [10]. It has been documented that drinking PW instead of SSBs prevents weight gain and obesity in children [4]. However, the consumption of caloric beverages (mainly SSBs) is rising rapidly, particularly in low- and middle-income countries in Latin America [8].

In Mexico, school-age children are one of the population groups with the highest energy intakes from beverages as a proportion of the total energy intake and with a high prevalence of overweight/obesity (34.4%) [11,12].

The Institute of Medicine (IOM) in the USA established the adequate intake (AI) of total water, including all beverages and moisture found in foods (the latter accounts for approximately 20% of intake) [12]. The AI of water for children aged four to eight years was set at 1700 mL/day (which includes approximately 1200 mL for total beverages, leaving 500 mL for moisture). The AI of total water for children aged 9 to 13 years was set at 2100 mL/day (girls) and 2400 mL/day (boys); this includes 1600 mL/day (girls) and 1800 mL/day (boys) of total beverages [13].

In Mexico, school-age children consumed 1254 mL of beverages per capita, in 2006, representing 20.7% of the total energy consumption, including 607 mL of PW [11].

Little evidence exists on PW consumption and energy intake among Mexican school-age children. The aim of this study is therefore to evaluate the association between the consumption of PW and SSBs in relation to total energy intake in Mexican school-age children.

2. Materials and Methods

2.1. Design and Study Population

Data were obtained from the National Health and Nutrition Survey 2012 (ENSANUT-2012, by its acronym in Spanish), a survey with probabilistic stratified cluster sampling representative at national, regional and urban/rural levels. Data collection was done between October 2011 and May 2012 (details can be consulted elsewhere) [14].

Dietary data were available for urban and rural strata in three regions. The initial sample consisted of 2751 children between five and 11 years having the required dietary information. After running two cleaning efforts to eliminate implausible data, the final study population comprised 2536 children.

Ethical aspects. The survey protocol was approved by the Ethics Commission of the National Institute of Public Health (INSP by its Spanish acronym), with ethic approval code 1108, and informed consent was obtained from the parent or guardian of each participant.

2.2. Data Collection and Variable Construction

Dietary assessment. Dietary data were collected using a 24 h recall. Complete information on foods and beverages consumed the day before the interview was obtained following a multi-pass method: (1) compiling a preliminary list of foods consumed throughout the day; (2) reviewing the food list to ensure the inclusion of foods often overlooked; (3) completing details on the list of foods such as meal times and associated activities; (4) completing details on each food item, including portion size and recipes; and (5) performing a final review. The details of this method have been published previously [15].

In children younger than 10 years, reporting was done by the mother, caregiver or person in charge of feeding the child; in children 10 years and older, the report was completed by the child assisted by the person responsible for feeding him or her. This information was then supplemented by the child to account for food consumed outside of the home.

2.3. Formation of Beverage Groups

Grouping was based on caloric contribution and sugar content, with PW taken as a group despite its lack of energy contribution. A total of six groups was created: (1) PW: included just the water consumed alone (without another ingredient); (2) dairy beverages without sugar: whole milk from any animal species; (3) dairy beverages with sugar: *atole* and *pozol* (traditional Mexican beverages made from corn), among others; (4) non-dairy beverages with sugar: *aguas frescas* (a mixture of fruit or flower, sugar and water), industrialized juices, coffee and tea with sugar, and soft drinks, among others; (5) natural juices; and (6) non-dairy beverages without sugar, listed in Table 1.

Table 1. Classification of beverage groups among Mexican school-age children (five to eleven years old), ENSANUT 2012.

	Beverage Group	Beverage
Group 1	Plain water (PW)	Plain water
Group 2	Dairy beverages without sugar	Whole milk or soy milk without sugar High-fat dairy drinks Whole lactose-free milk Reduced-fat milk Light milk formula
Group 3	Dairy beverages with sugar	Whole milk with sugar *Atole* (base on milk, any flavor) Yogurt drinks Milk-based smoothies
Group 4	Non-dairy beverages with sugar	*Aguas frescas* (a mixture of fruit or flower, sugar and water) Energy and sports drinks Chocolate drinks made with sugar and water *Atole/pozol* (traditional Mexican beverages made with corn flour, water, and sugar) Coffee or tea with sugar Industrialized juices Soft drinks of any flavor
Group 5	Natural juices	Natural fruit juices Natural vegetable juices
Group 6	Non-dairy beverages without sugar	Light soft drinks of any flavor Mineral water Light flavored water Powdered sugar-free drinks Coffee or tea without sugar

All groups were established according to caloric contribution and sugar content.

2.4. Identification of Outliers

To reduce systematic errors, implausible data were excluded from analysis according to two criteria. The first was excessive consumption (mL): we used data distribution to determine the largest consumption amounts in the six beverage groups, and established these values as cutoffs. For the groups concerning PW as well as non-dairy beverages with sugar and natural juices, excessive consumption was defined as anything above 3000 mL; for dairy beverages without sugar, anything above 1000 mL; for dairy beverages with sugar, anything above 1400 mL; and for non-dairy beverages without sugar, anything above 900 mL. We excluded 22 children in this step of the cleaning process. The second criterion was energy consumption (kcal): we defined cutoffs as the mean energy consumption in each group plus three times its standard deviation. Cutoffs were 301.47 kcal for dairy beverages without sugar; 585.32 kcal for dairy beverages with sugar; 669.12 for non-dairy beverages with sugar; 494 mL for natural juices; and 66.51 kcal for non-dairy beverages without sugar. We excluded 193 children in this final step of the cleaning process.

Energy intake. We estimated consumption and the corresponding energy intake for the food items within each group, and calculated the total energy intake for each group as well as the proportion of intake pertaining to each participant. Energy values were based on the food-composition tables formulated by the National Institute of Public Health (Nutrient Data Base, Compilation of the National Institute of Public Health, unpublished material, 2012).

Socio-demographic variables. The age, sex, area of residence and socioeconomic status (SES) of the sample children were obtained by means of a household questionnaire.

Area of residence was defined as rural for localities with <2500 inhabitants and urban for localities with ≥2500 inhabitants.

An SES index was constructed based on housing conditions (flooring and roofing materials); ownership of home appliances (refrigerator, stove, washing machine, television, radio, video player, telephone, and computer); and the number of rooms in the house. We used the Principal Component Analysis to generate a continuous variable which we then divided into tertiles representing low, middle, and high SES categories.

2.5. Statistical Analysis

To describe our analytic sample, we estimated percentages for each demographic variable and divided the results into quartiles (p25, p50 and p75) representing the consumption (mL), energy contribution and energy percentage levels of each beverage group.

In view of the biased distribution of beverage consumption and the small size of our consumer sample, we traced the differences on box plots.

To better interpret the association between beverage consumption and total energy intake, we expressed beverage consumption as servings of 240 mL for both PW and SSBs. SSBs were taken from two groups: dairy and non-dairy beverages with sugar.

In addition, we divided beverage consumption quality into four categories: (1) low water (<two servings) and high SSB consumption (≥two servings); (2) high water (≥two servings) and high SSB consumption (≥two servings); (3) low water (<two servings) and low SSB consumption (<two servings); and (4) high water (≥two servings) and low SSB consumption (<two servings). We used two servings as the cutoff point because this value was the median consumption portion for PW and SSBs.

We used two linear regression models to analyze the association between beverage consumption and total energy intake, adjusting by age, sex, area of residence, SES and energy obtained from non-beverage foods. The first model included PW and SSB consumption as continuous variables. Because the relationship between SSBs and total energy intake is not linear, we included the quadratic term SSBs to the model. The second model included PW and SSB consumption in the four categories mentioned below.

In order to maintain the original representativeness levels, we performed all of the analyses using STATA 14.1 SVY module software for survey data.

3. Results

3.1. Sample Characteristics

After excluding the outliers in beverage consumption and applying the expansion factor, our final analytic sample reached 2536 school children aged five to eleven years, representing a universe of 18,448,445 individuals nationwide.

Characteristics of the sample subjects are described in Table 2. Their mean age was 8.18 ± 2 years (not shown in the Table). Approximately half were male and half were female. About a third (28%) lived in rural areas. Twenty-nine percent occupied the highest and 35% the middle and low SES tertiles.

Table 2. Socio-demographic characteristics of Mexican school-age children (five to eleven years old). National Survey of Health and Nutrition 2012, Mexico.

	n	%	95% CI
Sex			
Male	1289	50.1	47.4–52.9
Female	1247	49.8	47.0–52.5
Age (years)			
5	335	12.2	10.5–13.9
6	354	12.4	10.5–14.4
7	406	14.5	12.7–16.3
8	386	14.2	12.4–15.9
9	378	13.9	12.0–15.9
10	332	15.3	13.1–17.4
11	345	17.2	14.9–19.5
Area [1]			
Urban	1556	71.4	69.4–73.4
Rural	980	28.5	26.5–30.5
Socioeconomic Status [2]			
Low	977	35.3	32.4–38.1
Middle	899	35.1	32.3–38.0
High	670	29.5	26.3–32.6
Total simple [3]	2536		

[1] Rural: <2500 inhabitants; urban: ≥2500 or more; [2] Calculated using principal components analysis; includes household characteristics, goods and services; [3] N = 18,448,445, which represents 18,448,445 school-age children.

3.2. Beverage Consumption

Table 3 illustrates the total energy consumption by socio-demographic variable. The national median was 1633 kcal/day. Caloric intake among urban dwellers was 1225 kcal/day for the 25th percentile and 2187 kcal/day for the 75th percentile. Rural dwellers showed intakes of 1182 and 2090 kcal/day, respectively.

Table 3. Total energy intake according to socio-demographic variables *.

	Total Energy Intake (kcal/Day)		
	p25	p50	p75
National	1215.3	1632.8	2173.2
Area			
Urban	1224.9	1655.9	2187.2
Rural	1182.2	1582.5	2089.7
Socioeconomic status			
Low	1189.5	1561.3	2149.1
Middle	1269.4	1701.1	2264.1
High	1218.2	1647.7	2145.3

All values shown in this table apply to the total sample. * *n* = 2536, which represents 18,448,445 school-age children.

The median energy intakes in the three SES categories listed in ascending order were 1561, 1701 and 1648 kcal/day. The highest energy intake occurred in the middle SES category with 2264 kcal/day; the lowest intake fell into the low category with 1189 kcal/day.

Table 4 displays the percentage of consumers at the national level and consumption (mL) in medians as well as the 25th and 75th percentiles of each beverage group. It also shows the energy contribution and intake distributions of the groups among school-age children. More than 70% of the children reported consumption of PW, almost 80% consume non-dairy beverages with sugar and more than one-third consume dairy beverages with sugar. Just 2.2% of the children consumed natural juices. The median consumption for PW was 480 mL, or two servings/day, as opposed to barely over one serving/day for both the dairy beverages without sugar and dairy beverages with sugar groups. Consumption reached approximately two servings/day for the non-dairy beverages with sugar, and less than one serving/day for the non-dairy beverages without sugar group.

Dairy beverages with sugar contributed the highest percentage of energy at the national level with a median of 12.2% of total energy intake. However, SSBs (combining dairy and non-dairy beverages with sugar) contributed approximately 20% (data not shown in table).

School-age children in rural areas consumed the highest percentage of non-dairy beverages with sugar (448 mL/day), while their urban counterparts consumed the highest percentage (21.0%) of SSBs in general.

Similarly, as regards the SES of our sample children, children with middle SES had the highest consumption of non-dairy beverages with sugar (427 mL/day), while the high SES group had the highest consumption of dairy beverages with sugar (272 mL/day), as well as the highest percentages of energy from dairy and non-dairy beverages with sugar (14.7% and 8.7%, respectively).

No difference was observed between areas of residence regarding consumption, energy contribution or percentage of energy.

Table 5 presents the association between beverage consumption and total energy intake. PW consumption was not associated with energy intake, whereas SSB consumption showed a positive association amounting to a 69 kcal ($p < 0.05$) per serving increase. The association proved even higher on analyzing the beverage consumption categories. The association of high water–low SSB consumption was 230 kcal less than that of low water–high SSB consumption with regard to total energy intake ($p < 0.01$).

Table 4. Quartiles of consumption, energy contribution and percentage of energy of beverage groups by socioeconomic status and area of residence in Mexican school-age children (*n* = 2536).

| | | NATIONAL | | | AREA | | | | | | SOCIOECONOMIC STATUS | | | | | | | | |
| | | | | | Urban | | | Rural | | | Low | | | Middle | | | High | | |
	%*	p25	p50	p75	p25	p50	p75	p25	p50	p75	p25	p50	p75	p25	p50	p75	p25	p50	p75
Consumption (mL)																			
Plain water	74.1	240.0	480.0	720.0	240.0	480.0	720.0	240.0	480.0	720.0	240.0	480.0	720.0	240.0	480.0	720.0	240.0	480.0	600.0
Dairy beverages without sugar	27.0	240.0	246.7	370.4	240.0	246.7	370.0	240.0	246.7	411.2	240.0	246.7	400.9	240.0	246.7	380.0	240.0	246.7	370.0
Dairy beverages with sugar	33.2	223.0	258.0	368.0	225.2	259.0	361.2	212.1	256.5	369.4	220.0	255.7	369.4	196.6	250.0	342.4	230.4	272.0	308.7
Non-dairy beverages with sugar	78.9	240.0	408	663.8	240	402.8	625.2	240.0	448.6	705.6	235.0	379.4	703.1	240.0	426.7	643.0	240.0	416.0	605.0
Natural juices	2.2	193.0	252.0	252.0	210.0	252.0	252.0	131.2	252.0	262.5	126.0	252.0	262.5	210.0	252.0	262.5	210.0	252.0	252.0
Non-dairy beverages without sugar	10.1	188.0	225.6	295.2	156.5	225.6	295.2	196.8	225.6	285.7	164.0	225.6	360	196.8	225.6	240.0	123.0	225.6	295.2
Energy contribution																			
Plain water		-	-	-	-	-	-	-	-	-	-	-	-	-	-	-	-	-	-
Dairy beverages without sugar		118.3	143.3	177.5	118.3	143.3	177.3	135	143.3	179.2	118.6	143.3	179.2	118.3	143.3	179.2	118.3	143.3	170.4
Dairy beverages with sugar		148.8	209.1	311.9	158.7	218.9	311.8	117.4	184.4	311.9	114.0	184.4	267.5	131.2	196	279.4	184.4	251.3	349.2
Non-dairy beverages with sugar		89.0	140.7	230.0	89.7	145.6	227.1	76.8	128.8	241.0	74.8	126.2	240.5	89.7	145.4	229.9	98.6	147.6	224.5
Natural juices		74.8	113.4	113.4	94.5	113.4	113.4	56.7	113.4	118.1	56.7	113.4	118.1	113.4	113.4	118.1	94.5	113.4	113.4
Non-dairy beverages without sugar		0.0	0.0	2.4	0.0	0.0	2.4	0.0	0.0	2.5	0.0	0.0	3.2	0.0	0.0	2.4	0.0	0.0	2.4
Energy percentage†																			
Plain water		-	-	-	-	-	-	-	-	-	-	-	-	-	-	-	-	-	-
Dairy beverages without sugar		5.6	8.7	12.8	5.7	8.7	13.2	6.2	9.1	13	6.7	8.8	13	5.7	8.9	13.8	5.1	8.5	12.4
Dairy beverages with sugar		8.0	12.2	19.1	8.4	12.7	19.3	6.3	10.7	17.4	6.6	11.2	17.4	7.1	11.4	16.3	10.0	14.7	22.0
Non-dairy beverages with sugar		5.0	8.4	13.5	5.0	8.3	13.3	5.0	8.3	13.4	4.3	8.2	13.4	5.2	8.1	13.6	5.4	8.7	12.9
Natural juices		4.7	6.4	8.7	4.7	6.4	8.7	4.5	5.7	8.7	2.6	6.4	8.7	5.1	6.7	8.7	4.7	5.8	8.6
Non-dairy beverages without sugar		0.0	0.0	0.1	0.0	0.0	0.1	0.0	0.0	0.2	0.0	0.0	0.2	0.0	0.0	0.1	0.0	0.0	0.0

All values pertain only to consumers. * Percentage of consumers at national level. † Regarding total energy intake.

Table 5. Multivariate linear regression analyses showing the association between beverage consumption and total energy intake in Mexican school-age children (*n* = 2536).

	Variable	Coefficient (SE)	*p*
Model 1 [a]	PW consumption (servings)	−1.09 (2.21)	0.611
	SSB consumption (servings)	112.08 (5.75)	<0.001 *
	SSB consumption (servings) [2]	−6.66 (0.82)	<0.001 *
	Age (years)	−2.88 (2.00)	0.150
	Sex (boy = 1)	1.45 (7.18)	0.839
	Energy from food (kcal)	0.99 (0.01)	<0.001 *
	SES low [b]	Reference	
	SES Medium	18.37 (9.01)	0.042 *
	SES High	38.75 (10.49)	<0.001 *
	Area of residence (urban = 1)	30.36 (7.99)	<0.001 *
	Constant	73.96 (21.69)	
Model 2 [c]	Low water–high SSBs [d]	Refererence	
	High water–high SSBs	−1.009 (14.64)	0.940
	Low water–low SSBs	−218.72 (11.16)	<0.001 *
	High water–low SSBs	−228.71 (12.48)	<0.001 *
	Age (years)	−1.88 (2.15)	0.379
	Sex (boy = 1)	1.65 (7.86)	0.833
	Energy from food (kcal)	1.00 (0.05)	<0.001 *
	SES low	Reference	
	SES Medium	17.71 (9.07)	0.051
	SES High	36.03 (11.17)	<0.001 *
	Area of residence (urban = 1)	34.41 (8.69)	<0.001 *
	Constant	353.53 (23.75)	

[a] Model 1. Linear regression model with consumption of PW (plain water) and SSBs (sugar-sweetened beverages) as continuous variables, adjusted by age, sex, energy from non-beverage foods, socioeconomic status and area of residence. The quadratic term SSBs was included; [b] Socioeconomic status categories calculated using principal components analysis; includes household characteristics, goods and services; [c] Model 2. Linear regression model with consumption of water and SSBs as four categories of consumption, adjusted by age, sex, energy from non-beverage foods, socioeconomic status and area of residence; [d] Cutoff point for water and SSB consumption was: (1) low water (<two servings) and high SSB consumption (≥two servings); (2) high water (≥two servings) and high SSB consumption (≥two servings); (3) low water (<two servings) and low SSBs (<two servings) consumption; and (4) high water (≥two servings) and low SSBs (<two servings) consumption. * Significant difference (*p* < 0.05).

4. Discussion

Based on data from a nationally representative survey, our study sheds light on the relationship of PW and SSB consumption with energy intake among Mexican school-age children. The main finding was that the combination of low PW and high SSB consumption was associated with higher total energy intake. We found no association between PW consumption (independent of SSB consumption) and total energy intake.

The median energy intake (1633 kcal/day) was within the required range for school-age children: 1200–2200 kcal/day, depending on the age and physical activity level [16] of the particular child.

Malik et al. found that, in Mexico, all age groups combined received ≈10% of their total energy intake from SSBs. Since then, the proportion of SSB energy intake has increased considerably among individuals older than five years of age [17].

It is important to note that the higher association between beverage consumption and total energy intake was found when combined specifically with high water and low SSB consumption. It has been argued that replacing SSBs with non-caloric beverages or PW may be a useful strategy for weight reduction as a result of less energy intake [18,19].

Our findings are consistent with those of Martinez et al., whose samples of children and adolescents in Uruguay, Brazil and Mexico demonstrated that the highest contribution to the total fluid intake came from beverages containing sugar (i.e., juices and sweet beverages) [20].

As indicated in other studies, one explanation for the observed link between SSB consumption and higher total energy intake may lie in the fact that individuals do not sufficiently reduce their energy intake from other sources to offset the calories ingested from beverages [21,22].

A meta-analysis on the effects of soft drink consumption obtained similar evidence [23]. It also found that replacing sweetened caloric beverages with PW was associated with a sustained caloric deficit among women in a 12-month clinical weight loss trial [19].

A study of Brazilian students from 10 to 11 years old provided no evidence of PW consumption having a protective effect on Body Mass Index increase—children who reported high PW consumption also reported a high intake of other beverages [24]. However, the study did confirm that consumption of juice drinks was a risk factor for increased BMI [24].

According to another study of Mexican children in the same age group as ours, the trends obtained by several dietary intake surveys point to a sharp increase in caloric beverage consumption among pre-school and school-age children. The surveys also found that beverages such as whole milk and sugar-sweetened juices were important contributors to the increased energy intake among children. Mexican school children were found to consume 20.7% of their energy from caloric beverages. The three most commonly consumed were whole milk, fruit juice with various sugar and water combinations, and carbonated and noncarbonated sugared beverages [11].

Findings from several clinical trials, epidemiological studies and intervention initiatives suggest that PW plays a potentially important role in reducing energy intake and, consequently, in preventing obesity [8]. Similarly, the results of a meta-analysis by Popkin et al. on the effects of PW intake alone suggest that PW consumption is linked to reduced energy intake when replacing sugar-sweetened beverages, juice, milk and diet beverages. These findings come primarily from clinical feeding studies, a well-regarded random controlled school intervention, and several additional epidemiological and intervention studies [2].

Our study did not yield the same results in this area, a difference that may be attributable to differences in the methodology for assessing PW intake, as has been the case in other published studies.

Our study has the following limitations that should be addressed in future epidemiological studies: ENSANUT 2012 did not track physical activity for all age groups. Therefore, it was impossible to adjust the models constructed to assess the association between beverage consumption and total energy intake for physical activity, a variable which could be attenuating the association [25,26].

Variability in the consumption of beverages and water in our study might be related to season. The ENSANUT was conducted from October 2011 to May 2012, with varying weather (temperature) throughout the study period potentially contributing to different liquid intakes. Subsequent studies are therefore necessary to determine beverage intake by season.

Moreover, research on child caloric beverages suggests that caloric beverages consumed by school-age children may be underestimated, particularly those consumed at school (e.g., fruit juices and *aguas frescas*) [10].

Another limitation of our study concerns the fact that data analyzed on the consumption of SSBs and PW were collected only from one 24 h recall. Self-reported intake may have been affected by recall bias and/or reporting errors. Such measurement errors could be randomly distributed across the sample or might affect certain sub-populations systematically [27].

Nevertheless, our study also has its strengths, one of which is the fact that the data come from a survey representative at national, state, and urban/rural area levels. This provides a sample size adequate not only to offer precise outcomes and external validity, but also to allow for extrapolating the results to all Mexican school-age children.

Another strength lies in the fact that dietary information was collected using the multi-pass 24 h recall method, thereby increasing accuracy in estimating the usual intake distributions [28]. Additionally, the questionnaire included PW intake as part of the 24 h recall.

The past 30 years have witnessed a marked increase in SSB consumption around the world. As indicated by our study, SSB consumption may account for the increase in energy intake among school-age children and could also be associated with obesity.

Public health initiatives in various countries, Mexico among them [29], are actively promoting PW consumption to help control weight. A number of American associations and organizations recommend drinking water either in greater volume or in place of other beverages as a part of weight management [30].

Effective strategies are required to restrict the supply of sugar-sweetened beverages and other high-calorie, nutrient-poor food products in places frequented by children such as schools, parks and recreation areas. The government needs to implement measures such as taxation in its battle against consumption of these addictive foods and beverages. At the same time, free PW must be made widely available for public health purposes.

5. Conclusions

Slashing SSB consumption can provide an important strategy for eliminating excess caloric intake; however, the choice of a replacement beverage is crucial. Promoting PW consumption could be a useful public health policy in that it is clearly an appropriate SSB replacement choice that is also economical if tap water is used. It could also be an effective strategy for balancing energy/nutrient intake and preventing overconsumption among Mexican school-age children.

Author Contributions: The responsibilities of the authors were distributed as follows: T.S.-L. and S.R.-R. designed the study; C.G.G.-C. and S.R.-R. performed the statistical analysis; C.G.G.-C., S.R.-R. and T.S.-L. drafted the manuscript; all of the authors shared primary responsibility for the final content. All of the authors read and approved the final manuscript.

Conflicts of Interest: The authors declare no conflict of interest.

References

1. Illescas-Zarate, D.; Espinosa-Montero, J.; Flores, M.; Barquera, S. Plain water consumption is associated with lower intake of caloric beverage: Cross-sectional study in Mexican adults with low socioeconomic status. *BMC Public Health* **2015**, *15*, 405. [CrossRef] [PubMed]
2. Popkin, B. Water, Hydration and Health. *Nutr. Rev.* **2010**, *68*, 439–458. [CrossRef] [PubMed]
3. Senterre, C.; Dramaix, M.; Thiébaut, I. Fluid intake survey among schoolchildren in Belgium. *BMC Public Health* **2014**, *14*, 651. [CrossRef] [PubMed]
4. Muckelbauer, R.; Gortmaker, S.L.; Libuda, L.; Kersting, M.; Clausen, K.; Adelberger, B.; Müller-Nordhorn, J. Changes in water and sugar-containing beverage consumption and body weight outcomes in children. *Br. J. Nutr.* **2016**, *115*, 2057–2066. [CrossRef] [PubMed]
5. An, R.; McCaffrey, J. Plain water consumption in relation to energy intake and diet quality among US adults, 2005–2012. *J. Hum. Nutr. Diet.* **2016**, *29*, 624–632. [CrossRef] [PubMed]
6. U.S. Department of Agriculture; U.S. Department of Health and Human Services. Dietary Guidelines for Americans, 7th ed. 2010. Available online: http://www.health.gov/dietaryguidelines/dga2010/ (accessed on 1 September 2016).
7. Daniels, M.; Popkin, B. The impact of water intake on energy intake and weight status: A systematic review. *Nutr. Rev.* **2010**, *68*, 505–521. [CrossRef] [PubMed]
8. Popkin, B.; Hawkes, C. Sweetening of the global diet, particularly beverages: Patterns, trends, and policy responses. *Lancet Diabetes Endocrinol.* **2016**, *4*, 174–186. [CrossRef]
9. Drewnowski, A.; Rehm, C.D.; Constant, F. Water and beverage consumption among children age 4–13 years in the United States: Analyses of 2005–2010 NHANES data. *Nutr. J.* **2013**, *12*, 85. [CrossRef] [PubMed]
10. Malik, V.S.; Pan, A.; Willett, W.C.; Hu, F.B. Sugar-sweetened beverages and weight gain in children and adults: A systematic review and meta-analysis. *Am. J. Clin. Nutr.* **2013**, *98*, 1084–1102. [CrossRef] [PubMed]
11. Barquera, S.; Campirano, F.; Bonvecchio, A.; Hernández-Barrera, L.; Rivera, J.A.; Popkin, B. Caloric beverage consumption patterns in Mexican children. *Nutr. J.* **2010**, *9*, 47. [CrossRef] [PubMed]
12. Gutiérrez, J.P.; Rivera-Dommarco, J.; Shamah-Levy, T.; Villalpando-Hernández, S.; Franco, A.; Cuevas-Nasu, L.; Romero-Martínez, M.; Hernández-Ávila, M. Encuesta Nacional de Salud y Nutrición 2012. Resultados Nacionales; Instituto Nacional de Salud Pública (MX): Cuernavaca, Mexico, 2012.
13. Institute of Medicine. Dietary Reference Intakes for Water, Potassium, Sodium, Chloride, and Sulfate. 2004. Available online: https://www.nap.edu/read/10925/chapter/6#p2000cb269970073001 (accessed on 6 September 2016).

14. Romero-Martínez, M.; Shamah-Levy, T.; Franco-Núñez, A.; Villalpando, S.; Cuevas-Nasu, L.; Gutiérrez, J.P.; Rivera-Dommarco, J.Á. National Health and Nutrition Survey 2012: Design and coverage. *Salud Publica Mex.* **2013**, *55*, S332–S340. [PubMed]

15. Zimmerman, T.P.; Hull, S.G.; McNutt, S.; Mittl, B.; Islam, N.; Guenther, P.M.; Thompson, F.E.; Potischman, N.A.; Subar, A.F. Challenges in converting an interviewer-administered food probe database to self-administration in the National Cancer Institute automated self-administered 24-h recall (ASA24). *J. Food Compost. Anal.* **2009**, *22*, S48–S51. [CrossRef] [PubMed]

16. Institute of Medicine. Dietary Reference Intakes for Energy, Carbohydrate, Fiber, Fat, Fatty Acids, Cholesterol, Protein, and Amino Acids. 2002. Available online: http://www.nap.edu/read/10490/chapter/1 (accessed on 9 September 2016).

17. Malik, V.S.; Popkin, B.M.; Bray, G.A.; Després, J.P.; Hu, F.B. Sugar-sweetened beverages, obesity, type 2 diabetes mellitus, and cardiovascular disease risk. *Circulation* **2010**, *121*, 1356–1364. [CrossRef] [PubMed]

18. Hu, F.B. Resolved: There is sufficient scientific evidence that decreasing sugar sweetened beverage consumption will reduce the prevalence of obesity and obesity-related diseases. *Obes. Rev.* **2013**, *14*, 606–619. [CrossRef] [PubMed]

19. Stookey, J.D.; Constant, F.; Gardner, C.D.; Popkin, B.M. Replacing sweetened caloric beverages with drinking water is associated with lower energy intake. *Obesity* **2007**, *15*, 3013–3022. [CrossRef] [PubMed]

20. Martinez, H.; Guelinckx, I.; Salas-Salvadó, J.; Gandy, J.; Kavouras, S.A.; Moreno, L.A. Harmonized Cross-Sectional Surveys Focused on Fluid Intake in Children, Adolescents and Adults: The Liq.In7 Initiative. *Ann. Nutr. Metab.* **2016**, *68*, 12–18. [CrossRef] [PubMed]

21. DiMeglio, D.P.; Mattes, R.D. Liquid versus solid carbohydrate: Effects on food intake and body weight. *Int. J. Obes.* **2000**, *24*, 794–800. [CrossRef]

22. Almiron-Roig, E.; Chen, Y.; Drewnowski, A. Liquid calories and the failure of satiety: How good is the evidence? *Obes. Rev.* **2003**, *4*, 201–212. [CrossRef] [PubMed]

23. Vartanian, L.R.; Schwartz, M.B.; Brownell, K.D. Effects of soft drink consumption on nutrition and health: A systematic review and meta-analysis. *Am. J. Public Health* **2007**, *97*, 667–675. [CrossRef] [PubMed]

24. Sichieri, R.; Yokoo, E.M.; Pereira, R.A.; Veiga, G.V. Water and sugar-sweetened beverage consumption and changes in BMI among Brazilian fourth graders after 1-year follow-up. *Public Health Nutr.* **2013**, *16*, 73–77. [CrossRef] [PubMed]

25. Piernas, C.; Miles, D.R.; Deming, D.M.; Reidy, K.C.; Popkin, B.M. Estimating usual intakes mainly affects the micronutrient distribution among infants, toddlers and pre-schoolers from the 2012 Mexican National Health and Nutrition Survey. *Public Health Nutr.* **2016**, *19*, 1017–1026. [CrossRef] [PubMed]

26. Stookey, J.J. Negative, null and beneficial effects of drinking water on energy intake, energy expenditure, fat oxidation and weight change in randomized trials: A qualitative review. *Nutrients* **2016**, *8*, 19. [CrossRef] [PubMed]

27. Castro-Quezada, I.; Ruano-Rodríguez, C.; Ribas-Barba, L.; Serra-Majem, L. Misreporting in nutritional surveys: Methodological implications. *Nutr. Hosp.* **2015**, *31*, 119–127. [PubMed]

28. Montgomery, C.; Reilly, J.J.; Jackson, D.M.; Kelly, L.A.; Slater, C.; Paton, J.Y.; Grant, S. Validation of energy intake by 24-h multiple pass recall: Comparison with total energy expenditure in children aged 5–7 years. *Br. J. Nutr.* **2005**, *93*, 671–676. [CrossRef] [PubMed]

29. Mexican President Urges Citizens to Exercise to Fight Obesity. Available online: http://www.telegraph. co.uk/news/worldnews/centralamericaandthecaribbean/mexico/10419302/Mexican-president-urges-citizens-to-exercise-to-fight-obesity.html (accessed on 8 October 2015).

30. Wang, Y.C.; Ludwig, D.S.; Sonneville, K.; Gortmaker, S.L. Impact of change in sweetened caloric beverage consumption on energy intake among children and adolescents. *Arch. Pediatr. Adolesc. Med.* **2009**, *163*, 336–343. [CrossRef] [PubMed]

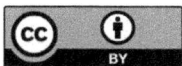

MDPI AG

St. Alban-Anlage 66

4052 Basel, Switzerland

Tel. +41 61 683 77 34

Fax +41 61 302 89 18

http://www.mdpi.com

Nutrients Editorial Office

E-mail: nutrients@mdpi.com

http://www.mdpi.com/journal/nutrients

www.ingramcontent.com/pod-product-compliance
Lightning Source LLC
Chambersburg PA
CBHW051717210326
41597CB00032B/5512